D1090765

Clinical Neurotherapy

Clinical Neurotherapy

Application of Techniques for Treatment

Edited by

David S. Cantor, PhD
Mind & Motion Developmental Centers of Georgia,
Johns Creek City, GA, USA

James R. Evans, PhD
Sterlingworth Center, Greenville, SC, USA

Amsterdam • Boston • Heidelberg • London
New York • Oxford • Paris • San Diego
San Francisco • Singapore • Sydney • Tokyo
Academic Press is an imprint of Elsevier

Academic Press is an imprint of Elsevier
32 Jamestown Road, London NW1 7BY, UK
225 Wyman Street, Waltham, MA 02451, USA
525 B Street, Suite 1800, San Diego, CA 92101-4495, USA

Notice
No responsibility is assumed by the publisher for any injury and/or damage
to persons or property as a matter of product liability, negligence or otherwise,
or from any use or operation of any methods, products, instructions or ideas
contained in the material herein.

Because of rapid advances in the medical sciences, in particular, independent
verification of diagnoses and drug dosages should be made.

British Library Cataloguing-in-Publication Data
A catalogue record for this book is available from the British Library.

Library of Congress Cataloging-in-Publication Data
A catalog record for this book is available from the Library of Congress.

ISBN : 978-0-12-396988-0

For information on all Academic Press publications, visit our
website at elsevierdirect.com

Typeset by MPS Limited, Chennai, India
www.adi-mps.com

Printed and bound in
14 15 16 17 18   10 9 8 7 6 5 4 3 2 1

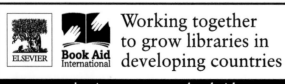

Working together
to grow libraries in
developing countries

www.elsevier.com • www.bookaid.org

CONTENTS

CONTRIBUTORS

Teresa Bailey
Private Practice, Los Altos, California, USA

Rex L. Cannon
University of Tennessee, Knoxville, Tennessee, USA

Thomas F. Collura
BrainMaster Technologies, Inc., Bedford, Ohio, USA
Brain Enrichment Center, Bedford, Ohio, USA

Jacques Duff
Behavioural Neurotherapy Clinic, Doncaster, Australia

Erbil Dursun
Physical Medicine and Rehabilitation Department, University of Kocaeli, Izmit, Turkey

Nigar Dursun
Physical Medicine and Rehabilitation Department, University of Kocaeli, Izmit, Turkey

Gerald Gluck
Center for Family Counseling and Biofeedback, Coral Springs, Florida, USA

D. Corydon Hammond
Physical Medicine & Rehabilitation, University of Utah School of Medicine, Salt Lake City, Utah

J. Lucas Koberda
Tallahassee NeuroBalance Center, Tallahassee, Florida, USA
Carrick Institute for Graduate Studies, Cape Canaveral, Florida, USA
Florida State University, College of Medicine, Tallahassee, Florida, USA

Lukasz M. Konopka
Yellowbrick Foundation, Evanston, Illinois and Loyola University Medical School Department of Psychiatry, Maywood, Illinois, USA

John K. Nash
Behavioral Medicine Associates, Inc., Edina, MN
St Mary's University of Minnesota, Minneapolis, MN, USA

Carlos A. Novo-Olivas
NeuroScopic Integrative Neurodiagnostics, Monterrey, Mexico

Estate M. Sokhadze
Department of Psychiatry and Behavioral Sciences, University of Louisville, Louisville, Kentucky, USA

Richard Soutar
NewMind Center, Roswell, Georgia, USA

M.B. Sterman
Geffen School of Medicine, UCLA, and ADD Centre, Toronto, Canada

Emily Stevens
Neurobehavioral Consulting, Stuart, Florida, USA

Tanju Sürmeli
Living Health Center for Research and Education, Istanbul, Turkey

Lynda M. Thompson
Geffen School of Medicine, UCLA, and ADD Centre, Toronto, Canada

Dagmar Timmers
Private Practice, Neuropsychological and Psychosocial Assessments and Treatment, Children, Adolescents, Adults, Oosterhout, The Netherlands

David L. Trudeau
ISNR Research Foundation

Elizabeth M. Zimmerman
The Chicago School of Professional Psychology, Chicago, Illinois, USA

PREFACE

It is interesting to note that when the first edition of *Introduction to Quantitative EEG and Neurofeedback* was published in 1999, no more than two other books dealing directly with neurotherapy had been published, whereas within the subsequent 14 years there have been at least 10, with a couple more in press. This is an indication of the rapid growth of the field.

In reviewing the names of contributing authors from several past books, it was noted that many of these authors were the true "pioneers" in the field, while others represented "rising stars." Sadly, some have passed on, including Margaret Ayers, Tom Budzynski, Joe Horvat and Hershel Toomim. However, 14 years later many of these authors are still shining brightly, and several are authors or coauthors of chapters in this book.

The prefaces of earlier texts usually provided some very basic descriptions of what the term neurotherapy (aka EEG biofeedback; neurofeedback) refers to. These terms are becoming more familiar to the general public, and certainly to most prospective readers of this book, and therefore this is probably no longer necessary. However, such definitions are provided by some of the present chapter authors. Not unexpectedly, other preface themes from the past remain relevant today. These include concerns about who is qualified to practice neurotherapy and for what conditions, along with continuing skepticism regarding the value of neurotherapy by mainstream medicine, psychology and education, and the general lack of insurance coverage for services, despite increasingly large amounts of related scientific research generally supporting its efficacy. The growth of publications exploring and demonstrating the utilization of various neurotherapy techniques has exploded geometrically over the past 14 years, with references on these topics in the hundreds of thousands in the Library of National Medicine. This growth in the scientific development of neurotherapies parallels the growing emphasis on protocols for neurotherapy to demonstrate treatment efficacy, much as evidence-based medicine protocols are becoming the standard of care in all areas of healthcare. This is no less true when it comes to the treatment of neurobehavioral disorders. However, the complexities of brain function as related to the subtleties of human cognition and human behavior across individuals may not yield simple "one size fits all" protocols for treatment. Recognition of this concept at once hampers the ready acceptance of neurotherapies into traditional medicine and proposes a paradigm shift toward optimizing individual recovery from a disorder, and, in fact enhancing the human condition in general.

With each passing year there have been major advances in equipment, development and refinement of normative databases, and software for accurately measuring and training increasingly more aspects of the EEG. For example, amplifiers are much smaller; wireless scalp-to-amplifier connection is being used by some practitioners; researchers can measure EEG activity simultaneously from over 100 scalp sites; and measures of connectivity (e.g., coherence and phase relationship) between signals from pairs of scalp electrode sites now are routinely considered along with EEG power measures in both diagnosis and neurotherapy. The availability of software for Z-score neurotherapy has been a relatively recent development enabling a client to simultaneously train multiple aspects of his or her EEG to approach age-adjusted average scores on the many EEG parameters involved in a database.

The aim of this book is to provide the reader with a review of neurotherapy techniques, not only of qEEG-based neurotherapy, including low-resolution electromagnetic tomography analysis, but also of transcranial magnetic stimulation, cranial electrotherapy stimulation techniques, auditory–visual entrainment, pharmacological manipulations and other forms of neuromodulation techniques in the treatment of many common neurobehavioral disorders. Additionally, there is growing interest in combining neurotherapy with other approaches, such as cognitive rehabilitation, metacognitive strategies, vision training and nutritional or integrative medicine methods. Thus, one goal of this book is to serve as a desk reference for the clinician and researchers as to what has worked and what has not when applying these methodologies toward treating disorders. A second goal that hopefully will be realized is to promote professional skills sufficient to exercise the freedom to design tailored treatment protocols in order to achieve optimized performance and function. In other words, professionals using these technologies will need to have a thorough understanding of their meaningfulness, and artful mastery in their application. Thus, the need for proper training, certification of such training, and methods of monitoring the quality assurance of professionals using such technologies is critical for the growth and mainstream acceptance of these methods. As evidenced by the varied professions represented by the authors in this book and their international representation, neurotherapy technology and its applications belong to the bigger universe of integrated health sciences, exploring and treating human behavior. In this context, the closing remarks from a 1999 preface remain relevant:

> *With proper foundations for the field, there are high expectations that NT will remain alive and well and continue to grow into its early promise of becoming one of the major treatment modalities for a very wide range of disorders.*

David S. Cantor
Jim Evans

FOREWORD

It is with great pleasure that I write the Foreword to this timely and eminently applicable textbook on the latest techniques and applications of neurotherapy across the spectrum of clinical neurology, psychiatry/psychology and medicine in general.

As opposed to the majority of medical/neurological literature and texts, which focus on aspects of "disease management" and "disease amelioration" (worthy as those goals are), this book expands on the 40+ year history of neurotherapy and its scientific foundations and widespread clinical/research applications.

As will be evident from the text, the underpinnings of current neurotherapies reveal a mechanism that is truly "health promoting" and that provides far more than allopathic "treatments." By accessing the fundamental connectomic properties of the brain's amazing neural networks, hubs, edges and borders, the field of neuromodulation – and EEG neurofeedback in particular – is demonstrating the ability to reverse and restore specifically targeted dysfunctional brain systems. Instead of having widespread, often nonspecific, pharmacological effects on the nervous system, often causing multiple comorbidities, clinical neurotherapy – correctly carried out by trained and experienced practitioners – treats the source(s) of symptoms, which may be highly focal and localized to specific networks or regions of the brain.

As is evident from the chapters and their authors, neurofeedback and related techniques are increasingly studied and applied both nationally and internationally. The techniques and principles reviewed here are currently being scientifically researched and successfully applied across virtually the entire spectrum of known human "diseases." The unprecedented history and increasing evidence for the efficacy of neurotherapy is supported by thousands of related peer-reviewed, scientifically substantiated articles and texts. The literature evidence for the clinical efficacy for neurofeedback in persons with intractable epilepsy, for example, rivals – and may exceed – that which exists for any other current "standard" treatments, including pharmacological, surgical and dietary.

Directed nonpharmacological, noninvasive neurotherapy can be used with increased diagnostic accuracy through the use of techniques of source analysis with tomographic quantitative electroencephalography. In fact, the resolution – approximately $3\,\text{mm}^3$ – provided by eLORETA, for example, is being demonstrated to be at least as accurate, if not more so, than current imaging techniques such as fMRI, MEG, SPECT, PET and high-resolution MRI.

Reading the sequence of chapters (though any individual chapter stands alone) demonstrates:

- the importance of high-quality training and certification required to be a clinician and/or researcher in this field, and to model the flawless ethical standards exhibited by qualified practitioners now, and over the past 40 years;
- the improved delineation of international standards created by the ISNR and AAPB to ensure the highest standards of patient safety and efficacy, and a thorough foundation for competent and compassionate practice and research;
- applications to the entire spectrum of brain-related dysfunctions and "diseases," with continued publication of verified studies and clinical efficacy; and finally,
- a view of the future of neurotherapy that promises even more application, effectiveness, research and growth than can be imagined in this age of pervasive use of pharmacological and invasive therapies, which often yield diminishing results coupled with increased mortality and morbidity.

The recent approval of biofeedback methodologies as a Level 1 treatment for ADHD by the American Academy of Pediatrics (resting on a 30+ year history of scientific research and clinical success in attentional dysfunctions) holds promise for the much overdue "approval" of these noninvasive, nonpharmacological therapies in the spectrum of the epilepsies and elsewhere (with even more evidence from the past 40+ years demanding its widespread application worldwide).

As a pediatric epileptologist and neurophysiologist, I have been transformed by the paradigm shift of experiencing electroencephalography no longer as only a **diagnostic** tool, but also as a **therapeutic** tool. To be able to offer these already scientifically validated techniques to the >20 million persons worldwide who suffer from the devastation of intractable epilepsy, to be able to use this technique as a first-line therapeutic trial prior to more invasive pharmacological or surgical treatments – that is what I long for in my daily practice of helping people transition from disease to health.

Now is the time, the "coming of age," of the field of neurotherapy, because it is now being shown to be the most comprehensive form of "integrative medicine," mechanistically, functionally, and clinically validated and applied.

Robert P. Turner, MD, MSCR

CHAPTER ONE

Definitions, Standard of Care and Ethical Considerations

D. Corydon Hammond

INTRODUCTION

It has become well known that problems with biological brain function are associated with a broad range of psychological and psychiatric conditions, as well as with the process of aging and a variety of medical conditions. Pharmacological approaches for influencing the brain are well known in the treatment of psychiatric conditions. However, as both professionals and the public become aware that psychopharmacology often produces only modest improvements over and above placebo effects in treating psychiatric disorders,[1–8] there is increasing interest in other methods that may be available for therapeutically influencing brain function. This chapter provides an introduction to the nature of these various neurotherapy modalities, as well as a review of ethical and standard of care issues in the field. Subsequent chapters will provide greater detail on various therapeutic modalities and their research support.

DEFINITIONS
Neurofeedback

Electroencephalographic (EEG) biofeedback, popularly known as neurofeedback, began to be researched in approximately 1970, first in animal studies and the treatment of uncontrolled epilepsy[9,10] and anxiety.[11] Typical neurofeedback training involves placing one or more electrodes on the scalp and one or two on the earlobes. EEG equipment then provides instantaneous real-time feedback about the brain's activity. Ordinarily one cannot reliably influence brainwave activity because there is no awareness of it, but when this awareness is provided to us a few thousandths of a second after it occurs, it provides us with an opportunity to gradually recondition brain activity. The mechanism

Clinical Neurotherapy.
Doi: http://dx.doi.org/10.1016/B978-0-12-396988-0.00001-5

by which this is accomplished is generally considered to be operant conditioning. Although the Food and Drug Administration (FDA) has approved neurofeedback only for producing relaxation, and hence manufacturers may legally advertise its use only for such, clinicians may use neurofeedback to treat any conditions within their scope of practice and training. Research has commonly shown that with ongoing practice sessions approximately 75–80% of persons can retrain how the brain is functioning, producing significant improvements in a wide range of conditions such as attention deficit disorder/attention deficit hyperactivity disorder (ADD/ADHD), learning disabilities, anxiety, depression, head injuries, insomnia, autism and addictions.[12]

Usually neurofeedback clinicians are seeking to inhibit certain brain-wave frequency bands (e.g., theta) while reinforcing other frequencies (e.g., beta). The computer display might be as simple as two bar graphs or as sophisticated as video animations. For example, one bar graph may represent inappropriate brainwave activity that we want to inhibit, while the other is associated with more appropriate activity that we want to increase. When the client concentrates on the computer screen and causes the inappropriate activity to decrease below a set threshold while the desired activity simultaneously increases mildly above a certain threshold, and these changes are maintained for half a second, clients both see this on the screen and are rewarded by a bell that rings or a tone that sounds. As this is repeated over and over, the client is basically gradually reconditioning how his or her own brain is functioning. When a trained therapist is present to actively coach the client, and when changes have been reinforced adequately through multiple sessions, healthier brain patterns become more enduring unless something happens to negatively affect brain function, such as drug abuse or a head injury.[13–17]

A variety of approaches to neurofeedback have evolved over the past 40 years. Each of these major approaches will now be described.

Traditional Neurofeedback and Symptom-Based Approaches

Traditional neurofeedback approaches have often used protocols where the electrodes were placed on the head over parts of the brain that were either intuitively or, based on available research, considered to be most likely associated with the client's problem. Thus because research[13,14] had found that ADD/ADHD is often associated with an excess of slow theta activity and a deficit in beta activity along the midline of the head, training typically occurred in these areas and focused on reducing theta/beta ratios. As the field has advanced, however, further research[18] has demonstrated that ADD/ADHD may also be associated with an excess of alpha or beta activity, and problems with coherence (how much of the brain is synchronously doing the same thing at the same time). Accumulating research[19] has documented that it is common for there to be a heterogeneity in the EEG patterns associated with most diagnostic conditions (e.g., anxiety, obsessive–compulsive disorder [OCD], insomnia, psychosis). Thus one cannot assume that a particular symptom is associated with only one EEG pattern. It has additionally become apparent, as will be discussed later, that when treatment is not individualized to the unique brainwave patterns of the patient, side effects of iatrogenic effects can occur.

A variety of treatment protocols have had encouraging results, for example in the treatment of depression when there is a frontal alpha asymmetry present,[20–22] with problems of physical balance,[23] with alcoholism and post-traumatic stress disorder (PTSD)[15,16] and insomnia.[24] However, as the field has evolved along with our knowledge that there is diversity and more complexity than originally realized in the EEG patterns associated with various symptoms, there has tended to be less use of fixed protocols unless there has been a pretreatment assessment of the EEG patterns of the individual patient.

qEEG-Guided Neurofeedback

Quantitative EEG (qEEG) is an assessment tool that allows clinicians to scientifically and objectively evaluate a person's brainwave function. The procedure usually takes about 60–75 minutes to gather data by the placing of a snug cap on the head with 20 electrodes to measure the brain's electrical activity. Data are gathered while the client rests quietly with the eyes closed, then open, and sometimes during a task. After data gathering the EEG is carefully examined to remove artifacts (e.g., from muscle tension, eye movement). Statistical analyses are then made where the data are compared to a normative database that provides scientifically objective information about how the brain is functioning compared to norms for the client's age. This assessment then allows the clinician to individualize neurofeedback treatment based on the objective data, reducing guesswork about what the brainwave patterns may be. Subsequent neurofeedback may then focus on reinforcing and/or inhibiting the magnitude of certain EEG frequencies, or modifying coherence (synchrony) or phase-lag (processing speed) between certain electrode sites.

Live Z-Score Training

Live Z-score training is a more recent methodology for neurofeedback where two, four or 19 electrodes are placed on the scalp. Continuous calculations are computed, comparing how the brain functions on different variables against a scientifically developed normative database. The feedback provided to the client is based on these moment-to-moment statistical comparisons to norms for the client's age. As with qEEG-guided training, the visual and audio feedback that is provided is designed to guide the brain toward normalized function. Preliminary results are very encouraging, although at present just one controlled study[25] and various case reports have been published.

LORETA and BrainAvatar Neurofeedback Training

LORETA refers to low-resolution electromagnetic tomography. It is a type of qEEG analysis that provides an estimate of the location of the underlying brain generators (e.g., in the anterior cingulate, fusiform gyrus, Brodmann areas) of the patient's EEG activity. LORETA neurofeedback and BrainAvatar—which is another method of doing LORETA neurofeedback—represent the most recent advances in the field. Live Z-score training and LORETA both allow feedback on multiple variables (e.g., power, coherence, asymmetries, phase-lag and phase-reset) simultaneously, as well as LORETA methods being able to target specific underlying areas of the brain. LORETA neurofeedback and 19-channel Live Z-score training do require definite extra effort for both therapist and patient (such as having to prepare and clean up an electrode cap, and the patient's hair, in every session), but the hope is that these methods will have the potential to reduce the number of overall treatment sessions required, or to provide another treatment approach for challenging cases that have not improved with other neurofeedback technologies.

The Low-Energy Neurofeedback System (LENS)

The Low-Energy Neurofeedback System (LENS) is a unique and passive form of neurofeedback that produces its effects through a very tiny electromagnetic field delivered to the scalp. The strength of this field (10^{-18} W/cm^2) is the equivalent of only 1/400th of the strength of the input received from holding an ordinary cell phone to the ear, equaling about the intensity of the output from a watch battery. The LENS updates the dominant frequency of the brainwave activity 16 times per second, and a feedback signal somewhat faster than the dominant frequency is provided and adjusted 16 times a second. Thus the feedback targets the dominant EEG frequency, seeking to disrupt it rather than reinforcing or inhibiting the magnitude of the EEG. LENS neurofeedback is done while the client simply sits still (usually with eyes closed) for very brief periods, which is an advantage when working with very young children, or persons who are less motivated or who lack the impulse control or stamina required by other neurofeedback methods. LENS has also been used to modify behavioral problems in animals.[26]

Slow Cortical Potentials Training

Slow cortical potentials (SCPs) are the positive or negative polarizations of the EEG in the very slow frequency range from 0.3 Hz to usually about 1.5 Hz. One can think of them as the DC baseline on which the AC EEG activity rides. There is generally a negative shift in DC potentials that occurs during cognitive processing, creating excitatory effects, and positive SCPs occur when cortical networks are being inhibited. As an example, during and prior to an epileptic seizure, the cortex is electronegative, and this same kind of hyperexcitability tends to be seen before many migraines. Following a seizure, when the cortex is fatigued, it tends to be electropositive. SCP neurofeedback training has been done particularly with epilepsy, ADHD and migraine, and has been most popular in Europe. During SCP training one electrode is placed in the center of the top of the head, and another electrode behind each ear, while the client focuses on changing a visual display on the computer.[27]

Hemoencephalography Training

There are two types of different hemoencephalography (HEG) systems[28] that are designed to provide neurofeedback to voluntarily influence cerebral blood flow. Near Infrared HEG (nirHEG) training, originated by Hershel Toomim, uses near infrared spectroscopy. This method uses a headband with closely spaced red and infrared light-emitting diodes (which are the light source), and an optode light receiver, separated from each other by about 3 cm. The light emitted is believed to penetrate the skull to a depth of about 1.5 cm into the highly vascular cortical tissue, where it is scattered and reflected, and a small amount of light that is modified by absorption returns to the surface and is measured. The red wavelength (660 nm) light source is less absorbed by oxygenated hemoglobin than by deoxygenated hemoglobin and reflects the energy demands of the tissue.

Passive Infrared HEG (pirHEG), innovated by Jeffrey Carmen, uses a small plastic box with a camera-like infrared detector that is placed on the forehead with an adjustable headband. It measures a heat signal from the underlying prefrontal cortex, and changes in this signal are believed to reflect the degree of engagement and increase in neural activity.

Both HEG systems are most easily used on the forehead, but the nirHEG system has a greater capacity to focus on small areas, whereas the pirHEG system focuses on larger areas. A series of case reports have focused on the treatment of migraines, with some reported use of HEG with ADD/ADHD and depression.

Infra-Low Frequency (ILF) Neurofeedback

This is an approach to neurofeedback that experiments on each individual, seeking to find an "optimal frequency" for reinforcement.[29] It is common for practitioners of this approach to reinforce frequencies in the range of 0.3 to 0.0001 Hz or lower. ILF theoretically proposes that reinforcing such low frequencies adjusts the "set-point" of a client's arousal level, facilitating stability in the arousal state through inducing a shift in coherence relationships in the resting state networks of the central nervous system. Only case reports[30] have been published on the effectiveness of this approach thus far, but critics[31] believe that neurofeedback systems cannot reliably measure frequencies this low and must, therefore, be measuring artifacts or something other than EEG activity.

fMRI Neurofeedback

Functional magnetic resonance imaging (fMRI) is a very sophisticated type of neuroimaging that measures changes in brain blood oxygenation levels. Studies have recently demonstrated the capacity for self-regulation of brain processes using fMRI neurofeedback in normal subjects, and some studies have shown potential for its use in stroke rehabilitation, management of pain perception and the treatment of tinnitus and psychological conditions. An advantage of fMRI neurofeedback is that it can influence functioning in deep subcortical areas of the brain, but a serious practical disadvantage is that it would be exceptionally expensive to use in routine clinical practice, requiring the use of million-dollar equipment with extremely high daily operating expenses.

Therapeutic Approaches to Brain Stimulation

A large number of techniques have evolved for therapeutically stimulating the brain. We will introduce them briefly, ranking them roughly from more intense to gentler methods. Later chapters will discuss many of these methodologies in more depth.

Electroconvulsive Therapy (ECT)

ECT became widely used in the 1940s and 1950s but continues to be used in psychiatry for treatment-resistant depression, and less commonly for mania and catatonia. In this treatment the brain of an anesthetized patient is shocked to induce a seizure. Electrodes are placed unilaterally (considered to be less effective but to produce fewer side effects) or bilaterally in the temporal area. Confusion and memory loss are common short-term side effects, and concerns are often expressed about the potential for more enduring cognitive and memory deficits following courses of ECT.[32–38] Although widely defended in psychiatry, a recent review[39] found that "placebo-controlled studies show minimal support for effectiveness with either depression or 'schizophrenia' during the course of treatment (i.e., only for some patients, on some measures, sometimes perceived only by psychiatrists but not by other raters), and no evidence, for either diagnostic group, of any benefits beyond the treatment period. There are no placebo-controlled studies evaluating the hypothesis that ECT prevents suicide, and no robust evidence from other kinds of studies to support the hypothesis" (p. 333). The review concluded: "Given the strong evidence (summarised here) of persistent and, for some, permanent brain dysfunction, primarily evidenced in the form of retrograde and anterograde amnesia, and the evidence of a slight but significant increased risk of death, the cost–benefit analysis for ECT is so poor that its use cannot be scientifically justified" (p. 333).

Repetitive Transcranial Magnetic Stimulation (rTMS)

Repetitive transcranial magnetic stimulation (rTMS) is a brain stimulation technology in that the patient is seated with a large coil positioned near the scalp that generates very strong (1.5–2 T, which is MRI intensity) magnetic pulses that induce an electrical field resulting in depolarization of the underlying area of the brain. Understanding of the mechanism by which rTMS stimulates neurons or interferes with cortical function is limited. Treatment often consists of the magnetic pulses being delivered for 5–10 seconds and then turned off for 30–60 seconds to prevent overheating and risk of seizures. It has been approved by the FDA for the treatment of depression and is perceived as offering an alternative to ECT. However, a review[40] concluded that "after 15 years of research, the general consensus is that rTMS treatment in depression has potential, but has not yet fully lived up to initial expectations" (p. 261).

Deep Brain Stimulation (DBS)

Although expensive, neurosurgical implantation of electrodes deep within the brain now allows for the electrical stimulation of deep neural structures. Deep brain stimulation (DBS) is being successfully used in the treatment of advanced Parkinson's disease to control tremors and dystonia, and may hold future potential in the treatment of psychiatric disorders.

Vagal Nerve Stimulation (VNS)

The vagal nerve stimulator is a small, neurosurgically implanted pacemaker-like battery-powered pulse generator that provides electrical stimulation to the vagal (tenth cranial) nerve. It is implanted in the upper left area of the chest with wires that are put through a tunnel and wrapped around the vagal nerve in the neck. The stimulation often occurs for a period whereby it is on for 30 seconds and then off for 5 minutes, but it can be individually programmed through an external wand, and turned on or off by the patient holding a magnet over the device. VNS has primarily been used in the treatment of partial-onset seizures, and more experimentally in the treatment of refractory depression. With stronger stimulation there are side effects that can include hoarseness, voice alteration, throat pain, cough and sleep apnea.

Transcranial Direct Current Stimulation (tDCS)

Low-intensity direct current stimulation of the brain is done through placing two saline-soaked sponge electrodes on the head, held in place by a rubber band. In contrast to the intensity of rTMS, tDCS uses a battery-powered device that delivers very small (often from 0.5 to 2 mA) currents that penetrate the brain and influence neuronal activity. In this neuro-modulation technique, stimulation by the anode sponge increases cortical excitability, and stimulation by the cathodal sponge reduces cortical excitability. Small studies have been carried out with problems of chronic pain, stroke rehabilitation, mood disorders and reduction of cravings in substance abuse.[41] Maximal improvements seem to occur when treatments take place four to five times a week. Generally side effects are mild and infrequent, and have included fatigue, skin irritation or pain under the electrodes, headaches and problems concentrating.

Cranial Electrotherapy Stimulation (CES)

Developed in the Soviet Union in the 1940s for the treatment of insomnia, CES today is usually done by placing small felt-covered ear clips, moistened with saline solution, on the earlobes. CES has been approved by the FDA for clinicians to use, or prescribe to patients to use, in the treatment of depression, anxiety and insomnia. Kirsch[3] provided abstracts on 29 animal studies, 31 published reviews, two meta-analyses and more than 100 studies on CES with insomnia, anxiety, depression, alcoholism and drug abuse withdrawal, cognitive dysfunction, fibromyalgia and other problems.

NeuroField

NeuroField is a pulsed electromagnetic device (pEMF) created by Nicholas Dogris and Brad Wiitala. It is able to generate frequencies ranging from 0.31 to 300 000 Hz with durations ranging from 100 milliseconds to 60 seconds at a time, which may be delivered via four small coils contained in small plastic boxes and attached to a cap. The pEMF output of NeuroField ranges from 1–400 mG, which is 10 million times weaker than the EMF output of rTMS, which was FDA approved as a safe and effective treatment for depression in 2008. NeuroField can be used as stand-alone equipment to provide stimulation in fixed frequency ranges (e.g., 40 Hz, 9–12 Hz etc.) and with programs designed to facilitate various effects (e.g., anxiety relief, concentration). It also uses pEMF biofeedback in combination with EEG and Z-score normative data designed to guide the brain to a more functional state. Preliminary case reports have suggested that NeuroField has the potential to help stabilize symptoms such as anxiety, depression and Parkinson's disease, but clearly controlled research is needed to demonstrate its promise.

Audiovisual Stimulation (AVS)

AVS, also known as photic driving and steady-state visual or auditory evoked potential, is a method of seeking to evoke different brainwave patterns using pulsing lights and/or audio signals. These stimuli are typically delivered through glasses (the center of which may in some cases be clear plastic with light-emitting diodes around the outside) and headphones where the person hears a tone beep. For example, photic or auditory stimulation at 10 Hz may be seeking to encourage an increase in 10 Hz alpha activity. Auditory stimulation may also be provided through binaural beats, where a different auditory stimulus is presented in each ear. As an example, the left ear may receive a beep at 133 Hz, while one is being presented in the right ear at 140 Hz, in the belief that there will be a steady-state entrainment of the EEG at the difference between the frequencies (e.g., 7 Hz). Numerous binaural beat CDs have been marketed, but not all research has verified this effect.[42]

At certain levels (most commonly in the 15–20 Hz range), photic stimulation has on rare occasions been found to induce a seizure. This has been verified in various studies as occurring in anywhere from 1 in 4000[43] to a conservatively estimated 1.1 in 100,000 persons annually.[44] By far the greatest proportion of persons who experience this seem to be between the ages of 7 and 19 years, and they will usually experience it first with the flickering light when watching television or using a computer screen. Thus, in that age group the chances of a seizure might be 1 in 4000, whereas such a risk has been estimated to only be one-fifth that great in adults over the age of 19.[44] However, Russell[45] used photic and auditory stimulation in the range of 14 Hz with more than 8000 children and reported never having a patient experience a seizure or negative reaction. Nonetheless, the literature cited above suggests this possibility, and therefore it is deemed wise for clinicians using AVS to present this possibility as part of the informed consent process, particularly with children.

Research[46,47] has demonstrated, however, that the effects of AVS alone can be complex, for instance in terms of eliciting harmonics, and increasing and reducing coherence in different parts of the brain. Thus harmonics of 10 Hz stimulation may also evoke activity at 5 and 20 Hz. Therefore, although studies have, for example, found positive effects from AVS with cognitive function,[48] seasonal affective disorder,[49] behavior problems[50] and various other conditions,[51] response to AVS alone is not entirely predictable or necessarily enduring.

However, there are some current (e.g., Brainmaster) and past technologies (e.g., Roshi I) where the AVS is EEG driven or contingent and thus provides more guidance to the brain's response, and that may have a greater likelihood of producing enduring changes.

GUIDELINES FOR ETHICAL PRACTICE AND LIABILITY PROTECTION

Several previous publications[52–55] have discussed issues of ethics and presented guidelines for best practice[56] in the field of neurofeedback that were designed to educate professionals and the public. These can be vitally important, because an increasing number of unlicensed persons have been seeking to practice neurofeedback, and because the technology is sufficiently powerful that, when misapplied, it can result in side effects and sometimes more serious iatrogenic adverse effects[28,57–64] that could lead to malpractice liability. The author considers the risk for iatrogenic effects to be greater when neurotherapy is not preceded by a thorough history, when treatment is not individualized based on an evaluation of brain function, sessions are not being supervised with an experienced clinician present for most of the session and when symptom changes are not being regularly monitored.

With what conditions can a neurofeedback clinician responsibly work? Licensing in biofeedback or neurotherapy does not currently exist, and therefore one must look to existing state statutes. Irrespective of the treatment modality being used, most states and provinces have laws requiring that when someone offers services to the public indicating that he or she qualified to work with conditions with DSM-V or ICD-10 diagnostic labels (e.g., ADD/ADHD, depression, PTSD, OCD, anxiety, learning disabilities, insomnia), he or she must be licensed in a recognized health sciences profession and be operating within that scope of practice and competence. However, unlicensed practitioners can certainly use neurofeedback with nonclinical conditions (e.g., optimal performance) or under the supervision of licensed practitioners. Recognized professions also require that clinicians document specialty training in various treatment modalities. In neurofeedback the only recognized certification is from the Biofeedback Certification International Alliance (www.bcia.org), because it is administered by an independent, nonprofit organization not affiliated with a specific vendor or training method. Many consider this certification as demonstrating minimal entry-level competency in neurofeedback. Likewise, practitioners using qEEG as an assessment tool should be able to document training in this methodology. Certification in the use of qEEG is available from the Quantitative Electroencephalography Certification Board and from the EEG and Clinical Neuroscience Society (ECNS).

In thinking about ethical practice, consider the following situations. A young man who had been variously diagnosed as having bipolar disorder and OCD was told by a psychologist that he would require at least 100 sessions of neurofeedback! He was introduced to a technician who would conduct sessions with the patient (and two other patients simultaneously) but was told that the psychologist would look in on the last couple of minutes of each session to track progress. No pretreatment assessment of brain function was conducted, and only once did the patient see the psychologist again—in a casual interaction as he was leaving the office. The technologist was not present for the majority of the time in the neurofeedback sessions. The man progressively deteriorated over the course of 19 sessions and then made a suicide attempt. He sought treatment elsewhere and, after a qEEG assessment and 30 individually supervised neurofeedback sessions, was symptom free and remained so at 1 year's follow-up. The young man documented that the psychologist had billed Medicaid for the 30-minute neurofeedback sessions (done by the technician) as if they were individual psychotherapy sessions with the psychologist. He filed complaints with the licensure board and for Medicaid fraud. Would any of us want to be in this position?

Two other recent cases will provide further information for the reader to ponder. An unlicensed technician, working for a physician, was doing neurofeedback treatment over the internet with equipment he rented to a man living in a distant state. Neither the physician nor the technician was licensed in the state where the patient resided, and now the patient is alleging harm done and has pursued actions against the company providing the distance treatment. In another situation a marriage and family therapist began doing neurofeedback and now operates what has been referred to as "neurofeedback mills" where he has three offices, with his unlicensed wife and college student son running offices where clients are left alone on equipment for significant periods of time because multiple sessions are taking place simultaneously. Some clients are reporting adverse effects and seeking help elsewhere. Would you want to have such malpractice liability?

The author is currently aware of neurofeedback malpractice lawsuits being pursued; a case where a psychologist was fined and lost his license for insurance fraud owing to billing neurofeedback sessions as individual psychotherapy rather than using biofeedback procedure codes; and of a physician in similar trouble for billing neurofeedback as medical office visits. There are many cases where state investigators have shut down the neurotherapy practices of unlicensed persons who were advertising their work with diagnostically labeled conditions. In one case the unlicensed person was arrested and successfully prosecuted for practicing psychology without a license. In light of such cases, neurofeedback clinicians are encouraged to think about practice guidelines not only in terms of quality of service, but also in terms of liability protection. In this regard, the following questions are posed to encourage thoughtful self-examination.

If you had to defend yourself in court in a malpractice lawsuit, how would the following elements of your practice appear to other professionals and members of the public serving on a jury if someone was challenging your quality of care? (a) The amount of pretreatment assessment of brain function and history gathering before seeking to modify someone's brain function? (b) The scope of practice of your license versus conditions you are treating? (c) The degree of independence versus supervision of technicians you employ? (d) Adequacy of your record keeping? (e) Accurate billing of services to insurance companies? (f) Documentation of a detailed informed consent process, especially with regard to neurotherapy techniques, procedures or conditions for which neurotherapy would be regarded as more experimental owing to limited controlled outcomes research? (g) Claims made in your advertising for the efficacy of treatment with various conditions? (h) The degree of pretreatment evaluation and ongoing supervision of home (remote) training? (i) Whether you have neurofeedback certification by BCIA, and certification in using qEEG from ECNS or the qEEG Certification Board?

Consider: is it appropriate, ethical or legal for a person to be doing distance training out of state with someone who resides in a state where the practitioner is not licensed? Is it appropriate, ethical or wise in terms of liability for a practitioner or company to rent equipment to home users without regular, ongoing supervision of what they are doing, and restrictions on whom the equipment may be used with and the manner in which it is to be used? Under what conditions does an introductory training course qualify a licensed practitioner to begin treating with neurotherapy methods? Should such a person be receiving ongoing mentoring? Is it appropriate, ethical or wise in terms of your liability to do qEEG analyses where you make neurofeedback treatment recommendations for unlicensed persons who may be treating diagnostic conditions?

Outcome research in neurofeedback has generally taken place with a trained therapist present in the room, supervising and coaching the client. Therefore, does it represent a high quality of care for therapists or technicians to attach clients to neurofeedback equipment and then leave them alone for most of the session? Cannot a person with attention problems "space out" as easily in neurofeedback as he or she does in school if not also being actively coached?

If you use a technician, is it wise to allow that person to conduct sessions without regular close supervision, or to run sessions all day in offices without a licensed person present? For liability protection, should licensed persons employing technicians have a document, signed by the technician, indicating their duties, responsibilities, types of services or conditions with which they can work, limits of their independent actions and responsibilities for reporting side effects or lack of progress to their supervisor?

How would you defend yourself in a malpractice lawsuit where someone indicated that he or she had experienced side effects or harm, and yet your website or informed consent suggested that neurofeedback was entirely safe?

For organizations and manufacturers, is it appropriate or ethical to train or to sell to unlicensed persons who are not going to be working under a licensed person's supervision? Should there be safety precautions in place for the management of side effects or adverse reactions in training workshops when large numbers of persons are simultaneously attached to equipment?

It is recommended for liability protection that practitioners engage in an informed consent process, documented in writing, that (a) identifies their qualifications; (b) notes areas of application that many persons would regard as experimental because there are no controlled studies; (c) identifies that there can occasionally be side effects or negative reactions, and how these should be reported to the clinician; (d) makes the client aware that there are other possible treatments (e.g., cognitive behavior therapy, medication); (e) indicates that significant improvement does not always occur; (f) indicates that medication needs and response to medications may change as neurotherapy progresses; and (g) addresses the Health Information Portability and Accountability Act, limits of confidentiality and fee policies.

REFERENCES

1. Jackson GE. *Rethinking Psychiatric Drugs: A Guide for Informed Consent*. Bloomington, IN: AuthorHouse; 2005.
2. Khan A, Khan S, Brown WA. Are placebo controls necessary to test new antidepressants and anxiolytics? *Int J Neuropsychopharmacol*. 2002;5:193–197.
3. Kirsch DL. *The Science Behind Cranial Electrotherapy Stimulation*. 2nd ed. Edmonton, Canada: Medical Scope Publishing Corporation; 2002.
4. Kirsch I. *The Emperor's New Drugs: Exploding the Antidepressant Myth*. New York, NY: Basic Books; 2010.
5. Kirsch I, Deacon BJ, Huedo-Medina TB, Scorbia A, Moore TJ, Johnson BT. Initial severity and antidepressant benefits. *PLoS Med*. 2008;5:260–268.
6. Kirsch I, Moore TJ, Scoboria A, Nicholls SS. The emperor's new drugs: an analysis of antidepressant medication data submitted to the U.S. food and drug administration. *Prev Treat*. 2002;5 Article 23. <http://www.journals.apa.org/prevention/>.
7. Moncrieff J. A comparison of antidepressant trials using active and inert placebos. *Int J Methods Psychiatr Res*. 2003;12:117–127.
8. Moncrief J. *The Myth of the Chemical Cure: A Critique of Psychiatric Drug Treatment*. New York, NY: Palgrave Macmillan; 2009.
9. Sterman MB. Basic concepts and clinical findings in the treatment of seizure disorders with EEG operant conditioning. *Clin Electroencephalogr*. 2000;3:45–55.
10. Sterman MB, LoPresti RW, Fairchild MD. Encephalographic and behavioral studies of monomethyl hydrazine toxicity in the cat. *J Neurother*. 2010;14:293–300.
11. Kamiya J. The first communications about operant conditioning of the EEG. *J Neurother*. 2011;15:65–73.

12. Hammond DC. What is neurofeedback: an update. *J Neurother*. 2011;15:305–336.
13. Lubar JF. Neurofeedback for the management of attention-deficit/hyperactivity disorders. In: Schwartz MS, ed. *Biofeedback: A Practitioner's Guide*. New York, NY: Guilford; 1995:493–522.
14. Monastra VJ, Monastra DM, George S. The effects of stimulant therapy, EEG biofeedback, and parenting style on the primary symptoms of attention-deficit/hyperactivity disorder. *Appl Psychophysiol Biofeedback*. 2002;27:231–249.
15. Peniston EG, Kulkosky PJ. Alcoholic personality and alpha-theta brainwave training. *Med Psychother*. 1991;2:37–55.
16. Peniston EG, Kulkosky PJ. Alpha-theta brainwave neuro-feedback therapy for Vietnam veterans with combat-related post-traumatic stress disorder. *Med Psychother*. 1991;4:47–60.
17. Strehl U, Leins U, Gopth G, Klinger C, Hinterberger T, Birbaumer N. Self-regulation of slow cortical potentials: A new treatment for children with attention-deficit/hyperactivity disorder. *Pediatrics* 2006;118:1530–1540.
18. Chabot RJ, di Michele F, Prichep L. The role of quantitative electroencephalography in child and adolescent psychiatric disorders. *Child Adolesc Psychiatry Clin North Am*. 2005;14:21–53.
19. Hammond DC. The need for individualization in neurofeedback: heterogeneity in QEEG patterns associated with diagnoses and symptoms. *Appl Psychophysiol Biofeedback*. 2010;35:31–36.
20. Baehr E, Rosenfeld JP, Baehr R. Clinical use of an alpha asymmetry neurofeedback protocol in the treatment of mood disorders: Follow-up study one to five years post therapy. *J Neurother*. 2001;2001(4):11–18.
21. Hammond DC. Neurofeedback treatment of depression and anxiety. *J Adult Dev*. 2005;12:131–138.
22. Hammond DC, Baehr E. Neurofeedback for the treatment of depression: current status of theoretical issues and clinical research. In: Budzynski TH, Budzynski HK, Evans JR, Abarbanel A, eds. *Introduction to Quantitative EEG and Neurofeedback: Advanced Theory and Applications*. 2nd ed. New York, NY: Elsevier; 2009:295–313.
23. Hammond DC. Neurofeedback to improve physical balance, incontinence, and swallowing. *J Neurother*. 2005;9:27–36.
24. Hoedlmoser K, Pecherstorfer T, Gruber G, et al. Instrumental conditioning of human sensorimotor rhythm (12–15 Hz) and its impact on sleep as well as declarative learning. *Sleep*. 2008;31:1401–1408.
25. Hammer BU, Colbert AP, Brown KA, Illioi EC. Neurofeedback for insomnia: a pilot study of Z-score SMR and individualized protocols. *Appl Psychophysiol Biofeedback*. 2011;36:251–264.
26. Larsen S, Larsen R, Hammond DC, et al. The LENS neurofeedback with animals. *J Neurother*. 2006;10:89–101.
27. Strehl U. Slow cortical potentials neurofeedback. *J Neurother*. 2009;13:117–126.
28. Toomim H, Carmen J. Hemoencephalography: photon-based blood flow neurofeedback. In: Budzyknski TH, Budzynski HK, Evans JR, Abarbanel A, eds. *Introduction to Quantitative EEG and Neurofeedback: Advanced Theory and Applications*. 2nd ed. New York, NY: Elsevier; 2009:169–194.
29. Othmer SF, Othmer S. Interhemispheric EEG. Training: clinical experience and conceptual models. In: Evans JR, ed. *Handbook of Neurofeedback, Dynamics and Clinical Applications*. New York, NY: Haworth Medical Press; 2007:109–136.
30. Legarda SB, McMahon D, Othmer S, Othmer S. Clinical neurofeedback: case studies, proposed mechanism, and implications for pediatric neurology practice. *J Child Neurol*. 2011;26:1045–1051.
31. Thatcher RW. *Handbook of Quantitative Electroencephalography and EEG Biofeedback*. St. Petersberg, FL: Anipublishing; 2012.

32. Breggin PR. *Brain Disabling Treatments in Psychiatry: Drugs, Electroshock, and the Psychopharmaceutical Complex*. New York, NY: Springer; 2007:237–239.

33. Coleman EA, Sackeim HA, Prudic J, Devanand DP, McElhiney MC, Moody BJ. Subjective memory complaints prior to and following electroconvulsive therapy. *Biol Psychiatry*. 1996;39(5):346–356.

34. Feliu M, Edwards CL, Sudhakar S, et al. Neuropsychological effects and attitudes in patients following electroconvulsive therapy. *Neuropsychiatr Dis Treat*. 2008;4:613–617.

35. MacQueen G, Parkin C, Marriott M, Begin H, Hasey G. The long-term impact of treatment with electroconvulsive therapy on discrete memory systems in patients with bipolar disorder. *J Psychiatry Neurosci*. 2007;32:241–249.

36. Philpot M, Collins C, Trivedi P, Treloar A, Gallacher S, Rose D. Eliciting users' views of ECT in two mental health trusts with a user-designed questionnaire. *J Ment Health*. 2004;3:403–413.

37. Sackeim HA, Prudic J, Fuller R, Keilp J, Lavori PW, Olfson M. The cognitive effects of electroconvulsive therapy in community settings. *Neuropsychopharmacology*. 2007;32:244–254.

38. Sussman N. In session with Charles H. Kellner, MD: current developments in electroconvulsive therapy. *Prim Psychiatry*. 2007;14:34–37.

39. Read J, Bentall R. The effectiveness of electroconvulsive therapy: a literature review. *Epidemiol Psychiatria Soc*. 2010;19:333–347.

40. Spronk D, Arns J, Fitzgerald PB. Repetitive transcranial magnetic stimulation in depression: protocols, mechanisms, and new developments. In: Coben R, Evans JR, eds. *Neurofeedback and Neuromodulation Techniques and Applications*. New York, NY: Academic Press; 2011:257–291.

41. Zaghi S, Acar M, Hultgren B, Boggio PS, Fregni F. Noninvasive brain stimulation with low-intensity electrical currents: putative mechanisms of action for direct and alternating current stimulation. *Neuroscientist*. 2010;6:285–307.

42. Wahbeh H, Calabrese C, Zwickey H, Zajdel D. Binaural beat technology in humans: a pilot study to assess neuropsychologic, physiologic, and electroencephalographic effects. *J Altern Complement Med*. 2007;13:199–206.

43. Harding GF. Video-game epilepsy. *Lancet*. 1994;35:1208–1216.

44. Quirk J, Fish DR, Smith SJ, Sander JW, Shorvon SD, Allen PJ. Incidence of photosensitive epilepsy: a prospective national study. *Electroencephalogr Clin Neurophysiol*. 1995;95:260–267.

45. Russell H. Intellectual, auditory, and photic stimulation and changes in functioning in children and adults. *Biofeedback*. 1997;25(16–17):23–24.

46. Frederick J, Lubar JL, Rasey H, Brim S, Blackburn J. Effects of 18.5 Hz auditory and visual stimulation on EEG amplitude at the vertex. *J Neurother*. 1999;3(3):23–27.

47. Frederick J, Timmerman DL, Russell HL, Lubar J. EEG coherence effects of audio-visual stimulation (AVE) at dominant and twice dominant alpha frequency. *J Neurother*. 2004;8(4):25–42.

48. Budzynski TH, Jordy J, Budzynski HK, Tang HY, Claypoole K. Academic performance enhancement with photic stimulation and EDR feedback. *J Neurother*. 1999;3:11–21.

49. Berg K, Siever D. A controlled comparison of audio-visual entrainment for treating seasonal affective disorder. *J Neurother*. 2009;13(3):166–175.

50. Joyce M, Siever D. Audio-visual entrainment program as a treatment for behavior disorders in a school setting. *J Neurother*. 2000;4(2):9–25.

51. Collura TF, Siever D. Audio-visual entrainment in relation to mental health and EEG. In: Budzynski TH, Budzynski HG, Evans JR, Abarbanel A, eds. *Introduction to Quantitative EEG and Neurofeedback*. New York, NY: Elsevier; 2009:195–224.

52. Striefel S. The role of aspirational ethics and licensing laws in the practice of neuro-feedback. *J Neurother.* 2000;4:43–55.
53. Striefe S. The applications of ethics and law in daily practice. In: Schwartz MS, Andrasik F, eds. *Biofeedback: A Practitioners Guide.* 3rd ed. New York, NY: Guilford; 2003:835–880.
54. Striefel S. *Practice Guidelines and Standards for Practitioners of Biofeedback and Applied Psychophysiological Services.* Wheat Ridge, CO: Association for Applied Psychophysiology and Biofeedback; 2004.
55. Striefel S. Ethics in neurofeedback practice. In: Budzynski TH, Budzynski HG, Evans JR, Abarbanel A, eds. *Introduction to Quantitative EEG and Neurofeedback.* New York, NY: Elsevier; 2009:475–492.
56. Hammond DC, Bodenhamer-Davis G, Gluck G, et al. Standards of practice for neurofeedback and neurotherapy: a position paper of the International Society for Neurofeedback & Research. *J Neurother.* 2011;15:54–64.
57. Hammond DC, Kirk L. First do no harm: adverse effects and the need for practice standards in neurofeedback. *J Neurother.* 2008;12:79–88.
58. Hammond DC, Stockdale S, Hoffman D, Ayers ME, Nash J. Adverse reactions and potential iatrogenic effects in neurofeedback training. *J Neurother.* 2001;4:57–69.
59. Lubar JF, Shabsin HS, Natelson SE, Holder GS, Whitsett SF, Pamplin WE. EEG operant conditioning in intractible epileptics. *Arch Neurol.* 1981;38:700–704.
60. Lubar JF, Shouse MN. EEG and behavioral changes in a hyperactive child concurrent with training of the sensorimotor rhythm (SMR): a preliminary report. *Biofeedback Self Regul.* 1976;1:293–306.
61. Lubar JF, Shouse MN. Use of biofeedback in the treatment of seizure disorders and hyperactivity. *Adv Clin Child Psychol.* 1977;1:204–251.
62. Matthews TV. Neurofeedback overtraining and the vulnerable patient. *J Neurother.* 2010;11(3):63–66.
63. Todder D, Levine J, Dwolatzky T, Kaplan Z. Case report: impaired memory and disorientation induced by delta band down-training over the temporal brain regions by neurofeedback treatment. *J Neurother.* 2010;14:153–155.
64. Whitsett SF, Lubar JF, Holder GS, Natelson S. A double-blind investigation of the relationship between seizure activity and the sleep EEG following EEG biofeedback training. *Biofeedback Self Regul.* 1982;7:193–209.

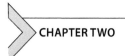

CHAPTER TWO

An Introductory Perspective on the Emerging Application of qEEG in Neurofeedback

Richard Soutar

The first efforts to develop a normative quantitative electroencephalographic (qEEG) database were by Matousek and Petersen.[1] Shortly following this publication, E. Roy John and his associates[2] also collected and developed their results. At about this same time, the first book on quantitative electrophysiology using normative reference EEG databases was written by E. Roy John and Robert Thatcher and published in 1977. At Harvard, Frank Duffy[3] had also been investigating this new approach to EEG analysis and, in parallel with John's work, in the 1980s developed a brain electrical mapping system (BEAM) to display electrical signals from electrodes into a color-coded map of the brain's electrical activity. Duffy's first major article, "Brain Electrical Activity Mapping (BEAM): Computerized Access to Complex Brain Function," was published in 1981. He formed Braintech, Inc in 1982 to develop, manufacture and distribute technology designed to convert EEG signals into topographic maps. Duffy and colleagues[4] also published a comprehensive volume on brain mapping entitled *Clinical Electroencephalography and Topographic Brain Mapping: Technology and Practice.*

John developed and marketed his first EEG database through a variety of enterprises, starting in the late 1970s and continuing into the early 1990s, which sold EEG acquisition systems with software on board to process and provide raw and Z-scored information about EEG variables. In an effort to increase the ability to calculate and produce age-adjusted Z-scored EEG information, John and associates then developed translators that would allow a wider variety of hardware acquisition systems. This software was sold and marketed under the name NxLink and achieved 510(K) status in 1998. However, it was soon withdrawn from the market because of a variety of business problems. This database was the first one generally used by a handful of neurofeedback practitioners and became the basis for the beginning of qEEG-guided neurofeedback.

Clinical Neurotherapy.
Doi: http://dx.doi.org/10.1016/B978-0-12-396988-0.00002-7

Robert Thatcher soon developed the Life Span Database from his work at the University of Maryland, which he initially marketed through Lexicor and eventually renamed Neuroguide. Neuroguide was quickly adopted as a major replacement for NxLink by the neurofeedback field, and in 2004 Robert Thatcher filed for 510(K) status.

These databases seemed initially destined for medical use, but the American Academy of Neurology opposed the consideration and use of Neurometrics in the field of medicine, and, under the leadership of Marc Nuwer,[5] published a position paper accordingly. It was an arguably flawed paper with respect to its analysis, as pointed out by responses from members of the Association for Applied Psychophysiology and Biofeedback and the International Society for Neurofeedback and Research (ISNR).[6] Instead of much medical use, these and other databases came to be progressively used by neurofeedback practitioners. The others included Bill Hudspeth's Neurorep Database and Barry Sterman and David Kaiser's database, The Skil Topometric Database. Some lesser known but widely used databases have eventually emerged in the field of neurofeedback, such as the Biological Records Centre database, reputed to be the largest and most comprehensive with respect to cognitive and neurophysiological measures (which filed for 510(K) status in 2005,[7] and Uri Kropotov's Human Brain Indices database system, which came somewhat later.[8] These later databases also include event-related potential data that can be used in assessment and task-based measures of EEG. In addition, several smaller referential databases emerged from the field of neurofeedback, such as Peter Van Deusan's TLC John Demo's MiniQ database and a still more extended version of the MiniQ in The New Mind Database System. These smaller databases were developed solely for neurofeedback users and typically did not involve the same statistical rigor and precision as those mentioned above. Nevertheless, they filled a void in neurofeedback, providing low-cost, simple-to-understand methods of qEEG assessment that provided a gateway to the use of the more sophisticated databases. To best use the more sophisticated systems clearly requires a good understanding of statistics and considerable training.

DATABASE CONSTRUCTION

The details of database construction are beyond the scope of this chapter, but a basic understanding of the methods used is important for the clinician to have in order to properly utilize them in a clinical neurofeedback setting. It is also important for clinicians to explain to other professionals the basic methods used to derive the databases and discuss the related research in a manner that demonstrates competence and inspires confidence.

The first step involves gathering and then carefully screening a sample of subjects for any signs of neurological or psychological problems in order to determine them as "normal." The databases provided by E. Roy John and associates, for example, screened all subjects by questionnaire for head injury, neurological or psychiatric disease, history of psychological problems, alcohol or drug abuse, use of psychiatric medication, and academic and social problems. Subjects were also psychometrically tested for evidence of cognitive or academic impairment.[2] Although a random sample of the entire normal population is desirable, this is obviously impractical, and other statistical techniques are employed to compensate for this. To offset this limitation, this original database was pooled from subjects in several places around the world. Subsequent statistical analyses showed that brain parameters were the same developmentally regardless of race or cultural upbringing.

Methodologically, EEG data are then collected from the sample of "normal" individuals using 19 or 21 locations on the scalp, utilizing the standard 10–20 system for EEG electrode placement developed by Jasper.[9] Medical-grade EEG amplifiers are used for this process and all electrodes are checked for proper impedance, typically at or below $5\,k\Omega$. The amplified EEG signals are digitized and then later computer processed, where they are filtered through a bandpass filter to eliminate noise and other frequencies (usually $>40\,Hz$) not relevant to analysis. They then are subjected to Fast Fourier analysis for further processing to derive the amplitude and power in each of five frequency bands. These bands are usually delta (0.5–3.9 Hz), theta (4.0–7.9 Hz), alpha (8–12.5 Hz) and beta (12.6–30 Hz). Recent developments have resulted in efforts to collect EEG up to 70 Hz as well in order to capture gamma frequencies (30–70 Hz) for inclusion and analysis. Some of these frequency bands are sometimes subdivided into low and high band components, for example alpha1 = 8–10 Hz and alpha2 = 10–12 Hz, etc.

Further computations are also performed to derive measures of peak frequency, phase, coherence and asymmetry. Peak frequency is defined as the peak within a broad band frequency at which the majority of the power falls. Phase is defined as the degree to which two waves from different sites are out of phase with each other. Coherence is commonly defined as the magnitude of waveform symmetry between active sites. Asymmetry, or power asymmetry, refers to the difference in power between two sites. This is done for each electrode location, or in the case of symmetry measures, from every pairwise comparison of electrode comparisons that can be made intra- or interhemispherically.

Further multivariate analysis (analyses of complex relationships between many variables) of these dimensions may be performed for purposes of reducing the variable set, for example collapsing all measures in the left hemisphere into one measure representing the deviation in the left hemisphere from a normed value; or more complex analyses such as developing discriminants to identify unique statistical features common to clinically identified categories of diagnosis, such as biopolar disorder or schizophrenia.

Factors such as age, gender and hand dominance require further consideration. Past research indicates that there is little difference between men and women.[2] Differences in EEG distribution related to hand dominance are found only in a very small percentage of the left-handed population that actually has reversed hemispheric dominance. Age difference has so far been dealt with in two basic fashions. One is to use age groups that show consistently similar mean values,[10] and the other is to adjust EEG values using linear or higher-ordered polynomial regression equations to correct such values caused by age effects.[2,11] The distribution of scores must be inspected to determine whether it is gaussian and thus appropriate for parametric evaluation. EEG scores typically exhibit some skewness and kurtosis. The use of a log-10 transformation has been found to be one of the better transformation functions to adjust for this deviance.

CONCERNS REGARDING NORMATIVE DATABASES

Niedermeyer and Lopes da Silva[12] note that perhaps as much as 15% of the population has globally low power. Little research has been done to determine the actual source of this phenomenon. Niedermeyer's citations on this topic are few, and he acknowledges many potential sources other than skull thickness, such as genetics, metabolic deficiencies and neurophysiological damage, such as that found in alcoholism. Thus, low power may be related to issues of both mental and physical health, and this population may be overrepresented in clinical settings. It has been argued that using normative measures on such a group (and perhaps others) may be a violation of statistical assumptions and parametric statistical theory. Some authors have expressed concern that a normative database may not accurately measure or represent abnormal populations.[13] However, the fact that databases such as that described by John et al.[2] have been cross-validated across laboratories around the world while meeting face, construct and convergent validity is a strong argument in support of the validity of this approach. In addition, the authors and developers of normative databases argue that indicators of test–retest and split-half reliability have shown that such measures are highly reliable in the same individuals over time, except when it begins to stretch across years (as with children, where changes are expected to happen as a result of growth and development).[14] The best of these databases have met the scientific standards of validity and reliability with respect to a general normal range of EEG activity and have been found to be very valuable measurement tools for research and clinical work.

The concept of "normal" is considered problematic by many critics of databases and will continue to be a challenge. Many ask, "Who defines normal, and is it the same across cultures and their subpopulations?" Clearly, many behaviors and possibly related physiological features that are considered unacceptable and abnormal in our Euro-American culture are accepted in other cultures. However, because the development of neurometric databases has been validated across different cultures, there is a high degree of confidence within the neurometric community that this issue has been laid to rest, and that brain development is generally the same regardless of race or culture. Those using neurometric databases are more likely to argue instead that accumulating research indicates that we now have a normative standard as a reference that better allows us to measure unique features of people, ranging from gifted individuals to those with disorders.

OTHER FACTORS AFFECTING DATA

Amplifier characteristics are an important consideration. EEG signals collected from the scalp are very weak – in the microvolt range – and require several stages of amplification before they can be processed and analyzed. Amplifiers vary in their construction and the efficiency with which they amplify different frequencies, and have the potential to distort values. Older analogue amplifiers used to collect EEG were often less efficient than more modern amplifiers, and more subject to noise and artifact because of low input impedance. The newer method of signal processing, on the other hand, requires the digitization of signals for computer analysis, and this can distort signals as well. Collection methods today typically require 256 samples per second of EEG data. Lower and higher rates tend to distort the amplitudes in the range of frequencies used in EEG analysis.

Signal processing differences can create differences in the way brain maps look. Many practitioners are disconcerted by the differences in amplitude and coherence they might find between qEEG map systems when mapping the same individual. Amplifier characteristics, filter types, filter settings, signal processing equations and significance settings for color representation can all affect map appearances.

Amplifiers vary in how evenly they amplify each frequency and typically display some bias: delta or theta frequencies may be amplified more than beta, or vice versa. This will have an effect downstream in the processing of the signal and may result in distortions in signal representation. Being sure the signal is processed in such a manner as to account for amplifier bias has been an important issue.[10] In contemporary times, however, amplifiers are rigorously tested by manufacturing companies to ensure they meet industry standards, and their findings are usually published in their specification manuals. Consequently, this is less of an issue at present.

The usual method for map analysis is to process the raw data through a band-pass filter to eliminate unwanted frequencies, submit the filtered data to Fast Fourier Transform analysis to derive the power in each frequency band, and then compute the remaining values of interest, such as magnitude and coherence. Even small coding errors can cause differences at each stage of this process. Equations may vary slightly for dimensions of interest, such as coherence and dominant or peak frequency, depending on user preference. This is one of the reasons the ISNR position paper on the uses of qEEG databases recommends using one database consistently for clinical analysis.[15] In spite of these factors, there is a fairly high degree of concordance between databases now being made commercially available.

Maps may have different color schemes, and these will vary depending on considerations of significance level selected for each color. Although deviation by two or more standard deviations (SD) from the norm may seem statistically reasonable as an indication of clinical deviance, the clinical population may demonstrate a different distribution pattern. For example, if 50% of that population is coming out of or going into a disorder, a significance level of 1 SD in some frequency bands may be more indicative of a problem than 2 SD. A client with a map having an absolute power deviance in the theta frequencies that is deviant by <1.5 SD may have neurological test scores which are significantly abnormal. The same could be true for delta frequencies. Such issues will require more research in the future to further define best settings. Also, they argue for a closer look into and increased use of the more subtle features of multivariate measures over univariate measures, which at present are more commonly inspected by practitioners in neurofeedback.

Maps also vary in their representation of the collected data. Some systems focus on the 10–20 locations specifically, whereas others use an interpolation technique to estimate the values that might exist between electrode locations. This approach produces a contour map that is more sophisticated in appearance but may not always be accurate in assumptions. Both John and Duffy generated their own solutions to this procedure,[16] and it is a popular method of representation in qEEG today.

ADDITIONAL ANALYSIS METHODS

At present the majority of normative databases use EEG collected using a linked ear reference. One of the two inputs from each of the amplifiers used to collect data are linked together and connected to both ears, and the remaining inputs are individually assigned and connected to each of the 19 scalp locations typically used to collect data. There are many other collection methods used in medical EEG, and these are referred to as montages. A few of the databases allow practitioners to reconfigure the montage through programming techniques. A popular one is the Laplacian montage, which is a form of weighted averaging. The weighted average reference compares each electrode to all other electrodes in a given array, and weighting factors are based on actual scalp interelectrode distances. Weighting factors are usually calculated as inverse linear distances: the longer the distance from the input, the less the surrounding electrodes will contribute to the reference. The Laplacian montage therefore uses the weighted average of electrodes surrounding the electrode of interest. But some electrodes at the edge of the array, such as F7, cannot be surrounded in the 10/20 system, and these edge effects can limit accuracy. Nevertheless, it is good for filtering out diffuse effects and emphasizing local waveforms, so that input to the electrodes from volume conduction is ignored in favor of local amplitudes.[16a] This can be useful, for example, when inspecting the maps for drug effects, which usually show up as diffuse elevations of specific frequencies.

LORETA

Low-resolution electromagnetic tomography analysis (LORETA) is a method of mathematically analyzing multiple EEG signals from across the scalp to determine their source from within the cortex. This method was developed by Roberto Pascual-Marqui in 1994.[17] The Physicist James Maxwell had long ago figured out how to compute where on the surface of a sphere a source of voltage from within the sphere would appear, but had never come up with a solution to do the reverse. In more recent times the mathematician Roberto Pascual-Marqui has figured out the solution to this dilemma, solving in mathematics what was known as the "inverse problem." Roberto's method based localization inference on the statistical parametric mapping of the EEG to the digitized Talairach Atlas from the Brain Imaging Centre at Montreal Neurological Institute. So, when an electrode is placed on a scalp site, we can estimate with fairly good accuracy where within the cortex EEG signals at that scalp site are originating. When a voltage is measured at the scalp, the other 19 locations can be used to determine its current source within the cortex. This technique is highly accurate and compares favorably with other imaging methods, such as positron emission tomography and magnetic resonance imaging (MRI), in terms of spatial accuracy, although, unlike the others, it is confined to the cortex.[18] In his 1999 paper Roberto argued that LORETA was capable of correct localization to within 1 voxel resolution on average. In 2002 he developed a new imaging method described as sLORETA, which reportedly yields images of standardized current density with zero localization error. There has been considerable experimental support for his findings from research using this imaging method. Still, more conservative experts in the field of medical EEG feel that inverse solutions should never be used in isolation to make important clinical decisions and should always be used adjunctively.[16a]

COLLECTION METHODS

A typical qEEG record length used in neurofeedback today is approximately 2 minutes of data derived from artifacting at least 5–10 minutes of data (assuming minimal artifact) for each condition of eyes closed and eyes open. The total length of time may be dictated by online monitoring of artifact to estimate whether there are sufficient EEG data to extract 2 minutes of artifact-free EEG. These data may be collected simultaneously using 19 channels, or sequentially using two or more channels from an amplifier. Each manufacturer has its own format, such as .eeg, .dat and .eas, and a standard appears to be emerging in .edf or European Data Format. The artifact-affected segments of data caused by such factors as eye blinks and movement can be edited out using special software that allows users to select the best EEG segments or epochs. Locations on the scalp that have the most artifact on average are the frontal and temporal leads Fp1, Fp2, F7, F8, T3 and T4, but all locations may be subject to contamination, even by weak muscle contractions.[19] In the 20–30 Hz range, contamination is most frequent at the frontal electrode sites, whereas temporal lobe leads are contaminated more by 40–80 Hz. After artifact-free selections are made, the record is knitted back together using mathematical techniques, and then processed using Fast Fourier analysis into groups of frequency bands that are usually analyzed for power, magnitude, phase, coherence and asymmetry. The "bands" may be 1 Hz in size and/or larger, such as a 4–8 Hz theta band. At this point the practitioner may write up a report analysis, send it out for analysis by a seasoned expert or load it into software that does automated report analysis. Experts vary somewhat in their interpretations, and on occasion more than one interpretation may be desirable. It is important to be properly trained in artifacting, but eliminating artifact from qEEG used for purposes of neurofeedback does not require great skill or time to learn. Individuals with medical backgrounds who are using qEEG for medical diagnosis and other applications, on the other hand, may want to acquire special extensive training for morphological analysis skills that pertain to their scope of practice. One of the best books on artifacting for neurofeedback therapists is the one published by ISNR and written by Cory Hammond and Jay Gunkelman.[20]

For many beginners the assumption is that "eyes open" is the obvious place to begin an analysis, and they struggle to understand that this assumption is incorrect. The primary analysis of a qEEG usually begins with the "eyes closed" map, because these data usually are the most artifact free and have proved to be the most reliable for interpretation and discriminant analysis.[21] In fact, NxLink did not provide eyes open map representations or discriminants, because they deemed it likely to be less reliable. Later database developers provided eyes open data to users with the understanding that it be used as additional data that may add information to the analysis.

Technical Aspects of Recording

Digitizing EEG to be processed by computers requires it to be diced up into bits that can be converted into numbers. This process must be done consistently at the correct rate of time to produce an accurate numerical representation of the waveforms. The minimum acceptable sampling rate is 2.5 times greater than the highest frequency of interest. If we are working with EEG up to 40 Hz, we should sample at somewhere close to 100 Hz minimum. Most of the neurofeedback equipment today typically samples between 120 and 256 samples per second. Sampling at rates lower than this will mean that when the signal is converted back to analogue form on the computer screen, it will not resemble the original waveform.

Input impedance, a measure of electrical resistance between the scalp and the electrode, is also important, and there is some dispute on just how rigorously it should be measured. The purpose of cleansing the skin with electrode gel before applying an electrode is to reduce impedance. Because this is a measure of resistance or opposition of a circuit to alternating current or EEG, the electrode and paste at the scalp represents the completion of such a circuit, and frequency measures can vary with the level of impedance. If it is incorrect, this can alter the amount of amplitude in each frequency band. There are medical standards for obtaining correct impedance. The current standard is $5\,\mathrm{k\Omega}$,[12] although the American Clinical Neurophysiology Society cites $10\,\mathrm{k\Omega}$ in its standards paper published in 2003. The standard of $5\,\mathrm{k\Omega}$ was established at a period in history when amplifier input impedance was limited by the technology of the time. Current equipment is capable of very high input impedances of $1\,\mathrm{G\Omega}$ or higher, and impedance levels up to $100\,\mathrm{k\Omega}$ can still provide good EEG readings[22,23,24]; however, at that level of impedance the signal is more subject to artifact. In a recent communication, Thatcher stated:

> Fluctuations in impedance (e.g., from 10 K to 100 K) are not relevant nor anything to be concerned about as long as you are using a modern amplifier that has high input impedance. High input resistance is important because small differences in electrode impedance will not result in differences in the output of the differential amplifier. If the impedance of a recording electrode is 10,000 ohms (1×10^4) as compared to 100,000 ohms (1×10^5) then this difference will be negligible, for example, if the input impedance is 100 giga-ohms (1×10^{11}) then (1×10^4)/(1×10^{11}) = 1×10^{-7} vs (1×10^5)/(1×10^{11}) = 1×10^{-6} and the difference between 0.00000001 vs 0.0000001 is very small and is therefore negligible.[22,23]

More recent efforts to establish international standards for qEEG recognize this change in technology, suggesting higher acceptable levels of scalp impedance.[24] Because there are considerable risks in breaking the skin from too much preparation, this should be balanced against zealous efforts to obtain perfect input impedance in a clinical setting.

There are a great number of publications demonstrating that qEEG is very stable over time if it is correctly recorded.[25] However, time of day can affect signal readings, and low circadian dips, such as between 2 pm and 5 pm, can lead to drowsiness possibly resulting in higher readings in the lower EEG frequencies.[10] Mornings tend to be better if good sleep is obtained; and a high-protein breakfast will help reduce blood sugar variations that may affect EEG. Poor sleep can also result in higher levels of slow-wave activity. Consequently, pre- and posttreatment maps are likely to be most accurate for comparison purposes if done at the same time each day. Time between food intake and qEEG acquisition can be important,[26] as can the type of food taken[27]; the last dosage of drugs being used is also important to consider.

ARTIFACTS AND CHALLENGES TO COLLECTING DATA

Client position during data collection is another important consideration, because EEG measures can vary between lying down and sitting up, and there is some controversy regarding the best positions. Medical EEGs are often collected in a prone position. However, because many of the databases were collected from individuals in a sitting position, it makes sense when these are used to record clinical EEGs in a sitting position. A chair that is too comfortable may put clients to sleep, whereas a rigid chair may result in discomfort and muscle tension, thereby increasing muscle artifact in the record. An electrode cap used to collect EEG data may also result in excessive muscle artifact if it is too tight. Dangling legs can introduce movement artifact, as can roving eyes. A room that is too hot or cold can affect recording, as can excess noise in the environment. A great number of individuals unconsciously grit their teeth, and this can introduce high levels of artifact into temporal lobe readings, and sometimes globally. Others have high muscle tension in their neck that generates excessive artifact in the posterior leads. Muscle artifact contaminates the record most clearly in the higher beta ranges, but can have considerable effect on frequencies as low as the 12 Hz range, and, in extreme cases, as low as 8 Hz.[19] Recent research using muscle paralysis techniques indicates that the majority of EEGs >20 Hz may be heavily contaminated with muscle artifact.[28] Fortunately, most of the EEG power is below roughly 26 Hz.

In spite of all of these problems, once a cap is placed on the head and gel is injected into the electrodes, an acceptable EEG usually can be collected within 45 minutes by a practiced technician.

READING A MAP

Watching an expert read a map is often fascinating and compelling. If done accurately, it inspires other clinicians with an intense desire to learn this skill. Unfortunately, like reading the raw EEG, it takes years of experience to learn. Beginning clinicians are encouraged to send their maps out for interpretation by experts. More recently, many of the database systems are providing symptom checklists that can be used in conjunction with the map to assist in interpretation. These systems also have discriminants based on multivariate analysis of the data that contribute significantly to the ease, accuracy and standardization of interpretation. These methods must be employed with caution, with a clear understanding of their limitations. They are not meant to be stand-alone diagnoses, but rather statistical probabilities that may be confirmatory in nature.[2,10,29]

THE CORTICAL WINDOW AND DEFAULT MODE

There is considerable evidence that an electrophysiological analysis of the cortex also can provide a robust picture of subcortical brain function, and this theory has been proposed by Kirk and Mackay.[30] Also, the discovery of the brain's default mode network reported by Buckner et al.[31] suggests that resting state analysis of the brain provides a good dynamic measure of overall cortical activity. Furthermore, recent research has emerged indicating that the default mode network can provide a clear picture of functional connectivity.[32–34] Relevant to the value of resting state brain analysis, prior to these discoveries, Thatcher[10] had already pointed out that assessments during active tasks likely involve too many confounding variables to provide a consistent, valid and reliable basis for qEEG evaluation. In addition, he pointed out that cortical, reticular and thalamocortical loops generate a high level of activity using at least 20% of the body's glucose in the eyes-closed state and consequently that it is a very brain-active state. Meehan[34] and others point out that the brain increases activity by only 5–15% under cognitive load. Hagemann's[35] work provides some evidence that using 10–20 locations may allow estimates of brain hub activity. In conjunction with eLORETA analysis, which is a genuine 3D distributed inverse solution with exact zero error localization in the presence of measurement and structured biological noise, the future of qEEG looks very bright with respect to its ability to provide an inexpensive and quick method of achieving a very accurate picture of brain dynamics with very high temporal and spatial resolution. Consequently, qEEG is being used more consistently in research today.[34,36] Its future use in the health field may be even more promising. At present the authors consider it to be an excellent tool for use in clinical neurofeedback.

Interpreting a brain map is a complex analytic process, and deriving treatment protocols is even more challenging because maps have so many dimensions of analysis. Consequently, intervention appears to be potentially useful in a variety of ways in each dimension.[10] It is of primary importance to understand all of these dimensions and the value of the information they provide in the analysis. In addition, in the process of evaluating the map one should review the actual values associated with the map, or "tabular information," in order to avoid overinterpretation of the map color changes. Sometimes a small increase in values can make values that are generally closer to 1 SD from normal appear as if they are reflective of 2 SD.

Power and amplitude are both measures of the energy in each frequency band of the EEG. Power is a universal value that is used extensively in physics, and useful in that it can be easily manipulated mathematically, especially for research purposes. It is a commonly used metric in databases. Some databases use amplitude or magnitude because it is the metric used clinically with most neurofeedback equipment. Power is amplitude squared. Magnitude is merely the average of amplitude over time. They mean roughly the same thing. Before qEEG as we know it today emerged, neurofeedback practitioners evaluated their clients, trained their clients, and communicated their findings to each other in terms of amplitude. The early work of Sterman[57] and Lubar[98] addressed levels of amplitude or magnitude in frequency bands such as SMR, beta and theta with respect to both research findings and clinical work. Consequently, the interpretation of brain function and symptomatology was in terms of spectral analysis with respect to amplitude. This continued to be an important dimension as qEEG migrated widely into the neurofeedback community. As user sophistication increased alongside clinical observation and access to measures of coherence and phase, other dimensions were observed to co-vary with symptomatology. A quick review of these dimensions can enhance an understanding of this evolution.

Power (or amplitude) is a measure of the waxing and waning of pre- and postsynaptic potentials.[4,16] This reflects electrophysiological activities of both excitation and inhibition. It can also be a proxy measure of hemodynamic response.[36–38] Power can vary by time of day as well as in response to metabolic changes in oxygen consumption and glucose consumption. Investigations into clamping blood flow to the brain indicate progressive slowing from alpha to theta to delta as resources diminish.[39] Niedermeyer and Lopes da Silva[12] note that low voltage is common in perhaps 7–12% of the population, and that "Low voltage records are categorically within broad normal limits of variability and do not represent an abnormality unless the frequency spectrum shows abnormal local or diffuse slowing, asymmetries, or paroxysmal events." It is unclear whether this is a genetic subtype or not, but some authors indicate that the prevalence of this lower voltage pattern seems to be more common after the age of 13, suggesting that the endocrine system may play a role. What is abnormal, according to Niedermeyer, is low-voltage EEG, which is dominated by either slow-wave activity or fast-wave activity. Ischemia, traumatic brain injury and alcoholism therefore also may be causally related to low power. Kaplan and Hammer[40] cite studies indicating that chronic excitotoxicity from stress and toxins can result in diminished EEG power. Power may also vary with respect to skull thickness,[35] but its effect is diminished to the point of irrelevance by statistical sampling in normative and reference database analysis.[10]

Delta

Recent research confirms that different frequencies to some degree reflect different general functions in the brain.[34,36,41] Delta reflects brain integration and white matter integrity,[42,43] although it appears we must use sub-delta frequencies to evaluate glial processes.[42] In a meta-analysis of the literature Knyazev suggests that delta <1 Hz is generated directly within cortical circuits, whereas higher-frequency delta rhythms are an intrinsic property of thalamacortical cells and intracortical network interactions. Delta may also reflect memory function[44] and general neurotransmitter activity with respect to acetylcholine and dopamine. Because of its activities in networks linking the brainstem and hypothalamus with the cortex, and especially the insula,[45] it is closely affiliated with the physiological interface between the brain and the body. In summary, it appears that slower delta frequencies relate to cortical integration with the body as well as regulation of the body in general, whereas higher delta frequencies relate to cognitive processes such as working memory.[44]

Theta

We should initially divide theta into functional theta and pathological theta.[46] Pathological tonic theta may result from cortical damage or hypoperfusion and may be diffuse or focal in any region. Elevated theta correlated with diminished blood perfusion, especially if it is focal, has been reported in a series of studies that have continued to support this since the 1970s.[39] Functional theta is generated in the septal hippocampal regions[13,46] but appears to be regulated in frequency by brainstem input from the reticular activation system. Whereas a general network generates basic rhythms in the 3–4 Hz range that predominate in the temporal regions, the supramammillary and entorhinal pathways enhance this process with output in the 5–7 Hz range, which finds its way through thalamic connections with the frontal midline.[30] These two thetas appear to be related to emotion[46] and memory[47] as well as spatial processing,[41] with the frontal theta relating to recognition and the left and right temporal theta relating to verbal recall and spatial orientation, respectively.

Frontal theta is sinusoidal in nature and high in amplitude as it generates 1–10 seconds bursts, and this phasic theta tends to be in response to events.[48] Hippocampal theta tends to be more tonic and diffuse and has been recorded in the posterior cingulate, entorhinal cortex, hypothalamus and amygdala.[46] Kahana et al.[49] and Mitchell et al.[46] found theta from areas all over the cortex using subdural electrodes that eliminate volume conduction issues. Sauseng et al.[47] agree that theta is related to encoding and retrieval, and appears to be predominantly in the 4 Hz range in young children and 5–6 Hz in older children. It is prominent in posterior regions in children and migrates forward with age.

The concept that hippocampal theta resonates with various cortical sites to elicit and coordinate memory has been proposed by leading theorists, and agrees with the perspectives regarding resonance proposed by Nunez and Srinivasan[50] and Buzsaki.[41] Meehan[34] reviews the current research to report strong support for the theory that globally active theta binds local gamma locations in autoassociative networks that appear ephemerally to generate longer-lasting beta networks involved in the actual cognitive processing operations. Because of conduction delays, theta may be well suited to synchronize global processing and integrate local cortical networks operating in gamma during the process in which cell ensembles form sensory and motor nodes in response to task demands.[51] Exactly who is master or slave in the theta and gamma dance is still unclear.[52] Interestingly, Bassette et al.[53] propose that frequency may code the channels of communication whereas phase modulations transmit the information. Phase-locking activities are likely the mechanism that integrates limbic emotional with cortical cognitive co-regulation.[22,23]

Alpha

Alpha appears to be related to resource allocation in the cortex. Although Anderson and Anderson[54] felt they had established alpha as emerging from the thalamus, subsequent work by others led Nunez[50] to conclude that alpha production is the result of a resonance process between the thalamus and the cortex. It has been observed more recently that alpha can indeed occur over any region of the brain,[12] just as theta activity can, but that it does seem closely tied to thalamic activity much as theta is closely tied to hippocampal activity. Interestingly enough, it also seems closely tied to reticular activation much as theta is tied to it[52] in order to participate in binding mechanisms and resource allocation with respect to orientation and task sequences.[55] Hughes and Crunelli[56] identify two major pathways of alpha production much in the manner that theta has two pathways. One is generated in the posterior region in the cuneus and dominates the posterior region, being the classic dominant eyes-closed alpha discovered by Berger that tends to operate between 9.5 and 10.5 Hz. The other pathway is in the motor strip, occupies a higher frequency range and is often called Mu. There appears to be a pathological diffuse alpha that occurs as well and is especially prominent in hepatic dysregulation, which has been common knowledge among EEG specialists and neurologists for decades.

Alpha diminishes while on task, and this is referred to as desynchronization.[12] It also diminishes during sleep onset,[57] and often can be observed when collecting EEG data as clients increase in drowsiness. Alpha slowing is a normal consequence of aging, and slowing, combined with increased frequency theta, often is an indicator of pathologically slowed high-amplitude alpha associated with cognitive decline and Parkinson's disease, as seen in the early studies of E. Roy John.[11] This pattern is usually seen in connection with global hypercoherence.[58] It likely reflects growing metabolic inefficiency as myelination degrades and cell death increases in the cortex.[12,40,42]

Beta

The higher EEG frequencies require greater energy for their production and place a greater metabolic demand on the brain's support system.[50] Beta appears to be most correlated with cognitive processing and is stimulated into activity by gamma.[34] Beta appears to be recruited locally from groups of cell ensembles, and its range of activity is confined to short distances. Beta is often divided into subcomponent bands of beta 1, beta 2, beta 3 and gamma, and opinions vary over how their territory is carved up. The higher beta frequencies are more correlated with arousal and vigilance functions, but some authors have made a convincing case that they are mostly a result of muscle artifact.[28] Heller et al.[59] found that elevated right hemisphere beta correlated highly with anxiety, and more recent work by Perlis et al.[60] found higher temporal lobe frequencies of beta associated with insomnia, whereas Walker[61] found central high beta correlated with migraines.

Gamma

The gamma range is also controversial, with some arguing that it extends up to 100 Hz,[52] whereas others extend it up to 150 Hz.[51] For more practical applications gamma is often defined in databases such as Neuroguide as 30–40 Hz. Gamma interacts with theta to recruit neurons stimulating local cell column activity.[34,50] Consequently it is especially associated with cortical processing related to cognitive functions. There has been much excitement about its relationship to meditative states,[62] but the exact nature of its function in these states is very vague. It was at one time popular to evaluate and train Sheer rhythms in this frequency domain to attempt to enhance academic performance.[63] More recently, Keizer et al.[64] have again begun investigating gamma training as a possible approach to enhancing intelligence and report promising results. Unfortunately, there has long been an ongoing argument among researchers regarding whether gamma can actually be effectively measured using current EEG technology because of muscle contamination, and previously mentioned recent research appears to strongly argue against it. Until this issue is resolved, this frequency domain will continue to be of limited clinical value.

CONNECTING FREQUENCY FUNCTION TO LOCATION FUNCTION BY SYMPTOM

The 10–20 system is the standard electrode location method used to collect EEG data and is the standard for most current databases. It was devised at a time when equipment was generally more limited in its capacity to record data and was not based on any anatomical considerations relating to function or structure, such as underlying Brodmann areas. The first effort in the neurofeedback community to generate a correlation between the 10–20 system, the Brodmann areas and brain functions based on MRI research was apparently by Soutar.[65,66] More recently there have been many more detailed efforts to correlate the two for purposes of qEEG-guided neurofeedback. There is a fair degree of correlation between many of the Brodmann locations and the 10–20 system; however, there are many more Brodmann locations than 19, and so it is a biased sample. Nonetheless, the results have been useful. The identification by Hagmann et al.[67] of key hubs in the brain has allowed further useful correlations with the 10–20 system and functions, but hubs are likely to tie together many important functions into one location. The scale-free small-worlds structure of brain connectivity results in six to eight key "rich club hubs" serving a large number of nodes with diverse functions,[34] thus allowing for a good measure of general levels of functionality but underestimating specific levels of various functions. Training key hubs may enhance general function, but these hubs must also rely on extensive network inputs being locally functional in order to respond to efforts at increasing general neuronal regulation. There is, in addition, the problem of consistency of the relationship between the 10–20 system and underlying locations. Homan et al.[68] investigated this relationship using cadavers and found about a 10% variance between the 10–20 system and anatomical locations in general. Fortunately, the diffuse nature of EEG analysis owing to the large dipole areas generating EEG likely tends to compensate for this disparity.

The use of LORETA to localize current sources frees qEEG as an evaluation method from the local constraints of the 10–20 system, and enhances spatial accuracy to the point where any of the Brodmann areas can be sampled for cortical dysregulation. This poses the dilemma of deciding which domain of analysis to employ: (1) architecturally constrained definitions of function and location derived from anatomical studies and Brodmann areas; (2) activation-constrained definitions from MRI research, and graph theory analysis of hub and node connectivity; or (3) electrophysiological considerations of excitation and inhibition. Fortunately, there is considerable correlation between MRI and EEG,[36] and the two are increasingly being used together in research. The MRI picture initially provided a simple model of local activation based on function, but progressive investigation found patterns of co-activation of multiple sites relating to function. The concept of simple function begins to degrade upon inspection, and co-activation as a measure becomes increasingly suspect.[69] Simply relating function to location using EEG or MRI or magnetoencephalography appears insufficient for the purpose of analysis. Meehan and Bressler,[34] following Bassette et al.,[53] have suggested a more complex multilevel approach involving network analysis. Laird et al.[70] have begun isolating general meta-network patterns through analysis of existing MRI research and identifying 18–20 functional networks.

Although the "Rich Club Hub" approach to analysis can provide guidelines to strategies of analysis, the complexity of contribution from supporting networks diminishes the reliability of a simple function-to-location approach. Furthermore, the definition of function itself is multileveled in the psychometric arena as well, and hints at the dilemma from the other direction of analysis. This creates a more urgent need for a clear understanding of patterns of connectivity.

Connectivity

The primary measures of connectivity in qEEG are phase and coherence. To understand coherence it is necessary to understand phase. Phase describes the temporal relationship between two waveforms at any moment in time, and in terms of qEEG between waveforms from any two 10–20 locations. Sometimes the peaks and troughs of waves as they cycle up and down in power or amplitude match up–i.e., coincide, or have perfect phase relationship–but sometimes they increase and decrease in power or amplitude at different rates. The rate at which they differ is measured in degrees. When this occurs, we say one site leads or lags the other site by a certain number of degrees, meaning one site peaks in power before the other or after the other. Two sites that match perfectly in their cycles are said to be synchronous, with 0 degree phase difference. When they are completely out of step, with one reaching its peak while the other reaches its trough, they are said to be 180 degrees out of phase.

Coherence measures generally take the relationship between any two sites one step further by looking at how much time they spend at roughly the same phase differential. If two sites remain at 45 degrees phase difference for around 500 ms, we might consider them as having a meaningful relationship that we term coherence. This is sometimes calculated using Pearson's correlation coefficient of power between sites but is sometimes calculated by one of several other methods. Current research suggests that coherence is a measure of communication between two sites,[71] in that it reflects changes in the mean coupling constants between two sites with respect to axonal connectivity. This reflects the number and strength of connections between neural assemblies at a given point in time.[10] It must be kept in mind, however, that coherence is not a measure of specific small networks or groups of neurons in communication, but the relationship between two large dipole layers of 60,000,000 neurons working together in an indeterminate number of cell ensembles.[50] It is a very general measure of communication between large areas of the brain. It does not distinguish which of thousands or millions of small networks are participating.[72]

Until recently the methods generally used to measure coherence were at best two-dimensional, and in addition subject to considerable distortion because of volume conduction, i.e., the collective background noise of electrical activity in the brain.[73] Nunez[50] notes that this is especially true for site-to-site distances of <8 cm. This conclusion indicates that shorter runs of coherence in brain maps may be somewhat unreliable, which might give one pause when considering training them with neurofeedback. These shorter runs represent more local activity, as indicated by Thatcher's[71] two-compartment model. Methods for reducing this background noise by first transforming the data with Laplacian analysis have been recommended by Nunez and Srinivasan.[50] Thatcher, however, argues that this would distort the phase measures to the point where the resulting coherence values would be completely unreliable.[74] The issue, for some, remains unresolved.

Other aspects of coherence are also of concern. Thai et al.[69] note that "any correlation found between two or more brain regions even if statistically significant may not be neurobiologically significant" (p 29). Many of the locations presented as connected in the coherence maps have different levels of actual physical cortical connectivity that are not included in the connectivity calculations. David Kaiser[75] brought into question the viability of training, and perhaps even of assessing, across nonhomotopic sites. Not all locations have equal potential for connectivity, and many areas are not connected across the corpus callosum.[76,77] For example, the locations T3 and T4 have direct pathways across the corpus callosum, but P3 and F3 might require a journey through the thalamus. Pascual-Marqui[73] argues that this further confounds the coherence calculations because this third dimension is not accounted for in simple two-dimensional correlations of values. Bill Hudspeth attempted to overcome this problem using a special method of principal components analysis.[78]

In the final analysis, longer runs of intra- and interhemispheric coherence are likely to be most reliable as long as we keep in mind that we are dealing with fairly large focal areas of the brain. Both Gomez et al.[58] and Teipal et al.[79] argue that interhemispheric coherence is a reliable measure of global connectivity, including thalamic and cerebellar integration with the cortex. McIntosh[32] sees intrahemispheric coherence to be more reflective of the degree of effective connectivity. Low coherence appears to reflect diminished integrity of the neuronal fibers.[79] Gomez[58] found that measures of low posterior temporal interhemispheric alpha coherence in particular were good at predicting mild cognitive decline. High coherence on the other hand is often considered evidence of a lack of differentiation between locations with respect to function. This could very well indicate a compensatory process between locations, and Pascual-Leone et al.[80] provide considerable evidence to validate this argument. With this in mind we might consider high coherence an adaptive response to more local and regional cortical dysregulation. Whether this occurs prior to or after local problems is still in debate. By matching symptoms to the functions of the locations involved in coherence pairs, we might begin to determine the level of functionality of large network components. Indeed, the work of Laird et al.[70] seems to show that many of the larger networks do work bilaterally in tandem across the corpus callosum.

DOMINANT FREQUENCY

There are many methods of calculating dominant or peak frequency, but the mathematical details are beyond the scope and intention of this chapter. The process of digital analysis of EEG results in the ability to determine just how much power is in each individual frequency band. When looking at a group of frequencies such as alpha, we can determine which frequency band, such as 9 Hz or 10 Hz, has the most power and is thus dominant in that band. We can also look at the entire spectrum from 1 to 40 Hz and make the same determination. This can be valuable, because different subcomponents of various traditional component bands can provide valuable insights. Slower dominant alpha frequency has been associated in the medical literature with liver function difficulties.[12] Cantero et al.[72] found alpha slowing of as little as 0.5 Hz to be significant in mild cognitive impairment (MCI) and Alzheimer's disease, with patients showing a slowing of 1 Hz difference from controls. Their analysis argued that thalamocortical alpha is the source of difference, as opposed to corticocortical alpha sources, which showed no significance. These and other studies predict that important links are to be found between various metabolic conditions and EEG activity. Other studies find links between dominant frequency and cognitive performance. Faster than normal alpha (>10.5 Hz) typically is associated with cognitive readiness in some recent research literature.[48,81] Jann et al.[82] continue to support these findings and report that individual (peak) alpha frequency is an accurate correlate of cognitive readiness. In normal adults, the higher the peak frequency of alpha, the better the cognitive performance. Gloor et al.[43] found that white matter damage in general resulted in elevated amplitude of delta frequencies in the lower range of 0.5–2.5 Hz. In addition, these delta frequencies may reflect cortical disconnect from the brain stem. Kirk and Mackay's work[30] suggests future possibilities of distinguishing between emotion-related lower-frequency theta and memory-related higher-frequency theta activity. These and other studies predict further important links to be found between various metabolic conditions, trauma, psychological disorder and specific EEG activity.

ASYMMETRY

The distribution of power or magnitude across the scalp can provide valuable insights into a client's general level of stress and emotional status. For instance, when theta is far higher in the frontal region than the posterior region, symptoms of attention deficit hyperactivity disorder (ADHD) are usually present. This makes sense physiologically, because reduced activation of the frontal regions would reduce the efficiency of frontal networks, which typically are engaged in activities related to attention, working memory, and socioemotional evaluation and planning.[83] Research by Spalletta et al.[84] and others before them found that imaging of the frontal regions of individuals with ADHD did show blood perfusion deficits. This would correspond to lower astrocyte activity and less metabolic activity, as well as reduced glycogen use. The outcome in this scenario is initially more slow-wave activity, starting in the theta range and eventually migrating into the delta range.[85] This correlation does not exist with respect to white matter; in fact, the correlation overall is very low compared to gray matter.[86] Richard Davidson's[87] findings that the left side of the brain appears to be naturally more activated than the right side in normal adults with right-hand dominance would lead to expectations that reduced fast-wave activity and increased alpha on the left side may be a strong indicator of mood. Heller et al.[59] found a similar relationship with respect to beta asymmetry and anxiety. Elsa Baehr and colleagues[88,89] published articles about using techniques to reduce asymmetry to effectively reduce symptoms of depression. More recently, these findings have been supported by research on alpha asymmetry and depression by Choi et al.[90] and Avram et al.[91] There is controversy regarding how this differential is best calculated, e.g., whether it should be based on linked ears references midline references, or intrahemispheric calculations using standard ear references. Peter Rosenfeld[92] felt confident enough in the method to patent a neurofeedback protocol in 1998 to remediate depression based on this body of research.

MAP ANALYSIS THEORY

In analyzing maps it is often useful to begin by cross-correlating the function of frequency with the function of location. Frequencies do tend to be associated with broad categories of functions in the brain.[36,41] Teipal,[79] Thai,[69] Sauseng et al.[47] and Knyazev[42] all find that frequency has a very important relationship to function. Sauseng et al.[47] cite Von Stein and Sarnthein,[93] stating that "brain rhythms of different frequency can help dissociating specific brain networks." They further emphasized "that the classical EEG brain rhythms show different neural generators and also different functionality" in most instances.

An example of matching function to frequency abnormality by location might be the observation of excess parietal theta at Pz. This location around the posterior cingulate was recognized by Posner and Raichle[94] as being a key location for the release of attentional focus on a stimulus. The neurology literature also records case studies of individuals with lesions in this region who are obsessive in their thinking. These findings appear to correlate with respect to function, and we might expect to find individuals with high focal theta in this region (suggesting reduced cortical function and perfusion) who exhibit obsessive thinking and related behaviors. The addition of coherence abnormalities involving the Pz region might add weight to this conclusion. Temporal T3 elevations of slow-wave activity in delta or theta may indicate difficulties with declarative memory, because these are frequencies related to memory function and this is a location related to declarative and episodic memory functions. Coherence abnormalities linked to this region again might support a hypothesis of functional problems related to this location. Theta dominant frequency analysis possibly could provide additional insights as to whether the problem is related more to emotional valancing and indexing, or to memory images and word processing. These kinds of insights can be useful in linking reported deficits with locations of abnormal EEG activity. Most of the qEEG databases likewise have developed, or are developing, methods that integrate a symptom checklist with qEEG. A danger with this approach is drifting into an electronic phrenology of sorts. Newcomers to the field are often seduced by the apparent simplicity of matching symptoms to regions of brain dysfunction and should be cautioned, as previously mentioned, that the general thrust of recent research is in the direction of even greater complexity, such as interlocking neural network functions and compensatory patterns of effective connectivity.[34]

We have previously introduced the concepts of networks, hubs, nodes and graph theory for analyzing brain networks. This is the cutting edge of qEEG analysis. Networks are diffuse, dense and complex, and mathematical modeling of network interactions is in its infancy.[34,95] Turner et al.[96] report that network redundancy allows damaged networks to access alternative resources, thereby making clear pronouncements about network function very difficult. *Estimating* probabilities of network function seems, realistically, to be the best approach, although the danger remains that many users may use this type of interpretation as a final diagnostic rather than a probability. The qEEG databases designed for neurofeedback have proved to be fairly valuable in making these kinds of estimates, but, pending supporting research, will not be recognized as valid by the larger scientific community. This appears to be the case, even though the majority of medical research supporting commonly used interventions is internationally recognized as questionable in itself.[97]

DISCRIMINANT ANALYSIS

John et al.[11] had developed what at first glance appeared to be a powerful ability to discriminate between various disorders using multivariate analysis, i.e., to consider the interaction of many variables at the same time. These multivariate sets appeared to form unique clusters that defined abnormal brain function in various *Diagnostic and Statistical Manual of Mental Disorders* (DSM) categories. qEEG discriminants use power, amplitude, dominant frequency, coherence, phase, asymmetry, co-modulation, unity and a host of other dimensions to achieve statistically significant measures of complex multidimensional patterns that correlate consistently with a category of disorders. Statistical accuracy is, of course, likely to vary with how orthogonal the present DSM categories of disorder actually are in terms of physiological variance from a recognized functional norm. Disorders such as Parkinson's, depression and obsessive–compulsive disorder may have a fairly robust and consistent set of markers, but distinguishing Parkinson's from MCI or early dementia may prove more difficult. Thatcher (1989) in Cantor[16] and others have found discriminants useful in assisting in the diagnosis of traumatic brain injury. However, ADHD, for example, has so many features that overlap with other disorders and is typically so comorbid in its presentation that it may not be reasonable to expect clear discrimination without articulating many subtypes.[98,99] Of incidental relevance here is that, in addition to such factors as the increasingly complex electrophysiological measures being used in qEEG research and clinical work, one of the difficulties with gaining broader acceptance for qEEG is that its very implementation and findings, even at a clinical level, call into question the entire paradigm behind the DSMs. Clients and most practitioners are interested in a DSM diagnosis because it allows for third-party payment for services, but they also may be interested in locating a physiological correlate of behavior that could assist in determining a clear course of therapeutic action. DSM diagnostic labels often do not do this and may provide small comfort compared to the stigmas and paperwork they generate. Such reasoning can be threatening to some established practitioners.

Thatcher[10] emphasizes the value of univariate statistics with respect to simplicity as well as to frequency variables and anatomical localization strengths. These can guide the therapist to a location or region relevant to treatment, whereas a more complex multivariate analysis can lead to confusion regarding intervention points because of such factors as inferential "inflation," or increased statistical error resulting from excessive multiple comparisons. Multivariates are useful for discriminant functions but currently limited in their value for determining treatment protocols, because software for neurofeedback does not yet enable derivation of which specific ones of the multivariates to consider. However, Thatcher and others may be close to resolving this issue. As network analysis research advances, we may find methods to aggregate networks related from a functional perspective,[70] and statistically calculate key relationship features between contributing networks that can be modified through neurofeedback. This seems likely to involve phase-reset analysis in a novel fashion, such as within Pascual-Marqui's three-dimensional connectivity model.

In the final analysis, discriminants, by universal agreement within the field of qEEG,[10,11,15,29] should be used only to support a diagnosis and not to make a diagnosis. This position can never be overemphasized in view of the excitement and confusion revolving around this valuable tool.

MORE ON NETWORK ANALYSIS

Freeman et al.[36] propose that brain regions may tend to specialize function around specific frequency domains, and that these regions share information through global frequency transfer and perhaps even volume conduction. "The most widely held hypothesis of cortical function is that each module generates its characteristic signal; that these signals intermingle by volume conduction; that separation might be achieved by decomposition with independent component analysis; and that intermittent transmission among modules is manifested by transient phase-locking of microscopic and mesoscopic oscillations with zero phase lags despite axonal propagation delays on temporary connections."[36] Bassette[53] develops this idea with further observations: "Frequency may code the channel of communication in neural circuits, and phase modulations may transmit information in specific channels." The research of Buzsaki and others continually moves us in this direction. Thatcher's focus and development of statistical tools for analysis of phase reset opens the door to qEEG analysis in this theater of investigation as well.

Cell ensembles are the basic unit of network genesis, and these ensembles emerge and dissipate in autocorrelative patterns suggesting nonlinear adaptive and self-organizing features.[41] They include neurons that participate across cell columns and vary in size and distribution across local, global and regional cortical territories. They also recruit and integrate subcortical networks. Buzsaki has outlined some basic rules of such connectivity: networks are reciprocal, hierarchy is determined by computational solution with no top-down or bottom-up solution, function is highly distributive, and synaptic weighting emerges from autoassociative attractor networks. In addition, circuits can sustain autonomous self-organizing activity, and connectivity is a combination of modular and small world design; consequently, not all routes between neurons are equal. Gamma synchrony is likely the key to network activation over long distances. Order is a function of environmental attachment. These rules appear to be consistently supported in the literature to date.[34]

WHERE IS IT GOING?

We should look to the future, bearing in mind the caution stated by Paul Nunez[50]: "...We are not generally justified in assuming that scalp EEG primarily records specific neural network activity, perhaps in contrast to hopeful views of some scientists." The work of John, Thatcher, Prichep, Chabot, Cantor and others has resulted in a form of statistical multivariate analysis that may provide the basis for large complex network analysis. This may be more than enough for clinical applications in neurofeedback. The additional work of Pascual-Marqui on LORETA has provided a potential means to calculate pathway functions with great specificity. Innovative methods such as Granger analysis and bayssan analysis may lead to effective connectivity estimates between large functionally associated networks, as identified by Laird and others.[34] This combination promises to provide a statistical basis for future research in qEEG and neurofeedback.

This chapter will conclude with some practical observations and advice that should prove useful, especially for beginning users of qEEG technology as it relates to neurofeedback. Some content is a repeat of information presented earlier but is considered sufficiently important to warrant repeating it in the course of demonstrating how it might be implemented.

APPROACHES TO READING A qEEG MAP

Analysis with a map can begin almost anywhere a diagnosis or symptom might direct you, based on clinical experience and the published literature. Many practitioners begin with an analysis of magnitude (or power, depending on the report system being inspected). One should assess the overall level of EEG power to determine whether the individual is an outlier and therefore may not be easily evaluated by the statistical system. Those with very low power can be evaluated for frequency distribution by interpreting the data tables or relative power, even though they show as only all low power in the visual head maps. Nunez[50] suggests that coherence may suffer under these conditions and should be interpreted cautiously as well. The reason it is important to know the distributional dynamics lies in the observation by Niedermeyer that these dynamics still hold under low-power conditions, but they are relatively invisible in the coloration of the normed head maps and must be sought in the numerical tabulations or tables. For example, knowing where delta or theta is high is still important under these conditions, because there are many individuals with low power who present symptoms of ADHD and have *relatively* high frontal theta. Clinicians may not be able to up-train (increase power in) the other frequencies owing to metabolic limitations, but they can still down-train the slow-wave activity and generate positive changes. With this in mind we can evaluate the functional relationship of frequency to location with respect to power or magnitude.

Asymmetry is a dimension that is frequently of value to inspect next, because it extends and refines understanding in a more subtle manner than power distribution. The research to date, as previously discussed, suggests that finding high levels of beta in the right hemisphere is likely to indicate an overaroused nervous system with symptoms of anxiety, whereas high levels of alpha in the left hemisphere are likely to indicate depressive features. In comparing these features with Beck Depression Inventory scores we have found these conclusions fairly consistent. So, bilateral asymmetry can indicate a general state of the central nervous system with respect to mood and anxiety. Anterior to posterior asymmetries may suggest problems with attention (in delta or theta bands), or features of excessive worry (in beta.).

Much remains to be known about dominant frequency, but slowed alpha is an example of a potentially valuable indicator. It is not unusual to find correlations between elevated slowed alpha and thyroid problems, and consequently it is often present in depression as well. When combined with some alpha hypercoherences, this condition may relate to difficulty shifting state, which can negatively affect task performance. This is useful to know as well when trying to down-train high-amplitude alpha. If the client's intake indicates thyroid issues, the alpha may be unresponsive to neurofeedback because of metabolic limitations. This is another example of why a detailed history is so valuable for map interpretation.

As time goes by, coherence appears to many in the clinical setting, as well as the neuroimaging community, as being a compensatory dimension. That is, it can reflect the response of the brain to dynamic functional stress as different regions and nodes are compromised by physical or emotional trauma.[95] In this view, the brain increases coherence in an effort to enhance communication between compromised locations and thereby compensate for loss of processing efficiency in those locations.[34,80,95,96] For instance, our clinical data on 91 clients with filtering difficulties show a high correlation between reports of difficulty filtering out background noises and coherence problems at parietal locations and the posterior temporal/parietal junction. This makes sense based on our understanding of the network activity in these regions and the functions they perform.[100] It appears that the brain is attempting to enhance the management of perceptual inputs to cope with overwhelmed networks "downstream". In the case of someone with elevated slowed alpha, it is not uncommon to find increased global alpha hypercoherence as the brain attempts to stabilize resource allocation globally. The consequence is a neural rigidity with respect to ability to shift resources when changes of state are demanded by environmental inputs. A left hemisphere asymmetry (relatively more left than right hemisphere alpha power) also may often be associated with this pattern, because it results in avoidant behaviors and the emergence of depressive features. Individuals with this type of pattern often complain of a loss of ability to multitask, or issues with task transitions in addition to frequent negative self-evaluations.

Matching symptoms to coherence pairs in different frequencies may be approached from the same perspective as power or magnitude analysis. Network functions in which coherence pairs have been found to participate can be considered, along with the functions of the frequencies in which the client shows abnormality. For instance T3–T4 has been found to be associated with a meta-network related to declarative memory and auditory processing (as identified by Laird et al.[70] and noted in much MRI research). If the coherence issues are in theta frequencies, we might speculate that loss of function is in memory processing, whereas coherence issues in beta may be related to auditory processing. Thus awareness of the functions of frequencies (as described earlier) may assist in diagnostic reasoning concerning potential loss of functions in multifunctional nodes.

Although phase is the basis for much of what occurs dynamically in the brain, it operates at timescales that appear to be mismatched to the time averaging done in a typical qEEG. Thatcher[10] cautions clinicians against attempting to interpret this dimension without expert assistance. As a result of artifacting procedures, events occurring in seconds become lost in EEG averaged over minutes from selected and discontinuous segments. In this scenario, key shifts in phase that could predict changes in network affiliations are lost in discarded segments or averaged time domains. Analysis of this dimension clearly requires sophisticated statistical analysis. Nevertheless, in spite of such considerations, Thatcher et al.[101,102] have reported value in studying aspects of phase reset as an important approach to measuring IQ using qEEG.

PROTOCOL DERIVATION

If qEEG analysis suffers from lack of standardization, protocol derivation for purposes of neurofeedback suffers even more. The same map can result in a large number of different training recommendations, depending on who interpreted the report. To a large degree this is a result of the nature of neurofeedback itself. The brain is the most complex structure in the universe, with massive parallel processing in nested networks unfolding in nonlinear dynamic patterns that are autocorrelative in nature, with neither top-down or bottom-up determination. The number of solution sets resulting in enhanced integration of function and improved signal-to-noise ratio in signal processing in such a complex system is bound to be very large. We should expect that multiple solutions will enhance system integration, and do so at different timescales. The consequence of this is that there will be no one "right" protocol, but only a "best-estimate" protocol. Statistically the odds are against us in determining the "best" protocol based purely on the map, because we do not yet understand enough about brain function to make that determination. We might reasonably expect to come up with a *group* of protocols that are likely to enhance function, and it seems reasonable to expect that through systematic observation of their subsequent impact on EEG distribution we can determine their relative effectiveness. Watching for the movement of different dimensions of EEG analysis toward the statistical mean of a normative reference is likely an effective method of evaluating the value of a given protocol. This could be done by inspecting either Z-scores or raw data if the general range of normative values is known. In fact, both of these approaches are highly used in neurofeedback. A main caveat here is that such approaches should allow for compensatory adaptive patterns in which values may periodically move into abnormal ranges for given periods of time. There are many conditions in biological systems that reflect this type of adaptive response in the healing trajectory.

One emerging popular solution has been to determine "worst" location/frequency scores with respect to deviance from normal that functionally correlate with the symptoms the client is experiencing, matching symptom to location. The clinician inspects the map to determine which dimensions – i.e., power, phase, coherence – are most deviant, and then trains the client toward the normative standards based on a dynamic linked library designed for that purpose. This has become known as Z-score training and is unique to qEEG-guided neurofeedback. With this approach, in spite of its globally applied and automated regulation of thresholds, it is still incumbent upon the therapist to closely inspect and track changes and be on guard for the limitations placed upon compensatory responses of the brain that might work against normalization of function. Regardless of the protocol method used or the method of protocol derivation employed, occasional repeats of the qEEG are highly useful in periodically assessing the efficacy of a given protocol with respect to moving the brain toward higher levels of integration.

qEEG REPORTS

There are currently few clear standards in qEEG report writing. Many reports provide lengthy detailed technical introductions with 30–40 pages of data and detailed analysis. This is quite opposite to existing standards in medical EEG, and those in this emerging field must ask themselves if such data density is of value in the clinical setting. In looking at MRI or computed tomography reports, one will rarely see such generous amounts of detail, because they do not involve the detailed quantitative analyses typical of qEEG. Most professionals in other fields are likely to find such lengthy data reports difficult to interpret and not very informative, despite the impressive detail. Thatcher (personal communication), who has contributed significantly to the field of forensic use of qEEG, has suggested including in a report only the specific information pertinent to the interpretation. Further detail can always be forwarded upon request. In this model a brief introduction explaining the equipment used, the sampling rate and a brief explanation of the meaning of each section of the report for purposes of orientation is useful. The date of the recording, record length, the client's name, gender and handedness should be included, as well as a list of medications the client is using. The context of the recording (i.e., eyes closed or eyes open) and length of recording time is typically part of the report, as well as the recording technician's impressions of the client's states, such as drowsiness. A basic summary page of the EEG head maps, a page or two of relevant statistics, and perhaps a few additional pages specifically depicting the abnormal features reported can be valuable. These bits of information, along with a paragraph on impressions, or, in some cases, a more detailed analysis involving a few paragraphs, should be all that is needed to provide other professionals with a simple yet clear picture of the issues at hand. As yet, however, there is no clear consensus on even this suggestion. It is also important to tie any clinical measures, such as scores from memory tests, continuous performance tests and other psychometrics as well as symptom history, to the features of the map with the greatest specificity possible. With this approach you are likely to be of more assistance to other professionals and generate a higher estimation of professionalism for our field of endeavor. The American Clinical Neurophysiology Society, among others, provides detailed guidelines for reporting that can be very helpful in setting up one's own report format.

REFERENCES

1. Matousek M, Petersen I. Frequency analysis of the EEG in normal children and adolescents. In: Kellaway P, Petersen I, eds. *Automation of Clinical Electroencephalography*. New York, NY: Raven Press; 1973:75–102.
2. John ER, Karmel B, Corning W, et al. Neurometrics: neurometrical taxonomy identifies different profiles of brain functions within groups of behaviorally similar people. *Science*. 1977;196:1393–1410.
3. Duffy FH. Brain electrical activity mapping (BEAM): Computerized access to complex brain function. *Int J Neurosci*. 1981;13:55–65.
4. Duffy FH, Iyer VG, Surwillo WW. *Clinical Electroencephalography and Topographic Brain Mapping: Technology and Practice*. New York: Springer-Verlag; 1989.
5. Nuwer M. Assessment of digital EEG, quantitative EEG and EEG brain mapping: Report of the American Academy of Neurology and the American Clinical Neurophysiology Society. *Neurology*. 1997;49:277–292.
6. Hoffman DA, Lubar JF, Thatcher RW, et al. Limitations of the American academy of neurology and American clinical neurophysiology society paper on QEEG. *J Neuropsychiatry Clin Neurosci*. 1999;11:401–407.
7. Gordon E, Cooper N, Rennie C, Hermens D, Williams LM. Integrative neuroscience: the role of a standardized database. *Clin EEG Neurosci*. 2005;36(2):64–75.
8. Kropotov JD. *Event-Related Potentials and Neurotherapy*. San Diego: Elsevier; 2009.
9. Jasper H. The ten-twenty electrode system of the International Federation. *EEG Clin Neurophysiol*. 1958;10:371–375.
10. Thatcher RW. EEG database guided neurotherapy. In: Evans JR, Abarbanel A, eds. *Introduction to Quantitative EEG and Neurofeedback*. San Diego, CA: Academic Press; 1999.
11. John ER, Prichep LS, Fridman J, Easton P. Neurometrics: computer assisted differential diagnosis of brain dysfunctions. *Science*. 1988;293:162–169.
12. Niedermeyer E, Lopes da Silva FH. *Electroencephalography: Basic Principles, Clinical Applications, and Related Fields*. New York, NY: Lippincott Williams & Wilkins; 2011.
13. Romano-Micha J. Databases of specific training protocols for neurotherapy? A proposal for a "clinical approach to neurotherapy." *J Neurotherapy*. 2003;7(3/4):69–85.
14. Kaye H, John ER, Prichep L. Neurometric evaluation of learning disabled children. *J Neurosci*. 1981;13(1):15–25.
15. Hammond D, Walker J, Hoffman D, et al. Standards for the use of quantitative electroencephalography (QEEG) in neurofeedback: A position paper of the international society for neuronal regulation. *J Neurotherapy*. 2004;8(1):5–27.
16. Cantor DS. An overview of quantitative EEG and its applications to neurofeedback. In: Evans JR, Abarbanel A, eds. *Introduction to Quantitative EEG and Neurofeedback*. New York, NY: Academic Press; 1999:3–27.
16a. Fisch BJ, Spehlmann R. *Fisch and Spehlmann's EEG Primer: Basic Principles of Digital and Analogue EEG*. New York, NY: Elsevier; 1999.
17. Pascual-Marqui RD, Michel CM, Lehmann D. Low resolution electro-magnetic tomography: a new method for localizing electrical activity in the brain. *Int J Psychophysiol*. 1994;18:49–65.
18. Pascual-Marqui RD. Standardized low resolution brain electromagnetic tomography (sLORETA): technical details. *Methods Find Exp Clin Pharmacol*. 2002;24D:5–12.
19. Goncharova II, McFarland DJ, Vaughan TM, Wolpaw JR. EMG contamination of EEG: spectral and topographical characteristics. *Clin Neurophysiol*. 2003;114:1580–1593.
20. Hammond DC, Gunkelman J. *The Art of Artifacting*. San Rafael, CA: ISNR Research Foundation; 2011.
21. John ER, Prichep LS, Easton P. Normative data banks and neurometrics. Basic concepts, methods, and results of norm constructions. In: *Methods of Analysis of*

Brain Electrical and Magnetic Signals. EEG Handbook. Revised ser. vol. 1, Gevins AS, Remond A. eds. Oxford: Elsevier Science Publishers; 1987:449–483.

22. Thatcher R. *Calculations and statements made on the Neuroguide Listserve.* 2012:17.

23. Thatcher RW. Coherence, phase differences, phase shift, and phase lock EEG/ERP analysis. *Dev Neuropsychol.* 2012;37(6):476–496. http://dx.doi.org/10.1080/8756564 1.2011.619421

24. Jobert M, Wilson FJ, Ruigt GéSF, Brunovsky M, Prichep LS, Drinkenburg, WHIM. Guidelines for the recording and evaluation of pharmaco-EEG data in man: the international pharmaco-EEG society (IPEG) guidelines committee. *Neuropsychobiology.* 2012;66:201–220.

25. Chu CJ, Kramer MA, Pathmanathan J, et al. Emergence of stable functional networks in long-term human electroencephalography. *J Neurosci.* 2012;32(8):2703–2713.

26. Fishbein D, Thatcher RW, Cantor DS. Ingestion of carbohydrates varying in complexity produce different brain responses. *Clin EEG.* 1990;43:21–36.

27. Cantor DS, Thatcher RW, Ozand P. Choline supplementation in Downs Syndrome: a case study. *Psychol Rep.* 1986;58:207–217.

28. Whitham EM, Pope KJ, Fitzgibbon SP, et al. Scalp electrical recording during paralysis: quantitative evidence that EEG frequencies above 20 Hz are contaminated by EMG. *Clin Neurophysiol.* 2007;118:1877–1888.

29. Johnstone J, Gunkelman J, Lunt J. Clinical database development: characterization of EEG phenotypes. *Clin EEG Neurosci.* 2005;36(2):99–107.

30. Kirk IJ, Mackay JC. The role of theta-range oscillations in synchronizing and integrating activity in distributed mnemonic networks. *Cortex.* 2003;39:993–1008.

31. Buckner RL, Andrews-Hanna JR, Schacter DL. The brain's default network: anatomy, function, and relevance to disease. *Ann NY Acad Sci.* 2008;1124:1–38.

32. McIntosh AR, Korostil M. Interpretation of neuroimaging data based on network concepts. *Brain Imaging Behav.* 2008;2:264–269. http://dx.doi.org/10.1007/s11682–008–9031–6

33. Honey CJ, Kotter R, Breakspear M, Sporns O. Network structure of cerebral cortex shapes functional connectivity on multiple time scales. *Proc Natl Acad Sci USA.* 2007;104:10240–10245.

34. Meehan TP, Bressler SL. Neurocognitive networks: findings, models, and theory. *Neurosci Biobehav Rev.* 2012;36(10):2232–2247.

35. Hagemann D, Johannes H, Christof W, Ewald N. Skull thickness and magnitude of EEG alpha activity. *Clin Neurophysiol.* 2008;119:1271–1280.

36. Freeman WJ, Ahlfors SP, Menon V. Combining fMRI with EEG and MEG in order to relate patterns of brain activity to cognition. *Int J Psychophysiol.* 2009;73(1):43–52. http://dx.doi.org/10.1016/j,ijpsych0.2008.12.019

37. Raichle ME, MacLeod AM, Snyder AZ, Powers WJ, Gusnard DA, Shulman DL. A default mode of brain function. *Proc Natl Acad Sci USA.* 2001;98:676–682.

38. Logothetis N. What we can do and what we cannot do with fMRI. *Nature.* 2008;453(7197):869–878.

39. Sharbrough FW, Messick Jr JM, Sundt Jr. TM. Correlation of continuous electroencephalograms with cerebral blood flow measurements during carotid endarterectomy. *Stroke.* 1973;4:674–683.

40. Kaplan GB, Hammer RP. *Brain Circuitry and Signaling in Psychiatry: Basic Science and Implications.* Washington, DC: American Psychiatric Publishing; 2002.

41. Buzsaki G. *Rhythms of the Brain.* New York, NY: Oxford University Press; 2006.

42. Knyazev GG. EEG delta oscillations as a correlate of basic homeostatic and motivational processes. *Neurosci Biobehav Rev.* 2012;36:677–695.

43. Gloor P, Ball G, Schaul N. The cortical electromicrophysiology of pathological delta waves in the electroencephalogram of a cat. *Electroencephalogr Clin Neurophysiol.* 1977;43(3):346–361.

44. Alper KR, Prichep LS, Kowalik S, Rosenthal MS, John ER. Persistent QEEG abnormality in crack cocaine users at 6 months of drug abstinence: thesis of neural sensitization in cocaine dependence. *Neuropsychopharmacology.* 1998;19:1–9.

45. Craig AD. How do you feel-now? The anterior insula and human awareness. *Nat Rev Neurosci.* 2009;10:59–70.

46. Mitchell DJ, McNaughton N, Flanagan D, Kirk IJ. Frontal-midline theta from the perspective of hippocampal "theta". *Prog Neurobiol.* 2008;86:156–185.

47. Sauseng P, Hoppe J, Klimesch W, Gerloff C, Hummel FC. Dissociation of sustained attention from central executive functions: Local activity and interregional connectivity in the theta range. *Eur J Neurosci.* 2007;25:587–593.

48. Klimesch W. Memory processes, brain oscillations and EEG synchronization. *Int J Neurosci.* 1996;24:61–100.

49. Kahana MJ, Sekuler R, Caplan JB, Kirschen M, Madsen JR. Human theta oscillations exhibit task dependence during virtual maze navigation. *Nature.* 1999;399:781–784.

50. Nunez PI, Srinivasan R. *Electric Fields of the Brain: The Neurophysics of EEG.* 2nd ed. New York, NY: Oxford University Press; 2006.

51. Jensen O, Colgin LL. Cross-frequency coupling between neuronal oscillations. *Trends Cogn Sci.* 2007;11(7):267–269.

52. Schroeder CE, Lakatos P. The gamma oscillation: master or slave? *Brain Topogr.* 2009;22:24–26.

53. Bassette DS, Meyer-Lindenberg A, Archard S, Duke T, Bullmore E. Adaptive reconfiguration of fractal small-world human brain functional networks. *PNAS.* 2006;103(51):19518–19523. http://dx.doi.org/10.1073/pnas.0606005103

54. Anderson P, Anderson SA. *Physiological Basis of the Alpha Rhythm.* New York, NY: Appleton Century Crofts; 1968.

55. Peterson SE, Posner MI. The attention system of the human brain: 20 years after. *Annu Rev Neurosci.* 2012;35:73–89.

56. Hughes SW, Crunelli V. Thalamic mechanisms of EEG alpha rhythms and their pathological implications. *Neuroscientist.* 2005;11(4):357–372.

57. Sterman MB. Physiological origins and functional correlates of EEG rhythmic activities: implications for self-regulation. *Biofeedback Self Regul.* 1996;21:3–33.

58. Gomez C, Stam CJ, Hornero R, Fernandez AZ, Maestu F. Disturbed beta band functional connectivity in patients with mild cognitive impairment: An MEG study. *IEEE Trans Biomed Eng.* 2009;56(6):1683–1690.

59. Heller W, Nitschke JB, Etienne MA, Miller GA. Patterns of regional brain activity differentiate types of anxiety. *J Abnorm Psychol.* 1997;106(3):376–385.

60. Perlis ML, Smith MT, Andrews PJ, Orff H, Giles DE. Beta/Gamma EEG activity in patients with primary and secondary insomnia and good sleeper controls. *Sleep.* 2001;24(1):110–117.

61. Walker JE. QEEG-guided neurofeedback for recurrent migraine headaches. *Clin EEG Neurosci.* 2011;42(1):59.

62. Davidson RJ, Kabat-Zinn J, Schumacher J, et al. Alterations and immune function produced by mindfullness meditation. *Psychosom Med.* 2003;65:564–570.

63. Sheer DE. Biofeedback training of 40-Hz EEG and behavior. In: Kamiya J, et al. *Biofeedback and Self-Control 1976/1977: An Annual Review.* Chicago, IL: Aldine; 1977.

64. Keizer AW, Verschoor M, Verment RS, Hommel B. The effect of gamma enhancing neurofeedback on the control of feature bindings and intelligence measures. *Int J Psychophysiol.* 2010;75(1):25–32.

65. Soutar R. *Doing Neurofeedback, a Workshop Manual.* NewMind Publications; 1999.

66. Soutar R, Longo R. *Doing Neurofeedback: An Introduction.* San Rafael, CA: ISNR Research Foundation; 2012.

67. Hagmann P, Cammoun L, Gigandet X, et al. Mapping the structural core of human cerebral cortex. *PLoS Biol.* 2008;6(7):1479–1493.

68. Homan RW, Herman J, Purdy P. Cerebral location of international 10–20 system electrode placement. *Electroencephalogr Clin Neurophysiol.* 1987;66:376–382.

69. Thai NJ, Longe O, Rippon G. Disconnected brains: What is the role of fMRI in connectivity research?. *Int J Psychophys.* 2009;73:27–32.

70. Laird AR, Fox PM, Eickhoff SB, et al. Behavioral interpretations of intrinsic connectivity networks. *J Cogn Neurosci.* 2011;23(12):4022–4037.

71. Thatcher RW, Krause PJ, Hrybyk M. Cortico-cortical associations and EEG coherence: A two-compartmental model. *EEG Clin Neurophysiol.* 1986;64:123–143.

72. Cantero JL, Atienza M, Gomez-Herrero G, et al. Functional integrity of thalamocortical circuits differentiates normal aging from mild cognitive impairment. *Hum Brain Mapp.* 2009;30:3944–3957.

73. Pascual-Marqui R. Time-frequency components of brain connectivity: Methods and examples. 16th ISNR Annual Conference, San Antonio, TX; 2008.

74. Thatcher RW. Validity and reliability of quantitative electroencephalogy (qEEG). *J Neurotherapy.* 2010;14:122–152.

75. Kaiser D. Synchrony measures and non-homotopic: do synchrony measures between non-homotopic area make sense?. *J Neurotherapy: Investigations in Neuromodulation, Neurofeedback, and Applied Neuroscience.* 2005;9(2):97–108.

76. Schmahmann JD, Pandya DN. *Fiber Pathways of the Brain.* New York: Oxford University Press; 2009.

77. Kandel ER, Schwartz JH, Jessel TM. *Principles of Neural Science.* 4th ed. McGraw-Hill Professional; 2000.

78. Coben R, Hudspeth W. Introduction to advances in EEG connectivity. *J Neurotherapy.* 2008;12(2–3):93–98.

79. Teipal SJ, Pogarell O, Meindl T, et al. Regional networks underlying interhemispheric connectivity: An EEG and DTI study in healthy ageing and amnestic mild cognitive impairment. *Hum Brainmapping.* 2009;30:2098–2119.

80. Pascual-Leone A, Amedi A, Fregni F, Merabet LB. The plastic human brain cortex. *Annu Rev Neurosci.* 2005;28:377–401.

81. Klimesch W, Schimke H, Pfurtscheller G. Alpha frequency, cognitive load and memory performance. *Brain Topogr.* 1993;5:241–251.

82. Jann K, Koenig T, Dierks T, Boesch C, Federspiel A. Association of individual resting state EEG alpha frequency and cerebral blood flow. *NeuroImage.* 2010;51(1):356–372.

83. Chow TW, Cummings JL. Frontal-subcortical circuits. In: Miller BL, Cummings JL, eds. *The Human Frontal Lobe.* New York, NY: Guilford Press; 1998:3–44.

84. Spalletta G, Pasini A, Pau F, Guido G, Menghini L. Prefrontal blood flow dysregulation in drug naive ADHD children without structural abnormalities. *J Neural Transm.* 2001;108:1203–1216.

85. Nagata K. Topographic EEG in brain ischemia–correlation with blood flow and metabolism. *Brain Topogr.* 1998;1(2):97–106. http://dx.doi.org/10.1007/BF01129174

86. Ingvar DH. "Hyperfrontal" distribution of the cerebral grey matter flow in resting wakefulness: On the functional anatomy of the conscious state. *Acta Neurol Scand.* 1979;60(1):12–25.

87. Davidson RJ. Anterior asymmetry, affective style, and depression (abstract). *Psychophysiology.* 1992;29(4A, suppl 4).

88. Baehr E, Rosenfeld JP, Baher R. The clinical use of an alpha asymmetry protocol in the neurofeedback treatment of depression: Two case studies. *J Neurotherapy.* 1997;3:12–23.

89. Baehr E, Rosenfeld JP, Baehr R, Earnest C. Clinical use of an alpha asymmetry protocol in the treatment of mood disorder. In: Evans JR, Abarbanel A, eds. *Introduction to Quantitative EEG and Neurofeedback.* San Diego, CA: Academic Press; 1999.

90. Choi SW, Chi SE, Chung SY, Kim JW, Ahn CY, Kim HT. Is alpha wave neuro-feedback effective with randomized clinical trials in depression? A pilot study. *Neuropsychobiology*. 2011;63:43–51.

91. Avram J, Baltes FR, Miclea M, Miu AC. Frontal EEG activation asymmetry reflects cognitive biases in anxiety: evidence from an emotional face stroop task. *Appl Psychophysiol Biofeedback*. 2010;35:285–292. http://dx.doi.org/10.1007/s10484-010-9138-6

92. Rosenfeld JP. An EEG biofeedback protocol for affective disorders. *Clin Electroencephalogr*. 2000;31(1):7–12.

93. Von Stein A, Sarnthein. Different frequencies for different scales of cortical integration: from local gamma to long-range alpha/theta synchronization. *Int J Psychophysiol*. 2000;38:301–313.

94. Posner MI, Raichle ME. *Images of Mind*. New York, NY: Scientific American Library; 1997.

95. Alstott J, Breakspear M, Hagmann P, Cammoun L, Sporns O. Modeling the impact of lesions in the human brain. *PLoS Comp Bio*. 2009;5(6):e1000408. http://dx.doi.org/10.1371/journal.pcbi.1000408

96. Turner GR, McIntosh AR, Levine B. Prefrontal compensatory engagement in TBI is due to altered functional engagement of existing networks and nonfunctional reorganization. *Front Syst Neurosci*. 2011;5(9):2.

97. Ioannidis JPA. Why most published research findings are false. *PLoS Med*. 2005;2(8):e124.

98. Lubar JF, Lubar J. Neurofeedback assessment and treatment for attention deficit/hyperactivity disorders. In: Evans JR, Abarbanel A, eds. *Introduction to Quantitative EEG and Neurofeedback*. New York, NY: Academic Press; 1999:243–310.

99. Chabot RJ, Merkin H, Wood LM, Davenport TL, Serfontein G. Sensitivity and specificity of QEEG in children with attention deficit disorder or specific developmental learning disorders. *Clin Electroencephalogr*. 1996;27:26–34.

100. Rabinovich MI, Afraimovich VS, Blick C, Varona P. Information flow dynamics in the brain. *Phys Life Rev*. 2011;9:51–73.

101. Thatcher RW, North D, Biver C. EEG and intelligence: univariate and multivariate comparisons between EEG coherence, EEG phase delay and power. *Clin Neurophysiol*. 2005;116(9):2129–2141.

102. Thatcher RW, North DM, Biver CJ. Intelligence and EEG phase reset: a two compartmental model of phase shift and lock. *Neuroimage*. 2008;42(4):1639–1653. http://dx.doi.org/10.1016/j.neuroimage.2008.06.009

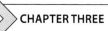

CHAPTER THREE

Neurofeedback and Psychopharmacology

Designing Effective Treatment Based on Cognitive and EEG Effects of Medications

Lukasz M. Konopka and Elizabeth M. Zimmerman

A patient seeking treatment with neurofeedback may do so for several reasons, one of which may be as an alternative to psychotropic medication. Many situations exist in which neurofeedback treatment is indicated without concurrent medications. In certain cases, however, patient symptoms are severe and difficult to manage, so much so that they may interfere with the neurofeedback process. Successful engagement in neurofeedback has a number of basic requirements of the patient (Figure 3.1), and in mental illness these are often disrupted. At least during the early stages of neurofeedback, certain patients may benefit from psychotropic medications that can curb disturbances from potentially interfering symptoms. Therefore, providers must have an awareness of how medication may influence neurofeedback treatment.

Neurofeedback is based on electroencephalographic (EEG) frequencies, which are unique to each patient and also influenced by the introduction of psychotropics. This requires the neurofeedback provider to have a clear understanding of EEG frequencies and their behavioral correlates, as well as EEG effects introduced by psychotropics. This chapter is designed to provide an overview of cognitive and EEG effects of broad classes of medications, as well as to offer implications for the neurofeedback provider in incorporating these effects in order to optimize treatment design.

The chapter begins with an introduction to pharmaco-EEG, which involves objective measurement of drug-induced electrophysiological changes that relate to cognition, behavior and EEG. It then provides an overview of certain medications and their acute and long-term influence on areas of cognitive function related to neurofeedback. Medication

Clinical Neurotherapy.
Doi: http://dx.doi.org/10.1016/B978-0-12-396988-0.00003-9

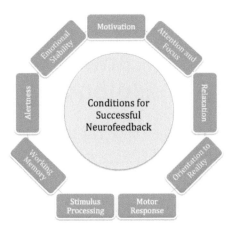

Figure 3.1 General patient characteristics required for successful engagement in neurofeedback.

influences on EEG patterns are explored in terms of their acute and long-term impact on absolute power in various frequency bands (delta, theta, alpha, beta), with a focus on anxiolytics, stimulants, antidepressants and antipsychotics. The chapter is not intended to provide recommendations for medication use, but instead aims to highlight major trends in medication-related shifts in cognition and EEG that may affect neurofeedback design and progress. Each section contains a table summarizing potential cognitive/behavioral and EEG effects from broad medication classes (Figure 3.2).

PHARMACO-EEG

An emergent area in electroencephalography known as "pharmaco-EEG" examines the impact of centrally acting psychotropic medications on EEG patterns. It allows the assessment of the functional bioavailability of these drugs in individual patients and objective evaluation of their impact on brain waves.[1] Pharmaco-EEG involves comparison of brain waves at a drug-free baseline, followed by EEG measures conducted after medication administration. Differences in EEG before and after medication can then highlight electrophysiological changes induced by a particular psychotropic agent. These effects vary based on a multitude of factors, including pharmacokinetic and pharmacodynamic drug properties affected by individual patient differences such as age, gender, weight, genetic makeup, drug–drug interactions, acute versus repetitive administration and fluctuating states of conscious activity.[2]

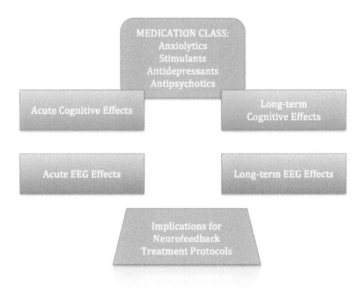

Figure 3.2 Chapter approach to neurofeedback and psychopharmacology.

Various classes of psychotropic medications typically induce similar changes in EEG, and often there are clear differences between classes.[1] According to current literature, anxiolytics have the most clearly identifiable EEG changes, followed by stimulants, then antidepressants and antipsychotics.[1] Familiarity with the EEG changes of these classes of drugs is crucial to the design of effective neurofeedback. Treatment paradigms must target areas of individual deficit while avoiding too much focus on medication-induced brain patterns. At the same time, neurofeedback clinicians must also consider medication side effects on cognition, which may critically affect a patient's ability to attend, focus and learn throughout treatment. Therefore, a combination of behavioral measures and assessment of EEG patterns is needed at several points throughout treatment (Figure 3.3). Ongoing assessments can then help the clinician and the patient to track progress and design future treatment based on objective measures.

ANXIOLYTICS

Patients in neurofeedback treatment are often those who suffer from anxiety and are seeking ways to improve focus, enhance relaxation and manage disruptive tension and worry. A patient's anxiety may be so high that he

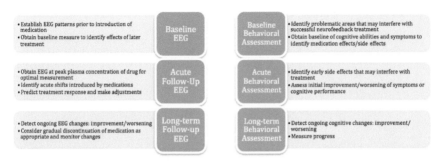

Figure 3.3 Purpose of ongoing behavioral and EEG assessments throughout treatment.

or she is unable to concentrate and remain calm and/or motorically steady. Anxiolytic medications may provide a transient reduction in these symptoms, thereby allowing patients relief from symptoms that might interfere with successful neurofeedback treatment. At the same time, anxiolytics may introduce a new set of side effects that could potentially interfere with the learning process and/or alter EEG patterns, so that the provider might design ineffective protocols based on EEG patterns driven by the medications themselves. This section reviews cognitive and EEG changes induced by benzodiazepines, with a brief overview of anxiolytic alternatives.

Background and Uses of Benzodiazepines

Benzodiazepines are among the most widely used psychotropic drugs in the treatment of anxiety disorders and are also used to treat depression and psychoses.[3] Therapeutic efficacy has been demonstrated for their use as anxiolytics, sedatives and hypnotics, antidepressants and anticonvulsants.[4] Additional uses include anesthetics and muscle relaxants, as well as the management of agitation in acute alcohol withdrawal.[3] Clinicians will likely encounter patients using benzodiazepines to manage a variety of symptom presentations. Benzodiazepines may interfere with cognitive processes or result in global EEG changes that affect the approach to protocol design, thus possibly hindering success.

Acute Cognitive Effects of Benzodiazepines

There are three classes of benzodiazepines: long-acting, intermediate-acting and short-acting (Table 3.1 for selected benzodiazepines). Common side effects of benzodiazepines have direct implications for performance in neurofeedback therapy. These side effects are related to dose-dependent

Table 3.1 Selected Benzodiazepines

Generic Name	Single-Dose Dosage Range (mg)
Long-Acting Agents (t^a=10–80)	
Clorazepate	3.75–15
Chlordiazepoxide	10–50
Diazepam	2–10
Prazepam	5–30
Intermediate-Acting Agents (t = 15–80)	
Clonazepam	0.5–2.0
Lorazepam	0.5–2.0
Short-Acting Agents (t = 2.5–12)	
Alprazolam	0.25–2.0
Oxazepam	10–30

[a]t = mean elimination half-life in hours.

depression of the central nervous system, which can result in cognitive and motor impairments. Dose-dependent cognitive side effects include drowsiness and sedation, which may progress to mental confusion, disorientation, slurring of speech and/or induction or exacerbation of dementia-related symptoms.[5] Elderly patients are particularly sensitive to these side effects at lower doses.[5,6] Benzodiazepines are also effective in producing anterograde amnesia, and surgery settings use drugs such as lorazepam and midazolam for this purpose.[5] Benzodiazepines are often used as muscle relaxants and/or sleep aids, and impair an individual's ability to perform complex motor tasks.[5] With acute administration benzodiazepines can occasionally introduce paradoxical symptoms, including excessive talkativeness, restlessness, anxiety, aggression, sleep disturbances, and even mania and acute rage reactions.[5] Cognitive side effects are common to most benzodiazepines, although some are drug-specific and differ in severity.[7]

The design of neurofeedback training protocols requires consideration of acute side effects that may significantly impair a patient's ability to progress successfully in treatment. If patients experience cognitive/motor impairments and are consequently unable to concentrate, neurofeedback likely will not yield beneficial results. On the other hand, if patients are unable to attend or concentrate because of excessive agitation or anxiety, short-term use of benzodiazepines concurrent with initial neurofeedback treatment may be indicated. Clinicians must carefully balance the costs and benefits of benzodiazepines, particularly in the initial stages of their use. Depending on a patient's tolerance, cognitive side effects of benzodiazepines may subside after a period of time, enabling relief from debilitating anxiety during the neurofeedback process.

Long-Term Cognitive Effects of Benzodiazepines

Research indicates that there are several long-term effects across many cognitive domains that may emerge in patients who have used benzodiazepines for longer than 1 year.[3] Many of the acute side effects that affect patients early in benzodiazepine treatment do not seem to be problematic in the long term,[7] yet specific cognitive dysfunctions may remain or emerge with chronic use.[8] Impairments of memory, attention and concentration, visuospatial skills, conceptual tracking, motor speed and speed of information processing have been reported with long-term use.[7]

Although the results of previous research are considered equivocal and limited because of methodological issues, meta-analytic findings suggest that cognitive function in long-term benzodiazepine users compared to control populations is often significantly impaired across the following 12 domains: sensory processing, nonverbal memory, processing speed, attention/concentration, general intelligence, working memory, psychomotor speed, visuospatial ability, problem solving, verbal memory, motor control/performance and verbal reasoning.[3] Results also indicate that cognitive effects may increase with duration of benzodiazepine use.[3] However, neuroimaging studies of long-term benzodiazepine users with computed tomography scanning do not support significant differences in brain structure compared to control groups.[3,8]

Cognitive improvement has been shown to occur after discontinuation of benzodiazepine in long-term users.[3] Therefore, when working with patients with cognitive difficulties related to chronic benzodiazepine use, clinicians might consider neurofeedback as a tool to support improvement and recovery from cognitive impairments after cessation of benzodiazepines. A critical assessment tool to aid clinicians in deciding the appropriate balance of neurofeedback and benzodiazepines is the individual patient's EEG.

EEG Effects of Acute and Long-Term Use of Benzodiazepines

Benzodiazepines act as facilitators of the inhibitory neurotransmitter gamma-aminobutyric acid (GABA) by binding at $GABA_A$ receptor sites.[9,10] GABA binding on receptors within the amygdala, hippocampus and frontal cortex is associated with the alleviation of anxiety, agitation and fear.[11,12] GABA binding on receptors in the spinal cord, cerebellum and brain stem is associated with mild muscle relaxation, and action at receptors in the cerebrum and hippocampus is associated with anticonvulsant effects.[9] Given the widespread presence of GABA receptors throughout the brain and the role of GABA in the generation of various brain rhythms, broad changes in brain waves occur at cortical and subcortical levels with the introduction of benzodiazepines. Replicable EEG changes have been identified based on plasma concentrations of certain benzodiazepines[13] causing alterations in EEG markers of wake activity and suggesting concentration-dependent effects underlying optimal function.[14]

A consistent alteration to EEG patterns introduced by anxiolytic medication is augmented beta activity.[15] Benzodiazepines have also been found to enhance both theta and beta frequencies during waking,[16] and to enhance delta frequencies at high concentrations.[17] Mandema and Danhof[17] review previous studies demonstrating that alpha decrease and beta increase are the most sensitive markers of benzodiazepine activity and reflect moderate sedation.[17] These authors note that EEG changes induced by benzodiazepines appear similar to EEG shifts that occur in the transition from sleep to wake. Furthermore, Mandema and Danhof[17] suggest that shifts in alpha and beta reflect moderate sedation and anxiolytic properties, whereas delta enhancement may indicate heavier sedation and hypnotic properties of benzodiazepines.

The enhancement of beta activity with benzodiazepines is directly related to decreased psychomotor performance,[13] and in patients taking benzodiazepine medication this change may reduce motor responses during neurofeedback treatment. Beta frequencies in particular appear to be influenced by the levels of plasma accumulation of benzodiazepines,[18] and thus clinicians must also consider the optimal timing of neurofeedback following benzodiazepine administration. Greater impairment in psychomotor function and enhancement of beta activity typically correspond with peak plasma levels, so neurofeedback treatment may be more strongly indicated either prior to or several hours following drug intake, depending on the drug's half-life.

Lasting EEG effects of long-term benzodiazepine use have not been as closely studied as acute EEG shifts. Benzodiazepines have been demonstrated in EEG activity to result in tolerance, both acute and chronic. Acute tolerance in some of these medications can develop in as little as 1 to

2 weeks with intermittent administration. Acute tolerance to alprazolam, for example, results in increased beta activity, decreased psychomotor performance and a tolerance to sedative but not anxiolytic effects after repetitive intake.[1,15] Longer-term effects also require further study and are often affected by several confounding factors, such as individual differences, concurrent treatments, interactions with other drugs, and more. Thus, neurofeedback providers must be aware of drug presence as well as pattern and length of intake, and their consequent impact on EEG patterns in individual patients.

Effects of Withdrawal from Benzodiazepines

Benzodiazepines are often used inappropriately, and clinicians must be careful when designing neurofeedback treatment to consider how its efficacy will be affected by benzodiazepine abuse. Physical dependence can result from prolonged use, and neurofeedback practitioners must be sensitive to cognitive and affective symptoms that emerge as patients are slowly withdrawn from benzodiazepines and progress toward discontinuation. Initial withdrawal symptoms can include rebound anxiety, agitation, insomnia, irritability, muscle tension and restlessness, and in very severe cases hallucinations, psychoses and seizures.[5] Although benzodiazepines are no longer recommended for long-term use (>4 weeks), they are often prescribed in repeat doses, particularly for elderly patients who are vulnerable to cognitive side effects.[6] Neurofeedback providers must therefore consider withdrawal symptoms, which generally appear between 6 and 12 hours after discontinuation, peak between 2 and 4 days, and subside after 3 weeks.[7] With severe symptoms, neurofeedback treatment may not be beneficial during the withdrawal period, particularly if the symptoms interfere significantly with the patient's cognitive abilities related to concentration and learning. A summary of acute and long-term effects of benzodiazepines is given in Table 3.2.

OTHER ANXIOLYTICS

Nonbenzodiazepine medications are often indicated for treatment of anxiety, including unique agents such as serotonin $5HT_1$ partial agonists. Buspirone is a weak $5HT_{1A}$ agonist that exerts its influence on both pre- and postsynaptic $5HT_{1A}$ autoreceptors. This agent is unique in that its anxiolytic properties are present without the emergence of significant cognitive

Table 3.2 Summary of Possible Effects of Benzodiazepine Use Related to Neurofeedback Treatment

Summary of Benzodiazepine Effects	
Acute Effects	
Cognitive Effects/Side Effects	**EEG Effects**[a]
Motor impairments	Increased theta activity
Agitation	Increased beta activity: associated with
Amnesia	impairments of psychomotor function
Anxiety	
Ataxia	
Behavioral disinhibition	
Cognitive deficits: interference with learning, memory consolidation and academic performance	
Delirium/symptoms of dementia/disorientation	
Drowsiness/lethargy/sedation	
Hostility/Aggression	
Reported Long-Term Effects	
Cognitive Effects/Side Effects	**EEG Effects**
Attention and concentration difficulties	Acute EEG tolerance after intermittent
Insomnia	administration
Memory impairment	Increase in beta activity
Reduced motor speed/performance	
Reduced speed of information processing	

[a]EEG changes are noted in absolute frequency bands and do not include other EEG measures, such as relative power, unless otherwise specified.[1,3,7,13,14]

impairment, memory difficulties, or sedative or hypnotic side effects that often accompany benzodiazepine use.[19] Whereas buspirone and benzodiazepines both demonstrate effects on serotonin, these medications affect other neurotransmitter systems differently.[1] Benzodiazepines appear to inhibit noradrenergic and dopaminergic neuronal activity, whereas buspirone increases the activity of both neurotransmitter systems.[1] In contrast to the nonselective action of benzodiazepines, the selective action of buspirone may explain its anxiolytic efficacy without the disruptive side effects of sedation or cognitive impairment.

Buspirone has a gradual onset and also is used for alleviation of concurrent anxiety and depressive symptoms.[20] This medication induces EEG changes that are generally characterized by a negative shift in the EEG frequency spectrum.[21] Such shifts are characterized by increases in theta power, a reduction in beta activity and acceleration of centroids, which refers to location of global field power within a given frequency spectrum, across delta, theta and beta frequency bands.[2] These EEG shifts differ greatly from those of benzodiazepines, even though both medications exert anxiolytic effects.

Implications for Anxiolytics and Neurofeedback

If a patient's anxiety adversely affects cognitive performance, benzodiazepines may be useful to transiently reduce symptoms that would otherwise interfere with neurofeedback. Neurofeedback protocols must also recognize that enhanced fast frequencies may be derived from the use of medication and design protocols so as not to counteract or work against intended medication effects. Other anxiolytic medications with more selective mechanisms may serve as an alternative for treating anxiety-related symptoms concurrent with neurofeedback, because those medications are not accompanied by the cognitive impairments commonly present with benzodiazepine use. The neurofeedback clinician must consider EEG changes by different types of anxiolytic medications and design optimal treatment accordingly, using ongoing cognitive and EEG assessments to measure progress and make appropriate adjustments at different points in treatment.

STIMULANT MEDICATIONS

Stimulants and ADHD

Another set of patients who seek neurofeedback includes individuals with attention deficits, hyperactivity or both. These patients may require intervention with stimulant medications. Stimulants are the leading treatment for attention deficit hyperactivity disorder (ADHD) and have been reported as a prescribed treatment in 4% of children aged 6–19 years old with this diagnosis.[22] ADHD is a commonly diagnosed psychological disorder with prevalence rates ranging from 3% to 7% in school-aged children.[23] Patients with these symptoms are often difficult to treat with neurofeedback because of their characteristic behaviors of impulsivity, hyperactivity and inattention.

ADHD is a complex clinical disorder, in terms of both behavioral presentation and EEG phenotypes. Designing neurofeedback protocols according to baseline EEG features can present a challenge. ADHD has been categorized according to DSM-IV-TR criteria into three symptom clusters: inattentive, hyperactive and combined.[23] However, these categories represent a wide range of problematic behaviors that include impaired working memory, decision-making and planning skills.[24] Patients with ADHD also have different EEG phenotypes that do not closely correspond to behavioral subtypes.[25] Some previous research has identified five EEG subtypes of ADHD[25–28]; thus ADHD defined either by clinical presentation or by EEG profile constitutes a complex, heterogeneous disorder.[29–32]

Despite the heterogeneity of behavioral and electrophysiological subtypes, certain EEG features are commonly present across diagnostic subtypes and phenotypes. Some researchers have estimated that a common feature present in approximately 90% of individuals with ADHD is an abnormally increased theta/beta ratio.[33] The theta/beta ratio has consistently differentiated between ADHD patients and normal controls, and has demonstrated stability over time and across gender and age.[26,28,31,34] Other EEG characteristics also commonly present in ADHD include increased theta, particularly in frontal regions, and decreased or increased beta, particularly in posterior regions of the brain.[25–28,35–37] Given the heterogeneity of ADHD, treatment design requires consideration of both behavioral and EEG patterns.

Acute Cognitive Effects of Stimulants

Stimulants, particularly methylphenidate, have been labeled the "gold standard" for the treatment of ADHD because of their influence on impulsivity, hyperactivity and inattention.[38,39] Not all patients respond to stimulant medication; however, those who do respond have corresponding improvements in both cognition and EEG.[40] Improvements from stimulant medications are supported across several domains of cognitive function and may provide transient support to the neurofeedback process by enhancing various attentional and learning processes.

Stimulant medications in children with ADHD improve sensorimotor gating to unrelated (task-irrelevant) stimuli, allowing for enhanced attention to be directed at effortful cognitive processes.[41] Stimulants have been shown to reduce certain risk-prone behaviors,[42] enhance working memory in children[43] and adults,[44] and improve inhibitory control, performance accuracy and intellectual function.[45,46] Although stimulants have not demonstrated unequivocal improvements in executive function, these medications have consistently resulted in at least short-term performance and behavioral enhancement.[46]

Studies of stimulants in adults with and without ADHD have reliably demonstrated improvement in sustained attention, and in normal adults, improved attention for simple tasks as well as enhanced declarative memory and long-term memory consolidation. However, some acute cognitive impairments have been noted in adults, including possible impairment of short-term memory acquisition and cognitive flexibility.[47] Because stimulants may have either cognitive improvement or impairment effects, early monitoring of cognitive change is critical.

Long-Term Cognitive Effects of Stimulants

Current research indicates mixed findings on the cognitive impact of sustained stimulant use. Some research demonstrates that although long-term stimulant use does not result in cognitive impairment, neither does it improve baseline deficits.[48] On the other hand, chronic administration of methylphenidate has been shown to improve certain areas of neuropsychological functioning, particularly on cognitive tasks related to recognition memory.[49] Cognitive decline is not supported as a side effect of long-term stimulant use, and behavioral improvements addressing impulsivity, hyperactivity and emotional lability are sustained with long-term use.[35,49]

Reasons for nonmedical use of stimulants as potential drugs of abuse include cognitive enhancement, particularly among students, as well as the induction of euphoria and suppression of appetite and sleep.[50] Therefore, patients seeking neurofeedback treatment may be using medications for purposes other than attention difficulties and may hesitate to report their use. Overall, current research suggests that adverse effects from stimulants, both cognitive and somatic, are mild to moderate.[51] Some literature has indicated an increased risk of seizures and the development of tic disorders with the use of stimulant medications; however, such risks may be lower than previously thought.[51] Ongoing EEG and behavioral evaluations should be conducted during chronic stimulant treatment to detect the possible emergence of such symptoms.

EEG Effects of Acute Use of Stimulants

Acute changes in EEG derived from the administration of stimulants have been most widely studied in individuals with ADHD using methylphenidate. Findings have been divergent.[24,39,52] Some investigators have found that stimulant medication resulted in improvement in global EEG measures, whereas others showed improvement only in a set of patients identified as "responders," and yet others have found no global effects on EEG. Although there is some discrepancy, the larger trend in the literature suggests that stimulant medications result in global EEG shifts that often lean toward normalization of EEG patterns in patients with ADHD.

EEG changes that reflect enhanced cortical arousal with stimulants are characterized by increased beta and decreased slow waves.[53,54] Acute positive effects following stimulant medication on other EEG measures, such as phase, coherence and symmetry, suggest improvement in cortical communication.[55] Studies differentiating between medication responders and nonresponders have found acute EEG changes that have direct implications for behavioral performance. Individuals with a positive cognitive response to short-term medication use, as demonstrated by improved performance on a continuous attention task, had associated normalization in global EEG frequencies.[40] Medication responders with increased frontal beta activity following stimulant medication had closely correlated improvements in sustained attention.[37,55]

EEG Effects of Long-Term Use of Stimulants

Several studies offer support for a shift toward normalization in the EEGs of children with ADHD on long-term stimulant medication. In trials of 4 weeks or more, stimulant medication resulted in improvements in EEG patterns from baseline, particularly in patients with excess theta and deficit beta frequencies.[35,52,55,56] These shifts included absolute power decreases in theta and increases in beta, which research suggests may reflect enhanced cortical arousal.[52] Long-term use of stimulants has also resulted in significant reduction in theta/alpha and theta/beta power ratios with either methylphenidate or dexamphetamine.[52]

Improvements seen with long-term stimulant use are dependent on the pattern of baseline EEG. The majority of individuals with ADHD present with excess theta and reduced beta at baseline; however, a subset of patients with ADHD has been identified with initial patterns of excess beta. The latter patients demonstrate a different EEG shift with chronic stimulant use, characterized by a reduction in power but not a normalization of their EEG patterns.[27] Thus, baseline EEG is a critical component that can aid in the prediction of treatment response with high levels of sensitivity and specificity. It has been found that patients who do demonstrate EEG normalization have corresponding behavioral improvements.[35] Baseline EEG alone, however, is not enough for the prediction

Table 3.3 Summary of Possible Effects of Stimulant Use Related to Neurofeedback Treatment

Summary of Stimulant Effects	
Reported Acute Effects	
Cognitive Effects/Side Effects	**EEG Effects[a]**
Improved accuracy and performance	Decreased slow wave activity
Enhanced prepulse inhibition/reduced impulsivity	Increased alpha and slow beta activity
Enhanced working memory	Reduced fast beta activity
Improved sustained attention on simple cognitive tasks	Decreased theta/beta ratio
Impairment of short-term memory acquisition	
Reduced cognitive flexibility	
Somatic complaints that may distract from learning (headaches, nausea, insomnia)	
Reported Long-Term Side Effects	
Cognitive Effects/Side Effects	**EEG Effects**
Sustained performance across cognitive domains	Decreased theta activity
	Increased beta activity
Infrequently reported:[51]	Decreased theta/alpha ratio
Increased risk of motor tics	Decreased theta/beta ratio
Increased risk for seizures	
Psychotic symptoms	

[a]EEG changes are noted in absolute frequency bands and do not include other EEG measures, such as relative power, unless otherwise specified.

of treatment response to stimulants without objective behavioral measures.[33] The recommended approach with stimulants and other medications involves combined behavioral and EEG evaluations, both at baseline and during medication use, to predict and assess treatment response.[35] Acute medication challenge approaches, which involve the use of medications that have rapid onset of effects with measurements of EEG before and after medication administration, may also be useful in predicting long-term clinical response to stimulants.[29] A summary of acute and long-term effects of stimulant use is provided in Table 3.3.

Implications for Stimulant Medications and Neurofeedback

If patients are unable to focus, follow directions or respond appropriately because of inattention or hyperactivity, stimulant medication may provide transient support for neurofeedback treatment. Stimulants are the medications most often used for treatment of ADHD. However, ADHD is a heterogeneous disorder in terms of both behavioral problems and EEG patterns, and therefore a baseline assessment may provide guidance as to the specific type of medication intervention. Furthermore, a follow-up EEG should offer neurofeedback providers information concerning specific areas of ongoing EEG abnormalities. Neurofeedback can then be designed to address, for example, excess or deficit frequency patterns specific to each patient. Over time, stimulants may be withdrawn as patients practice neurofeedback. It is recommended that, in additional to clinical presentation, practitioners obtain objective behavioral measures, such as tasks of sustained attention, for example Test of Variables of Attention or Integrated Visual and Auditory Continuous Performance Test. Such measures would provide external validation in reaching treatment efficacy. These tasks could be used throughout therapeutic intervention to determine alterations in medication dosages and eventual termination of both medication and neurofeedback treatment.

ANTIDEPRESSANTS

Antidepressants represent a broad class of medications with varying mechanisms of action. They include, among others, selective serotonin reuptake inhibitors (SSRIs), selective norepinephrine reuptake inhibitors (SNRIs), and tricyclic and dual-action antidepressants. Neurofeedback protocols for the treatment of depression generally target EEG asymmetry patterns in alpha frequencies, which may or may not change over the course of treatment with medication. Studies have identified targets for treatment intervention that are implicated in depressive symptoms such as the subcallosal cingulate gyrus,[30] and which may have new implications for neurofeedback design. Many individuals seeking neurofeedback for difficulties with attention, concentration, anxiety or other symptoms also present with comorbid depressive symptoms. Therefore, neurofeedback providers should be familiar with the impact of antidepressant medications on cognition and EEG patterns.

Acute Cognitive Effects of Antidepressants

Cognitive impairments in patients suffering from major depression have been well documented and have been shown to exist apart from medication side effects.[57] Functions that are impaired include attention, executive function, learning and memory.[57] Medications may provide patients with remediation of these symptoms if they respond positively. At the same time, antidepressant medications can introduce a new profile of side effects that can adversely affect cognitive processes.

Antidepressants have differential effects on cognitive function, often depending on their activating or sedation properties. Tricyclic antidepressants have been shown to cause sedation and result in marked impairment of information processing and cognitive function.[58] SSRIs and SNRIs have been demonstrated to have a mixed impact on cognitive function in both healthy volunteers and depressed patients. For example, paroxetine, fluoxetine and fluvoxamine impair cognitive performance in certain healthy volunteers after a single administration. These deficits include impaired visual attention, recall, and response time and accuracy.[58] At the same time, SSRIs also have been reported to enhance performance in certain cognitive tasks.[58,59] The differential cognitive effects of antidepressants must take into account various pharmacological mechanisms of action, as well as individual patient characteristics, such as the severity of depressive symptoms and previous history of medication use.[60]

Long-Term Cognitive Effects of Antidepressants

Research on the cognitive effects of long-term use of antidepressants is mixed, with different impacts in healthy versus patient populations. For several classes of antidepressants, different studies of long-term use have demonstrated enhanced cognitive performance, cognitive impairment and no change from baseline. Tricyclic antidepressants have been shown to have lasting impairments on memory beyond deficits because of the initial sedating effects,[58] yet some tricyclic agents, such as amitriptyline, imipramine and clomipramine, have enhanced cognitive performance in areas such as memory, attention and reaction time.[59]

Cognitive performance in long-term users of SSRIs also is variable. After chronic administration to depressed patients, SSRIs have been shown to enhance memory, reaction time, attention and cognitive flexibility.[58] More specifically, in depressed patients it was demonstrated that fluoxetine and paroxetine had similar effects on cognitive improvement, which were greater than that shown by amitriptyline. Use of sertraline in depressed patients has demonstrated cognitive enhancement beyond that of fluoxetine, particularly on vigilance tasks.[58] A general conclusion drawn from previous studies of antidepressants is that cognitive improvement appears to parallel improvement in mood.[59] Patients taking antidepressants may therefore progress more rapidly in neurofeedback as their depressive symptoms subside.

EEG Effects of Acute Use of Antidepressants

Antidepressants have been divided into two main categories, based on their most clearly differentiated effects on EEG patterns: those with activating effects and those with sedative-like effects.[2,61] Activating antidepressants, for example fluoxetine, have resulted mainly in increases in power in alpha frequencies, as well as decreases in concomitant faster and slower waves.[39] Antidepressants with sedative effects, for example fluvoxamine, show the opposite pattern, with an increase in power in concomitant slower and faster frequencies and decreases in alpha waves.[2,39,61] Specific tricyclic agents and SSRIs belong in either one of these categories, depending upon their activating or sedative EEG effects. Acute neurobiochemical changes have been identified after a single dose.[61] EEG changes caused by different classes of antidepressants reflect alterations in arousal states of the brain, and thus can affect target frequencies for neurofeedback protocols.

EEG and Prediction of Long-Term Treatment Outcomes of Antidepressants

Conclusive data on EEG changes with long-term antidepressant use are limited; however, EEG has proven to be a useful tool in the prediction of treatment outcomes with antidepressants. Some studies have shown that EEG changes after long-term antidepressant use parallel acute EEG changes. Treatment with SSRIs lasting longer than 6 weeks has been associated with reductions in alpha activity and increases in the power of slow and fast frequencies. These changes are similar to the acute EEG shifts seen with imipramine-like sedative compounds.[62] Other studies have shown no EEG normalization in either medication responders or non-responders after chronic administration, particularly with regard to alpha asymmetries.[63] These findings suggest that certain frequency bands may be influenced by antidepressant medications, whereas others, such as alpha, represent more stable, state-independent EEG characteristics.[63]

A growing body of literature is exploring the prediction of long-term outcomes with antidepressant treatments based on EEG patterns present at baseline (medication-free) and during early treatment (2 or more days). The push to identify markers for treatment response is driven by response failure and/or low success rates of antidepressant treatment. Inadequate or partial responses to antidepressant treatment are common, with only 30–40% of patients achieving full remission, defined as 3 consecutive weeks of minimal symptoms.[64] Some studies have identified markers for treatment response based on early changes in EEG frequencies. EEG activity in the theta band, both at baseline and following the start of treatment, appears to be the most sensitive marker for successful prediction of treatment outcomes and improvement.[60,65] Medication responders to SSRIs and tricyclic medications have demonstrated significant theta abnormalities, often characterized by increased theta power at baseline compared to nonresponders.[62,65,66] Abnormalities in the alpha frequency band have also been used to predict treatment response,[65] albeit with less consistency.

One EEG measure employed in the prediction of treatment response is cordance. Cordance uses both absolute and relative frequency power ratios that reflect cerebral activity and perfusion.[67] Changes in cordance values, particularly decreases in prefrontal cordance in the early stages of treatment with SSRIs, SNRIs and atypical antidepressants, have successfully differentiated between responders and nonresponders.[68,69] Whereas medication use during early treatment may not yield obvious shifts in the absolute power of EEG frequencies, other EEG measures may detect improvement or change in cerebral activity and provide for a more accurate reflection of medication effects.[65] Thus, neurofeedback providers should be mindful that medication might have a significant impact on electrophysiology, even when not clearly identified by absolute power measures alone. A summary of acute and long-term effects of antidepressants is provided in Table 3.4.

Implications for Antidepressants and Neurofeedback

Antidepressants constitute a broad class of psychotropics with many pharmacological mechanisms of action. An antidepressant drug may initially enhance or impair cognitive performance, depending upon the drug itself and unique patient characteristics, and these changes may shift with chronic or repeated use.[60] Neurofeedback providers should conduct repeated assessments for both cognitive and EEG changes. These assessments would be most useful when acquired at baseline, 2–7 days following the start of medication, and 4 weeks after medication use. Providers may also wish to consider mood measures, because many cognitive improvements may parallel the alleviation of negative mood states.

Table 3.4 Summary of Possible Effects of Antidepressants Related to Neurofeedback Treatment

Summary of Antidepressant Effects

Reported Acute Effects

Cognitive Effects/Side Effects	EEG Effects[a]
Agitation	*Imipramine/Amitriptyline-like compounds:*
Inattention	(Sedative Effects)
Memory impairment	Increased slow frequencies (delta, theta)
Reduced psychomotor speed and	Increased fast frequencies (beta)
reaction time	Marked decrease of alpha frequencies
Improvements in attention	*Desipramine-like compounds:*
Enhanced memory	(Activating Effects)
Increased reaction time	Decreased slow frequencies (delta, theta)
	Decreased fast frequencies (beta)
	Increased alpha frequencies
	Across antidepressants:
	Decreased frontal cordance in the theta band in medication responders

Reported Long-Term Effects

Cognitive Effects/Side Effects	EEG Effects
Impairments in attention	Changes parallel to acute EEG alterations
Memory impairment	(different for sedating or activating agents)
Reduced psychomotor speed	
Treatment emergent-deficits	No correction for alpha asymmetry found
such as delirium	at baseline
Improvement in attention	
Enhanced memory	

[a]EEG changes are noted in absolute frequency bands and do not include other EEG measures, such as relative power, unless otherwise specified.

ANTIPSYCHOTICS

Antipsychotic medications historically have been used in the treatment of schizophrenia. However, with the advancement from first-generation antipsychotics (FGAs) to second-generation antipsychotics (SGAs), the use of antipsychotics in nonpsychotic disorders has increased rapidly.[70] FGAs, such as chlorpromazine (Thorazine) and haloperidol (Haldol), are effective in treating positive symptoms of schizophrenia, but they also carry the risk of significant side effects, including acute and long-term movement disorders, such as tardive dyskinesia.

SGAs, such as clozaril (Clozapine), risperidone (Risperdal), olanzapine (Zyprexa), quetiapine (Seroquel), ziprasidone (Geodon) and aripiprazole (Abilify), can serve as an alternative to first-generation medications without the same risk of serious side effects. Selected SGAs have been used to treat bipolar disorder, unipolar depression, dementia, autism spectrum and pervasive developmental disorders, aggression, posttraumatic stress and obsessive–compulsive disorders, borderline personality disorder and Parkinson's disease. Thus, while neurofeedback would not likely be used for patients experiencing acute psychotic symptoms such as sensory hallucinations, such treatment may be indicated for patients who are stable and/or treated with antipsychotics for other purposes, including affective and anxiety disorders.

Acute and Long-Term Cognitive Effects of Antipsychotics

Most studies focus on the long-term cognitive impact of FGAs or SGAs. In studies of acute administration, elderly volunteers showed slight motor impairment and impaired information processing with low doses of risperidone, but no other deleterious effects.[71] In first-episode patients suffering from acute psychosis, researchers found no cognitive impairment within the first 72 hours of treatment with haloperidol, risperidone or olanzapine, nor were impairments noted after 6 weeks of treatment.[72] Other research supported these results, finding no changes after acute administration of the second-generation olanzapine.[73]

With longer-term use of antipsychotics, first-generation medications introduce adverse extrapyramidal side effects that have also been found to impair performance on cognitive tasks.[74] SGAs appear to have fewer negative cognitive side effects, if any, and have even been implicated in cognitive enhancement. Olanzapine, clozapine and risperidone have been shown to moderately improve working memory and attention as well as verbal fluency, learning and memory in patients who are treatment responders.[73,75,76] These findings hold true of first-episode schizophrenic patients, with moderate cognitive improvement noted for both SGAs and haloperidol.[74] Cognitive benefits have also been found for nonschizophrenic patients using atypical antipsychotics to treat affective disorders.[77] Trends in the literature suggest the favorability of certain SGAs over first-generation drugs for cognitive functioning,[78,79] and provide support for cognitive improvement with SGAs.[80] Although these cognitive improvements may be a function of symptom remission,[74] SGAs in particular appear to offer cognitive benefits in long-term use.

EEG Effects of Acute Use of Antipsychotics

FGAs can be divided into two categories based on their quantitative EEG (qEEG) profiles: sedative, low potency versus nonsedative, and high potency.[39] Low-potency sedative FGAs include chlorpromazine-type medications, and their EEG effects are characterized by increased slow frequencies and decreased alpha frequencies. High-potency nonsedative FGAs such as haloperidol are associated with acute increase in slow alpha (7.5–9.5 Hz) and alpha-adjacent beta power with no change in slower frequencies.[78] In high-potency medications, the increase in slow alpha activity has been associated with a favorable clinical response.[82]

SGAs do not result in clearly identifiable EEG profiles.[39] Some congruent findings have pointed to frontal shifts in alpha power. Yoshimura and colleagues[80] conducted a single-dose study of effects of two FGAs and four SGAs on healthy volunteers. These researchers found that haloperidol enhanced power in alpha-1 frequencies, whereas quetiapine reduced alpha-1, suggesting that certain SGAs may have sedative-like qualities that overlap the profile of some first-generation drugs. As with some previous research,[84] Yoshimura et al.[83] reported that quetiapine and olanzapine resulted in similar shifts in centroid alpha frequencies in anterior regions. The researchers suggested that these localized findings may be related to mechanisms of action specific to frontal lobe function.

EEG profiles of other SGAs have been reviewed and found to involve discrepant findings. Some profiles appear similar to antidepressant EEG profiles, whereas others are more akin to FGA sedative medications.[39,81,85] The discrepancies may be explained by differing affinities for dopamine and serotonin across antipsychotic medications, as well as variable sample populations, which have included both healthy volunteers and patients with schizophrenia. Researchers have suggested that although consistent findings are available for FGAs in traditional approaches to pharmaco-EEG, studies of SGAs may need to revisit assumptions regarding acute administration, and possibly incorporate a broader range of qEEG measures.[39] Patients taking SGAs may therefore have very different EEG profiles, and treatment considerations must include patient variability and repeated assessment.

EEG Effects of Long-Term Use of Antipsychotics

Long-term use of FGAs has resulted in decreased delta activity and increased alpha activity.[86–88] Other noted shifts include decreased beta frequencies with the use of FGAs such as haloperidol and fluphen-azine.[83,87,89] Long-term treatment with SGAs such as clozapine often results in EEG changes characterized by slowing, with increased power in delta and theta bands.[90] Further research is needed to look into the EEG effects of long-term use of FGAs and SGAs in both healthy volunteers[83] and patients, but variability again highlights the importance of individualized and ongoing EEG assessment throughout treatment. A summary of acute and long-term effects of antipsychotics is given in Tables 3.5 and 3.6.

SUMMARY

Neurofeedback providers will be faced with several challenges when determining treatment protocols for individuals on medication. Psychotropic drugs have both short- and long-term cognitive and EEG effects that can reflect treatment progress as well as response to medication. Drugs have very different pharmacokinetic and pharmacodynamic profiles from each other, such as dose- and time-efficacies; even medications within the same class or subcategory have various properties. Furthermore, patient characteristics are unique and have a significant impact on medication response. Electrophysiological profiles of drug response depend on gender, age, genetics, severity of illness, previous treatment history, compliance and other unique patient characteristics, such as volume distribution, renal function and related physiological properties.

There are some important limitations to designing research and neurofeedback training protocols with the concurrent use of psychotropic medications. For example, although the literature has defined the EEG impact of individual centrally acting drugs, there are no studies addressing drug–drug interactions, and many patients are using polypharmacy for symptom management. Literature is also lacking regarding the chronic use of medication. Questions raised in this discussion point to the necessity of engaging in studies that address issues of chronic use and polypharmacy.

Additionally, EEG currently provides indicators of electrophysiological changes that lie beyond the scope of this chapter, but which offer important information about the impact of medications on brain activity. These methods include relative and absolute power variables and their reflection of cerebral perfusion,[67] measures of intra- and interhemispheric communication, such as phase, symmetry and coherence, and source localization of EEG with low-resolution brain electromagnetic tomography.[91,92] Such

Table 3.5 Summary of Possible Effects of Antipsychotics Related to Neurofeedback Treatment

Summary of Antipsychotic Effects

Acute

Cognitive Effects/Side Effects	EEG Effects[a]
FGAs:	*Low-Potency Sedative FGAs (chlorpromazine):*
Decreased psychomotor speed	Increase in delta and theta frequencies
Reducing information processing speed	Decrease in slow alpha frequencies
Potential between extrapyramidal side effects and performance on cognitive tasks	Decreased fast frequencies
	High-Potency Nonsedative FGAs (haloperidol):
SGAs:	Increase in delta and theta frequencies
Mild motor impairment	Increase in slow alpha, associated with positive clinical response
Mild decrease in processing speed	Decreased fast frequencies
Minimal cognitive impairments at time of acute administration	
	SGAs:
	Variable profiles in healthy controls & patients
	Clozapine/olanzapine: increased slow activity, decreased fast activity; reduction in alpha-2

Long-Term

Cognitive Effects/Side Effects	EEG Effects
FGAs (haloperidol):	*FGAs:*
Psychomotor speed	Decrease in delta
Information processing	Increase in alpha-1
	Decrease in beta
SGAs:	
Working memory and attention	*SGAs:*
Verbal fluency, memory, and learning	Increase in delta
Psychomotor speed	Increase in theta
Information processing	Increase in overall power

[a]EEG changes are noted in absolute frequency bands and do not include other EEG measures, such as relative power, unless otherwise specified.

methods allow the discovery of localized changes associated with use of psychotropics.[61]

Identification of localized medication effects is critical given recent data indicating that the human brain is not uniform in distribution. Based on recent investigations using measurement of neurotransmitter levels,

Table 3.6 Summary of General Pharmaco-EEG Drug Profiles

General Pharmaco-EEG Drug Profiles[a]

Drug Class	Examples	Pharmaco-EEG Profile
Neuroleptics		
Sedative neuroleptics	chlorpromazine, clozapine, dapiprazole, zetidoline, zotepine	↑ (increased) delta ↑ theta ↓ slow alpha (7.5–9.5 Hz) ↑ beta (less consistent finding)
Nonsedative neuroleptics	haloperidol	↑ delta ↑ theta ↑ slow alpha ↑ alpha–adjacent beta
Antidepressant drugs		
Sedative qualities − Imipramine/ amitriptyline-like effects	amitriptyline N-oxide, danitracene, doxepin, fluvoxamine, maprotiline, paroxetine	↑ slow and fast activities ↓ alpha
Activating qualities − Desipramine-like effects	diclofensine, fluoxetine, nomifensine, pirlindol, sercloremine, sertraline, tranylcypromine, zimelidine	↓ slow and fast activities ↑ alpha
Anxiolytic sedatives (both tranquilizers and hypnotics)		
Anxiolytic sedatives (General)		↑ alpha ↑ beta ↓ total power
Daytime tranquilizers/ low-dose benzodiazepines	bromazepam, clobazam, oxazepam, prazeplam	No augmentation of slow activity
Nighttime hypnotics/high–dose benzodiazepines	brotizolam, cloxazolam, flunitrazepam, flurazepam, lopirazepam, lorazepam, temazepam, triazolam	↑ delta
Psychostimulants[b]		
Pharmacological stimulants	D-amphetamine, methamphetamine, adrafinil, modafinil	↓ slow and fast activities ↑ alpha ↑ alpha–adjacent beta

[a]Profile is dependent on the baseline, type of patient and dose.
[b]Differences among studies are found based on states of vigilance: resting v. vigilance-controlled. For review see 1,2,17,37,58.

receptor mapping, functional brain imaging, performance tasks and electrophysiological tools, emerging evidence suggests hemispheric specialization in function based on differential impact of neurotransmitters between the left and right hemisphere.[93] Lateralized distribution in normal function, for example speech,[94] as well as focal lateralized abnormalities in receptor distribution,[95] for example in seizure activities, suggest that the brain is not uniform. Based on these findings, medication effects may be predicted to have focal and lateralizing actions; therefore, further research in pharmaco-EEG and medication use in neurofeedback treatment is needed to understand how medications may affect localized circuits. In light of the aforementioned complexities, other types of neuroimaging may also provide critical insight into complex clinical presentations to further clarify symptoms and guide treatment design.[96]

Despite limitations and wide-ranging variables, the provider can use certain practices to guide effective treatment design and obtain optimal outcomes. The most critical component to neurofeedback protocol design is personalized, ongoing assessment that objectively tracks cognitive abilities and EEG patterns over the course of treatment. By doing so, the provider can make adjustments when appropriate, and just as importantly, identify rate and specific areas of improvement. Measurable improvements are not only useful for guiding the practitioner, but also should be recognized by the patient. This introduction to the effects of psychotropic medications will hopefully provide the practitioner with basic guidelines for assessment and serve as a starting point for further exploration into relationships between concurrent pharmacological interventions and neurofeedback.

REFERENCES

1. Barbanoj MJ, Riba J, Morte A, Antonijoan RM, Jané F. Basics of PK-PD using QEEG: Acute/repetitive administration, interactions. Focus on axiolytics with different neurochemical mechanisms as examples. *Methods Find Exp Clin Pharmacol.* 2002;24C:67–83.
2. Saletu B, Anderer P, Saletu-Zyhlarz GM. EEG topography and tomography (LORETA) in the classification and evaluation of the pharmacodynamics of psychotropic drugs. *Clin EEG Neurosci.* 2006;37(2):66–80.
3. Barker M, Greenwood K, Jackson M, Crowe S. Persistence of cognitive effects after withdrawal from long-term benzodiazepine use: a meta-analysis. *Arch Clin Neuropsychol.* 2004;19(3):437–454.
4. Pollack MH. Innovative uses of benzodiazepines in psychiatry. *Can J Psychiatry.* 1993;38(suppl 4):122–126.
5. Buffett-Jerrott S, Stewart S, Finley G, Loughlan H. Effects of benzodiazepines on explicit memory in a paediatric surgery setting. *J Psychopharmacol.* 2003;168(4):377–386.

6. Curran H, Collins R, Fletcher S, Kee S, Woods B, Iliffe S. Older adults and withdrawal from benzodiazepine hypnotics in general practice: Effects on cognitive function, sleep, mood and quality of life. *Psychol Med.* 2003;33(7):1223–1237.
7. Stewart S. The effects of benzodiazepines on cognition. *J Clin Psychiatry.* 2005;66(suppl 2):9–13.
8. Bastien C, LeBlanc M, Carrier J, Morin C. Sleep EEG power spectra, insomnia, and chronic use of benzodiazepines. *Sleep.* 2003;26(3):313–317.
9. Haefly W, Kulscár A, Möhler H, Pieri L, Polc P, Schaffner R. Possible involvement of GABA in the central actions of benzodiazepines. *Adv Biochem Psychopharmacol.* 1975;14:131–151.
10. Möhler H, Okada T. Benzodiazepine receptor: demonstration in the central nervous system. *Science.* 1977;198(4319):849–851.
11. Bremner JD, Innis RB, White T, et al. SPECT [I-123]iomazenil measurement of the benzodiazepine receptor in panic disorder. *Biol Psychiatry.* 2000;47(2):96–106.
12. Geuze E, van Berckel B, Lammertsma AA, et al. Reduced GABA$_A$ benzodiazepine receptor binding in veterans with posttraumatic stress disorder. *Mol Psychiatry.* 2008;13(1):74–83.
13. Greenblatt DJ, Gan L, Harmatz JS, Shader RI. Pharmacokinetics and pharmacodynamics of single-dose triazolam: electroencephalography compared with the digit-symbol substitution test. *Br J Clin Pharmacol.* 2005;60(3):244–248.
14. Giménez S, Romero S, Mañanas M, Barbanoj M. Waking and sleep electroencephalogram variables as human sleep homeostatic process biomarkers after drug administration. *Neuropsychobiology.* 2011;63(4):252–260.
15. Barbanoj M, Urbano G, Antonijoan R, Ballester M, Valle M. Different acute tolerance development to EEG, psychomotor performance and subjective assessment effects after two intermittent oral doses of alphrazolam in healthy volunteers. *Neuropsychobiology.* 2007;55(3–4):203–212.
16. Kopp C, Rudolph U, Low K, Tobler I. Modulation of rhythmic brain activity by diazepam: GABA$_A$ receptor subtype and state specificity. *Proc Natl Acad Sci USA.* 2004;101(10):3674–3679.
17. Mandema JW, Danhof M. Electroencephalogram effect measures and relationships between pharmacokinetics and pharmacodynamics of centrally acting drugs. *Clin Pharmacokinet.* 1992;23(3):191–215.
18. Tan X, Uchida S, Matsuura M, Nishihara K, Kojima T. Long-, intermediate- and short-acting benzodiazepine effects on human sleep EEG spectra. *Psychiatry Clin Neurosci.* 2003;57(1):97–104.
19. Chamberlain S, Müller U, Deakin JB, et al. Lack of deleterious effects of buspirone on cognition in healthy male volunteers. *J Psychopharmacol.* 2007;21(2):210–215.
20. Casacalenda N, Boulenger J. Pharmacologic treatments effective in both generalized anxiety disorder and major depressive disorder: clinical and theoretical implications. *Can J Psychiatry.* 1998;43(7):722–730.
21. McAllister-Williams R, Massey A. EEG effects of buspirone and pindolol: a method of examining 5-HT1A receptor function in humans. *Psychopharmacology (Berl).* 2003;166(3):284–293.
22. Zuvekas SH, Vitiello B, Norquist GS. Recent trends in stimulant medication use among US children. *Am J Psychiatry.* 2006;163:579–585.
23. American Psychological Association. *Diagnostic and Statistical Manual of Mental Disorders.* 4th ed., text rev. Washington, DC: Author; 2000.
24. Rhodes S, Coghill D, Matthews K. Neuropsychological functioning in stimulant-naive boys with hyperkinetic disorder. *Psychol Med.* 2005;35(8):1109–1120.
25. Arns M, Gunkleman J, Breteler M, Spronk D. EEG phenotypes predict treatment outcome to stimulants in children with ADHD. *J Integr Neurosci.* 2008;7(3):421–438.

26. Clarke A, Barry R, McCarthy R, Selikowitz M. EEG-defined subtypes of children with attention-deficit/hyperactivity disorder. *Clin Neurophysiol.* 2001;112(11): 2098–2105.

27. Clarke A, Barry R, McCarthy R, Selikowitz M, Clarke D, Croft R. Effects of stimulant medications on children with attention-deficit/hyperactivity disorder and excessive beta activity in their EEG. *Clin Neurophysiol.* 2003;114(9):1729–1737.

28. Clarke A, Barry R, McCarthy R, Selikowitz M, Johnstone S. Effects of stimulant medications on the EEG of girls with attention-deficit/hyperactivity disorder. *Clin Neurophysiol.* 2007;118(12):2700–2708.

29. Konopka LM, Poprawski TJ. Quantitative EEG studies of attention disorders and mood disorders in children. In: Ivanenko A, ed. *Sleep and Psychiatric Disorders in Children and Adolescents.* New York, NY: Informa Healthcare USA, Inc; 2008:293–304.

30. Hamani C, Mayberg H, Stone S, Laxton A, Haber S, Lozano A. The subcallosal cingulate gyrus in the context of major depression. *Biol Psychiatry.* 2011;69(4):301–308.

31. Loo S, Barkley R. Clinical utility of EEG in attention deficit hyperactivity disorder. *Appl Neuropsychol.* 2005;12(2):64–76.

32. Martin C, Konopka L. Community-based electrophysiological abnormalities in children with ADHD: translating research findings into a clinical setting. *Act Nerv Super.* 2011;53(3–4):129–140.

33. Snyder SM, Hall JR. A meta-analysis of quantitative EEG power associated with attention-deficit hyperactivity disorder. *J Clin Neurophysiol.* 2006;23:440–455.

34. Lubar JF, Swartwood MO, Swartwood JN, Timmerman DL. Quantitative EEG and auditory event-related potentials in the evaluation of attention deficit/hyperactivity disorder: effects of methylphenidate and implications for neurofeedback training. *J Psychoeducational Assess.* 1996;14:143–160.

35. Chabot RJ, Orgill AA, Crawford G, Harris MJ, Serfontein G. Behavioral and electrophysiologic predictors of treatment response to stimulants in children with attention disorders. *J Child Neurol.* 1999;14(6):343–351.

36. Lansbergen M, Arns M, van Dongen-Boomsma M, Spronk D, Buitelaar J. The increase in theta/beta ratio on resting-state EEG in boys with attention-deficit/hyperactivity disorder is mediated by slow alpha peak frequency. *Prog Neuropsychopharmacol Biol Psychiatry.* 2011;35(1):47–52.

37. Loo SK, Hopfer C, Teale PD, Reite ML. EEG correlates of methylphenidate response in ADHD: association with cognitive and behavioral measures. *J Clin Neurophysiol.* 2004;21(6):457–464.

38. Hanwella R, Senanayake M, de Silva V. Comparative efficacy and acceptability of methylphenidate and atomoxetine in treatment of attention deficit hyperactivity disorder in children and adolescents: a meta-analysis. *BMC Psychiatry.* 2011;11:176–184.

39. Mucci A, Volpe U, Merlotti E, Bucci P, Galderisi S. Pharmaco-EEG in psychiatry. *Clin EEG Neurosci.* 2006;37(2):81–98.

40. Loo SK, Teale PD, Reite ML. EEG correlates of methylphenidate response among children with ADHD: a preliminary report. *Biol Psychiatry.* 1999;45(12):1657–1660.

41. Ashare R, Hawk L, Shiels K, Rhodes J, Pelham W, Waxmonsky J. Methylphenidate enhances prepulse inhibition during processing of task-relevant stimuli in attention-deficit/hyperactivity disorder. *Psychophysiology.* 2010;47(5):838–845.

42. DeVito EE, Blackwell AD, Kent L, et al. The effects of methylphenidate on decision making in attention-deficit/hyperactivity disorder. *Biol Psychiatry.* 2008;64(7):636–639.

43. Mehta MA, Owen AM, Sahakian BJ, Mavaddat N, Pickard JD, Robbin TW. Methylphenidate enhances working memory by modulating discrete frontal and parietal lobe regions in the human brain. *J Neurosci.* 2000;20 RC65(1–6).

44. Mehta M, Calloway P, Sahakian B. Amelioration of specific working memory deficits by methylphenidate in a case of adult attention deficit/hyperacitivity disorder. *J Psychopharmacol.* 2000;14(3):299–302.

45. Berman T, Douglas V, Barr R. Effects of methylphenidate on complex cognitive processing in attention-deficit hyperactivity disorder. *J Abnorm Psychol*. 1999;108(1):90–105.

46. Nazari MA, Querne L, De Broca A, Berquin P. Effectiveness of EEG biofeedback as compared with methylphenidate in the treatment of attention-deficit/hyperactivity disorder: a clinical outcome study. *Neursci Med*. 2011;2:78–86.

47. Advokat C. What are the cognitive effects of stimulant medications? Emphasis on adults with attention-deficit/hyperactivity disorder (ADHD). *Neurosci Biobehav Rev*. 2010;34(8):1256–1266.

48. Smith M, Farah M. Are prescription stimulants "smart pills"? The epidemiology and cognitive neuroscience of prescription stimulant use by normal healthy individuals. *Psychol Bull*. 2011;137(5):717–741.

49. van der Meere J, Gunning B, Stemerdink N. The effect of methylphenidate and clonidine on response inhibition and state regulation in children with ADHD. *J Child Psychol Psychiatry*. 1999;40(2):291–298.

50. Coghill D, Rhodes S, Matthews K. The neuropsychological effects of chronic methylphenidate on drug-naive boys with attention-deficit/hyperactivity disorder. *Biol Psychiatry*. 2007;62(9):954–962.

51. Graham J, Coghill D. Adverse effects of pharmacotherapies for attention-deficit hyperactivity disorder: Epidemiology, prevention and management. *CNS Drugs*. 2008;22(3):213–237.

52. Clarke A, Barry R, Bond D, McCarthy R, Selikowitz M. Effects of stimulant medications on the EEG of children with attention-deficit/hyperactivity disorder. *Psychopharmacology (Berl)*. 2002;164(3):277–284.

53. Song DH, Shin DW, Jon DI, Ha EH. Effects of methylphenidate on quantitative EEG of boys with attention-deficit/hyperactivity disorder in continuous performance test. *Yonsei Med J*. 2005;46(1):34–41.

54. Goforth HW, Konopka LM, Primeau M, et al. Quantitative electroencephalography in frontotemporal dementia with methylphenidate response: a case study. *Clin EEG Neursci*. 2004;35(20):108–111.

55. Lubar JF, White JN, Swartwood MO, Swartwood JN. Methylphenidate effects on global and complex measures of EEG. *Paediat Neurol*. 1999;21(3):633–637.

56. Hermens D, Williams L, Clarke S, Kohn M, Cooper N, Gordon E. Responses to methylphenidate in adolescent AD/HD: evidence from concurrently recorded autonomic (EDA) and central (EEG and ERP) measures. *Int J Psychophysiol*. 2005;58(1):21–33.

57. Porter R, Gallagher P, Thompson J, Young A. Neurocognitive impairment in drug-free patients with major depressive disorder. *Br J Psychiatry*. 2003;182(3):214–220.

58. Lane R, O'Hanlon J. Cognitive and psychomotor effects of antidepressants with emphasis on selective serotonin reuptake inhibitors and the depressed elderly patient. *Ger J Psychiatry*. 1999;2(1):1–42.

59. Amado-Boccara I, Gougoulis N, Poirier Littré M, Galinowski A. Effects of antidepressants on cognitive functions: a review. *Neurosci Biobehav Rev*. 1995;19(3):479–493.

60. Hunter AM, Cook IA, Leuchter AF. Does prior antidepressant treatment of major depression impact brain function during current treatment. *Eur Neuropsychopharm*. 2012;22:711–720.

61. Saletu B, Anderer P, Saletu-Zyhlarz GM, Arnold O, Pascual-Marqui RD. Classification and evaluation of the pharmacodynamics of psychotropic drugs by single-lead pharmaco-EEG, EEG mapping and tomography (LORETA). *Methods Find Exp Clin Pharmacol*. 2002;24(suppl C):97–120.

62. Knott V, Mahoney C, Kennedy S, Evans K. EEG correlates of acute and chronic paroxetine treatment in depression. *J Affective Disord*. 2002;69(1–3):241–249.

63. Bruder G, Sedoruk J, Stewart J, McGrath P, Quitkin F, Tenke C. Electroencephalographic alpha measures predict therapeutic response to a selective

serotonin reuptake inhibitor antidepressant: Pre- and post-treatment findings. *Biol Psychiatry*. 2008;63(12):1171–1177.

64. Rush AJ, Kraemer HC, Sackeim HA, et al. Report by the ACNP task force on response and remission in major depressive disorder. *Neuropsychopharmacology*. 2006;31(9): 1841–1853.
65. Iosifescu D. Electroencephalography-derived biomarkers of antidepressant response. *Harv Rev Psychiatry*. 2011;19(3):144–154.
66. Knott V, Telner J, Lapierre Y, Browne M, Horn E. Quantitative EEG in the prediction of antidepressant response to imipramine. *J Affective Disord*. 1996;39(3):175–184.
67. Leuchter AF, Cook IA, Lufkin RB, et al. Cordance: a new method for assessment of cerebral perfusion and metabolism using quantitative electroencephalography. *Neuroimage*. 1994;1(3):208–219.
68. Cook I, Leuchter A, Morgan M, Stubbeman W, Siegman B, Abrams M. Changes in prefrontal activity characterize clinical response in SSRI nonresponders: A pilot study. *J Psychiatric Res*. 2005;39(5):461–466.
69. Cook IA, Leuchter AF, Witte E, et al. Neurophysiologic predictors of treatment response to fluoxetine in major depression. *Psychiatry Res*. 1999;85(3):263–273.
70. Tremeau F, Citrome L. Antipsychotics for patients without psychosis? What clinical trials support. *Curr Psychiatry*. 2006;5(12):33–44.
71. Allain H, Tessier C, Bentué-Ferrer D, et al. Effects of risperidone on psychometric and cognitive functions in healthy elderly volunteers. *Psychopharmacology (Berl)*. 2003;165(4):419–429.
72. González-Blanch C, Crespo-Facorro B, Vázquez-Barquero J, et al. Lack of association between clinical and cognitive change in first-episode psychosis: The first 6 weeks of treatment. *Can J Psychiatry*. 2008;53(12):839–847.
73. Wagner M, Quednow B, Westheide J, Schlaepfer T, Maier W, Kühn K. Cognitive improvement in schizophrenic patients does not require a serotonergic mechanism: randomized controlled trial of olanzapine vs amisulpride. *Neuropsychopharmacology*. 2005;30(2):381–390.
74. Davidson M, Galderisi S, Weiser M, et al. Cognitive effects of antipsychotic drugs in first-episode schizophrenia and schizophreniform disorder: a randomized, open-label clinical trial (EUFEST). *Am J Psychiatry*. 2009;166(6):675–682.
75. Harvey P, Green M, McGurk S, Meltzer H. Changes in cognitive functioning with risperidone and olanzapine treatment: a large-scale, double blind, randomized study. *Psychopharmacology (Berl)*. 2003;169(3–4):404–411.
76. Sharma T, Hughes C, Soni W, Kumari V. Cognitive effects of olanzapine and clozapine treatment in chronic schizophrenia. *Psychopharmacology (Berl)*. 2003;169(3–4):398–403.
77. MacQueen G, Young T. Cognitive effects of atypical antipsychotics: focus on bipolar spectrum disorders. *Bipolar Disord*. 2003;5(suppl 2):53–61.
78. Ehlis A, Herrmann M, Pauli P, Stoeber G, Pfuhlmann B, Fallgatter A. Improvement of prefrontal brain function in endogenous psychoses under atypical antipsychotic treatment. *Neuropsychopharmacology*. 2007;32(8):1669–1677.
79. Purdon SE, Jones BD, Stip E, et al. Neuropsychological change in early phase schizophrenia during 12 months of treatment with olanzapine, risperidone, or haloperidol. *Arch Gen Psychiatry*. 2000;57(3):249–258.
80. Keefe R, Silva S, Perkins D, Lieberman J. The effects of atypical antipsychotic drugs on neurocognitive impairment in schizophrenia: a review and meta-analysis. *Schizophr Bull*. 1999;25(2):201–222.
81. Saletu B. The use of pharmaco-EEG in drug profiling. In: Hindmarch I, Stonier PD, eds. *Human Psychopharmacology: Measures and Methods*. New York, NY: Wiley; 1987:173–200.
82. Moore N, Tucker K, Brin F, Merai P, Shillcutt S, Coburn K. Positive symptoms of schizophrenia: response to haloperidol and remoxipride is associated with increased alpha EEG activity. *Hum Psychopharmacol*. 1997;12(1):75–80.

83. Yoshimura M, Koenig T, Irisawa S, et al. A pharmaco-EEG study on antipsychotic drugs in healthy volunteers. *Psychopharmacology (Berl)*. 2007;191(4):995–1004.

84. Hubl D, Kleinlogel H, Frölich L, et al. Multilead quantitative electroencephalogram profile and cognitive evoked potentials (P300) in healthy subjects after a single dose of olanzapine. *Psychopharmacology (Berl)*. 2001;158(3):281–288.

85. Galderisi S. Clinical applications of pharmaco-EEG in psychiatry: the prediction of response to treatment with antipsychotics. *Methods Find Exp Clin Pharmacol*. 2002;24(suppl):85–89.

86. Begić D, Hotujac L, Jokić-Begić N. Quantitative EEG in schizophrenia patients before and during pharmacotherapy. *Neuropsychobiology*. 2000;41(3):166–170.

87. Kemali D, Galderisi S, Maj M, Mucci A, DiGregorio M, Bucci P. Computerized EEG topography findings in schizophrenic patients before and after haloperidol treatment. *Int J Psychophysiol*. 1992;13(3):283–290.

88. Ramos J, Cerdán L, Guevara M, Amezcua C, Sanz A. Abnormal EEG patterns in treatment-resistant schizophrenic patients. *Int J Neurosci*. 2001;109(1–2):47–59.

89. Nagase T, Okubo Y, Toru M. Electroencephalography in schizophrenic patients: comparison between neuroleptic-naive state and after treatment. *Biol Psychiatry*. 1996;40(6):452–456.

90. Knott V, Labelle A, Jones B, Mahoney C. Quantitative EEG in schizophrenia and in response to acute and chronic clozapine treatment. *Schizophr Res*. 2001;50(1–2):41–53.

91. Pascual-Marqui R, Michel C, Lehmann D. Low resolution electromagnetic tomography: a new method for localizing electrical activity in the brain. *Int J Psychophysiol*. 1994;18(1):49–65.

92. Pascual-Marqui RD, Lehmann D, Koenig T, et al. Low resolution brain electromagnetic tomography (LORETA) functional imaging in acute, neuroleptic-naive, first-episode, productive schizophrenia. *Psychiatry Res, Neuroimaging*. 1999;90:169–179.

93. Kuji I, Sumiya H, Tsuji S, Ichikawa A, Tonami N. Asymmetries of benzodiazepine receptor binding potential in the inferior medial temporal lobe and cerebellum detected with 123I-iomazenil SPECT in comparison with 99mTc-HMPAO SPECT in patients with partial epilepsy. *Ann Nucl Med*. 1998;12(4):185–190.

94. Fink M, Wadsak W, Savli M, et al. Lateralization of the serotonin-1A receptor distribution in language areas revealed by PET. *Neuroimage*. 2009;45(2):598–605.

95. Fitzgerald PJ. Whose side are you on: does serotonin preferentially activate the right hemisphere and norepinephrine on the left? *Med Hypotheses*. 2012;79(2):250–254.

96. Zimmerman EM, Golla MA, Paciora RA, Epstein PS, Konopka LM. Use of multimodality imaging and neuropsychological measures for the assessment and treatment of auditory verbal hallucinations: a brain to behavior approach. *Act Nerv Super (Praha)*. 2011;53(3–4):150–158.

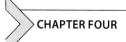

CHAPTER FOUR

Hidden Factors Thwarting Success

A Sociotechnical Field Theory Application for the Neurofeedback Therapist

Gerald Gluck

THINKING ABOUT THE FIELD OF TREATMENT

Despite the centrality of operant condition to biofeedback, biofeedback is not the mechanical application of conditioning. There is in fact no magic ghost in the box. Whereas the application of scientific principles to neurofeedback is a necessary condition for success, alone it may not be sufficient, not just in the treatment of clinical disorders, but even for simple temperature training. This chapter assumes that humans have a mind and a body and that they interact. Such an assumption is supported by the excellent literature review by Shellenberger and Green[1] and Elmer and Alyce Green's discussion of volition and mind–body interaction in *Beyond Biofeedback*.[2]

Mind and body interaction is key to understanding the success and failure of neurofeedback. To make sense of this we must understand the field of which neurofeedback is a part: the interaction between the person and the field. I do not mean the field – i.e., profession – within which it takes place, but rather the field in a Lewinian sense that makes it both an activity of the field and an active interactor in it. This is not because neurofeedback lacks specificity – just the opposite. It is true because it *is* specific.

For the purposes of this discussion, there are two types of specific effects, Newtonian (linear/individual) and systemic. Normally we think of specificity in the manner in which drug studies use that term, in a mechanistic one-to-one relationship between a chemical and a physiological effect. The concept of drug effects on a person assumes a lack of volition, e.g., given a properly sufficient amount and administration of lidocaine an

Clinical Neurotherapy.
Doi: http://dx.doi.org/10.1016/B978-0-12-396988-0.00004-0

anesthetic experience will result, irrespective of the will of most patients. However, neither is the patient likely to learn anything. The term placebo is used to demonstrate the opposite: causing the effect without the drug – and has led us astray to some extent. The use of the term placebo is unfortunate because it directs our attention to part of the field containing the inert substance (the dummy pill) rather than to an active ingredient that should perhaps be maximized in the interactional field,[3] which itself is healing even in allopathic medicine. Colloca and Miller[4] write:

> The effects following the administration of a placebo can be due to the general psychosocial context around the therapy. As a positive psychosocial context may induce a placebo effect, a negative context, including information about side effects, may lead to opposite expectations and outcomes, called the nocebo effect (p1922).

The field of interaction is an analogue of the psychosocial context. We know from the field of medicine that mere treatment stimulates the anterior cingulate, the dopaminergic system, the dorsal lateral prefrontal cortex and the basal ganglia.[5] It may be that, although we may be able to isolate *some* effects from the field, the placebo/nocebo effect may merely be an indication that the Newtonian mechanistic model of treating humans is incomplete, and the failure to consider systemic context limits successful treatment. It is a limitation because it likely leads to an incomplete definition of meaning, and meaning is defined by and encoded in the electro-encephalogram (EEG), the very parameter we seek to change.[6] Humans are meaning-creating organisms. Thus, to approach treatment with this misconception limits our success. Siegel points out that we create our meanings expressed as rates of neural firing. Changes are also expressed as a change in the rates of neural firing[7] and in phase changes across frequencies.[8,9] This leads to a greater need for anatomical and functional specificity (discussed below), but it also points the way to a redefinition and a correction in remodeling our field of treatment interaction. Remodeling occurs where social and technological variables meet to form a sociotechnical system, expanding where we should look for evidence of specificity.

Neurofeedback distinguishes itself from the current incomplete model of specificity because it is *volitional and involves learning*. It is more of a whole-brain systemic concept, because volition and learning involve many parts of the brain and are distributed across many networks. Thus to understand limitations on success in neurofeedback we must redefine specificity into a systemic specificity that would include the way in which we view drug effects. That is, one of the things that have limited our success is using the wrong definition for specificity. Shellenberger and Green, above, show in their discussion that biofeedback is not purely a matter of the specific effect of the machine, but of the information provided to the person who then processes it, which is exactly what Trist and Bamforth[10] showed, only in a work setting. We can measure the specificity of the effect of neurofeedback, challenging as it might be, even though it is embedded in the field and interacts with the field's components, as long as we use a definition of specificity that is isomorphic with the clinical reality of the construct we call neurofeedback. Once this methodological error is corrected, we will more clearly be able to see what is and what is not a limit on success, and more clearly define what standards of training and competency are necessary for practitioners. Thus to understand the successful or unsuccessful outcome of neurofeedback, the clinician must understand the components of the field, all of which are co-acting in the treatment process. In short, the unit of analysis is the sociotechnical field, of which neurofeedback and the manner in which it is conducted are the critical variables.

Neurofeedback training is a sociotechnical system. A sociotechnical system[10,11] is a set of organized behaviors and subsystems that integrate and manage social (cognitive and sentient) and technological boundaries, transactions and relationships for the purpose of producing an outcome. The term was first used to describe work environments in which social systems and technical or task requirements interacted. Lewin's work was combined with this to show how forces combined to manage social and task variables, and to explore methods of change of individual and systemic behaviors.

Lewin used field theory as a tool to conceptualize a sociotechnical system as a field, in order to understand and change forces that propel or restrain us from reaching a goal. Adapted to neurofeedback, the treatment field might look something like Figure 4.1.

Defining the Field

Driving or restraining forces are generally not categorical in nature, but are judged on whether or not they support treatment goals. Not all restraining forces should be avoided or attenuated. For example, forces that act to protect the patient may or should act as a restraining force in some situations. Treatment success is not treatment success at all risks or costs. In the same way, we must be anatomically and functionally correct in choosing the location or locations to train. When we are correct, this becomes a

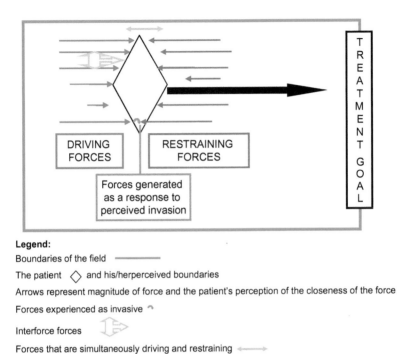

Legend:

Boundaries of the field ─────

The patient ◇ and his/herperceived boundaries

Arrows represent magnitude of force and the patient's perception of the closeness of the force

Forces experienced as invasive ⌐

Interforce forces

Forces that are simultaneously driving and restraining ←──→

Figure 4.1 Patient–therapist field of treatment.

driving force. If incorrect or partially correct, it becomes either a restraining force or an attenuated driving force, for example requiring a greater number of sessions for goal completion.

The thick black arrow in Figure 4.1 represents the resulting summed vectors of treatment. The Treatment Goal box lies inside and outside treatment boundaries to reflect that the effect of treatment is carried into the patient's life outside the treatment room, and because the treatment field is itself embedded in a larger macro social system. Each treatment goal would have its own field diagram. The lengths of the arrows represent the magnitude of the forces in the field. If the arrow crosses the patient's boundary and the patient perceives it as invasive, that invasion may itself produce other forces that affect the field. How many, their direction and magnitude will vary by individual differences and the nature of the systems of which the patient finds himself or herself a member.

A double-sided arrow reflects a force that is simultaneously both a driving and a restraining force. An example of this might be a therapist who anxiously wants to show results. New therapists are often anxious to show results and prove their competency, improve their confidence or gain the approval of a mentor. Clients are likely to see this as enthusiasm, and this likely would help treatment. On the other hand, it can also communicate the therapist's anxiety about gaining approval. This may create resistance to treatment. Or, a therapist who has more of a belief in the technique of treatment than in observing good scientific application and the clinical procedure of the treatment may provide extra motivation and empathy and commitment to the treatment relationship. However, at the same time such motives may impair the judgment and/or observational skills of the therapist and thus impair treatment. Thus, forces can act in both a restraining and/or a driving manner.

Some forces in the field do not directly act on the goal in the field but are interforce forces and are designated as ⬚. The vertical arrows represent the two forces that are interacting, and the thickness of the vertical arrows represents the magnitude or force involved in the interaction. The horizontal arrow represents its effect on the patient, i.e., whether in sum it is a driving or a restraining force. If it is a restraining force, the arrow would be pointed to the left. In the illustration it is a driving force, so it is pointed to the right. If the interaction of the two forces cancels the forces out, then the forces would essentially function neither as restraining nor as driving forces and would be represented by ⬚.

THE SOCIOTECHNICAL SOIREE: SENTIENT, PHYSICAL, TECHNICAL AND BOUNDARY FORCES WITHIN AND BETWEEN PATIENT AND THERAPIST

The Body as a Hidden Factor

Genes in the Field

Genetics is not destiny but does provide limits to our destiny. Genetics plays a role in neurodevelopmental disorders, neurodegenerative disorders and in learning, that is, changes in the brain as it adapts to its environment. With that in mind, our genetic codes may be expressed in perhaps an almost infinite variety of ways, such that destiny is a shared experience between biology, environment, intention and choice. Although identical twins may look and talk alike, they will marry different people, but their genetics seems only to influence occupational choices for males and not females.[12] In studies of monozygotic twins, although the impact of heritability on the incidence of schizophrenia is high, there still appears room for a healthy outcome.[13] Even stronger evidence of this combination position is detailed by Segalowitz and Schmidt,[14] in their discussion of Kagan's work, which reported that shy children, otherwise developing typically, exhibited "greater relative right frontal electroencephalographic (EEG) activity, high and stable heart rate at rest...and high morning basal cortisol levels" (p2). Yet despite this seemingly genetically connected EEG similarity, only the children whose mothers saw themselves as having low social support actually grew up to be shy. Mothers who saw themselves as having high social support had children who grew up without being shy. This demonstrates not only environmental effect on genetic expression, but also a degree of randomness. For who or what is to determine which child with this genetic predisposition is granted a mother with the perception of low or high social support?

There seems also to be a link between neurofeedback, circulating endorphins and alcohol abuse and posttraumatic stress disorder (PTSD). The cohort studied by Peniston and Kulkowsky[15] of nonrelapsing alcoholics who also suffered from PTSD did not experience an increase in circulating beta endorphins. The authors expressed interest in how that and other neuropeptides might influence or be influenced by neurofeedback, or a predisposition to disorders such as alcoholism or PTSD. Genetic factors may predispose to, as well as experience, PTSD. Individuals with PTSD appear to have reduce hippocampal volume,[16] not as a result of PTSD, but as a risk factor. Further, sufferers of PTSD have lower levels of cortisol than both normal controls and others exposed to trauma but not suffering PTSD.[17] Yet in their extensive examination of this area, although they conclude that genetics probably plays a role in the development of PTSD, and therefore would appear as an input into our field of training, they have difficulty declaring that it is the only effect and see other environmental variables as risk factors, as have previous authors.[16]

Genetics and randomness seem to determine how we are wired, but it is not yet determined how much contribution each makes and therefore how much of a limitation or force it is in our treatment field. But we are surely wired for pleasure,[18] and the results of exposure to pleasure-rewarding stimuli linked to neural events shapes the EEG[19] and in neurofeedback.[20]

"Genes determine the shape of a neuron, the region over which it extends branches...whether they actually connect is not determined by genes"[21] (p107). Seung goes on to argue that experience both destroys and creates synapses. The essence of Seung's argument is that change involves both creation and destruction in the connectome. He refers to change in the connectome as the four Rs: "reweighting, reconnection, rewiring and regeneration"[21] (p131). He points out that these processes and their limitations are not set in stone, but rather can be altered by manipulating molecules through the use of drugs, because it is changing certain molecules that changes the connectome. But he does not abandon the field entirely to pharmacology, because he concludes, "the four Rs are also guided by experience, so finer control will be achieved by supplementing molecular manipulations with training regimens"[21] (p132). This seems close to a suggestion that neurons and neuronal systems change and are limited by an interaction between genes and experience, which seems to this author quite close to the stage and field in which we enact neurofeedback training. It suggests that neurofeedback may not be an alternative field, but rather complementary to and an extension of the hard clinical sciences studying, changing and supporting the development of the genetic connectome. Speculatively, then, the genetically determined shape of neurons and basic wiring provides some boundary to neurofeedback. But neurofeedback interacts with genes as part of the experiential domain of a person. Neurofeedback therefore participates in both the creation and the pruning of synapses.

Our experiences and genes may leave us underaroused in response to appropriate stimuli, and this seemingly inborn limitation in the anterior cingulate can be altered by neurofeedback.[22] Further, it seems to correct what appears to be a dopamine deficiency in response to a task, because the posttraining functional magnetic resonance imaging (fMRI) showed increased arousal in the left caudate and the left substantia nigra, which is consistent with prior evidence that there is a relationship between "ADHD and polymorphism of the dopamine transporter gene, as well as the dopamine D4 and D5 receptor genes"[22] (p220).

Genetics appears to play a role of determining EEG characteristics associated with temperament in children as young as 9 months of age. Researchers were able to associate response to maternal separation, asymmetry and behavioral inhibition from EEGs taken during infancy and followed in children until 12 years of age.[23] Whether or not this plays a limiting role later in childhood or adulthood of our ability to change the EEG through neurofeedback is unknown, but it is useful for the practitioner to keep in mind that genetic heritage may indeed have a powerful role in shaping the temperament and personality associated with EEG asymmetric patterns of arousal.

In a study by Tye and colleagues[24] using very low frequency (VLF) (0.02–0.2 Hz), genetics was measured as a strong influence on VLF power, but "unique environmental influences contribute substantially to VLF power"[24] (p6). Nonetheless, genetics did not account for a significant difference between attention deficit hyperactivity disorder (ADHD) and control twins on measures of cognitive performance.

Peterson and Posner[25] said: "Genetic modulation by environmental factors is perhaps clearest for the dopamine 4 receptor gene (DRD4) which has been associated with the executive network…" (p84) Specifically, they reviewed evidence that, as children, individuals with the repeat 7 allele DRD4 gene were most responsive to changes in parenting and to the intervention of parenting courses. The interventions appeared to modify impulsivity, thrill seeking and "high-intensity pleasure"[25] (p85), but this sensitivity to environmental influence was *not* found in children without this allele. This is particularly of interest to neurofeedback professionals when we look at Monastra et al.'s study of attention deficit disorder (ADD)/ADHD children.[26] We do not know the allele distribution of children in this study, the design of which included parenting skill courses for *all* the parents of children included. Monastra wrote that parents reported that the children's behaviors improved at home, i.e., were responsive to the parent skills course intervention, which included behavioral interventions, skills in problem solving with preteens and teens, nutrition, and most importantly "the role of positive parental attention and systematic use of reinforcement strategies in reducing the functional impairments associated with ADHD"[26](p237). This occurred irrespective of whether the child was treated with neurofeedback or not. Only the children receiving neurofeedback also improved at school and maintained their improvement when withdrawn from Ritalin. Essentially the parents were educated to better understand their children and trained in how to use behavior modification and contingent reward to alter the behavior of their children. Interestingly, this replicates some of the conditions necessary in the treatment field of neurofeedback for these children, i.e., the use of positive attention and reinforcement for appropriate behavior. This is a demonstration of the need for the presence of this kind of specificity in the field of interaction, but to achieve permanent generalized results there must be EEG-specific treatment in the treatment field as well that has the same characteristics as Monastra's home training. The children responded at home to the same model of training that they were exposed to during neurofeedback treatment, except that no precise and repetitive EEG conditioning was taking place at home. The treatment at home produced field-specific effects (changes in behavior at home); however, without EEG modification in the field, treatment-specific effects did not persist or transfer outside the treatment field.

Neurofeedback encourages neuroplasticity and the growth of new connectivities, and thus it might be worthwhile to at least mention the role of genes in the growth of neurons and neuroplasticity.

Typically, any genetic inheritance that would affect the brain's ability to learn from operant conditioning may make neurofeedback more challenging, or even possibly thwart success. Probably the most succinct summary of the impact of genetics was given by Pinker,[27] when he wrote: "How the genes control brain development is still unknown, but a reasonable summary of what we know so far is that brain modules assume their identity by a combination of what kind of tissue they start out as, where they are in the brain, and what patterns of triggering input they get during critical periods in development" (p36). To the extent that neurofeedback requires the experience of pleasure, specifically in receiving the reward, one might consider a different view by Nelson, de Haan and Thomas,[28] who argue that the ability to experience pleasure is probably inborn and directed by genes, because this ability is necessary to bond to a caretaker, which is essential for survival. Indeed, we have found that humans can even bond to a band of wolves that nurture the child in the case of feral children, and that abused children will bond to their abusers for the sake of survival. Nelson et al. are reluctant to stake a total claim to this belief, because they assert that proof would require unethical research designs. But their view is not absolutist, as they point out, correctly, that failure to nurture and stimulate the brain and help it both develop and prune neural assemblies early in life can result in permanent deficits.

But does this affect the effectiveness of neurofeedback? The answer is that there is no solid peer-reviewed evidence to conclude one way or another, but we do know that children with reactive attachment disorder, despite Sebern Fisher's contribution, are difficult to treat and generally require treatment modalities in addition to neurofeedback. Consequently, it seems that early genetic development does influence our ability to treat but may not be a disqualifier for treatment, although it may be a limiting factor in the efficacy of neurofeedback treatment. People with these kinds of genetic predispositions will therefore probably require a multimodal approach for success.

Why a multimodal approach? Neurofeedback is a learning model for changing brain function based on operant conditioning.[29] One of the requirements of operant conditioning is that the reward is pleasurable. Pleasure is experienced through the release of dopamine, and that which amplifies or delivers high levels of dopamine will result in repeated acts.

Conditions associated with the repetition, before and after the act, will be bonded to the pleasure and result in increased incidence.[18,30] The anatomical areas involved in this circuit are the ventral tegmentum, "nucleus accumbens, prefrontal cortex, the dorsal striatum and the amygdala."[18] (p18). Any genetic condition that interferes with dopamine release or reception will thus likely impair one of the requirements of the operant conditioning model, and thereby reduce the effectiveness and success of neurofeedback.

One might expect that a disorder such as autism, which affects the development of the dopamine system,[31] would affect the outcome of neurofeedback. And, perhaps it is a limiting factor. This may be one reason that although neurofeedback can be effective with individuals on the autistic spectrum, its success rate is not as high as seen in the Peniston–Kulkowsky Protocol for addictions, or in neurofeedback treatment for ADDs. The genetic roots of autism are yet to be settled by science, but such a disorder does influence the duration of treatment and accessibility. Clinically, these children – and sometimes adults – require the application of good behavior management techniques from the therapist to make them able to access neurofeedback. This may be related in some cases to their ability to interpret facial expressions, tolerate sensory input, control impulsivity, and understand social context and emotional cues, as well as the impact the disorder has on the regulation of the amygdala.[28]

A genetic disorder determined by the FOXP2 gene that results in verbal dyspraxia has been documented in the KE family.[32] The authors' description of this disorder is devastating. "The core deficit…seriously interferes with the rapid selection, sequencing and execution of sounds that culminates in the production of articulate and intelligible speech [and] a plethora of expressive and receptive language problems and …difficulties with aspects of reading, writing, and nonverbal intellectual abilities as well as with perception and execution of rhythms"[32] (p169). There is no known neurofeedback treatment for the variant of this disorder known as chronic developmental verbal and orofacial dyspraxia, and thus the severity of this disorder stands at least as evidence that there is an outside genetic limit to neurofeedback treatment.

Chronic degenerative diseases such as Parkinson's and the various dementias, including early-onset and typical-onset Alzheimer's disease, have failed to show reversal of the disease process. There have been some case reports of slowing of the manifest symptoms of the disease, but no objective radiological or laboratory evidence of the slowing of the disease with the use of neurofeedback. The author has treated one person with Parkinson's in whom the progression of the tremor appears to have attenuated and even stopped, but the follow-up time is limited to several months and is confounded by the patient taking dopamine-promoting supplements after the several-month follow-up. Then, 9 months after nutriceutical dopamine was ceased, the tremor had worsened in intensity. After approximately 10 low-resolution electromagnetic tomography (LORETA) neurofeedback sessions, the tremor began to attenuate in intensity and amplitude, but the patient had to discontinue treatment, at least for the present.

With the increase in specificity in the use of LORETA neurofeedback, we may be able to push the boundaries of some of these disorders. It is a future worth contemplating and worth being curious and proactive about – dimensions that will be discussed below.

Drugs, Toxins, Hormones

The concealed use of illicit drugs is not news to most clinicians, but the ability to screen for such an event may not be as ubiquitous. Careful history-taking and, if necessary, psychometric testing may be necessary to reveal such use. Determine whether your scope of licensure permits urine testing for drugs. If not, arrange to have it done randomly by a physician. Even expensive sophisticated screens such as are used in pain management practices have rates of false positives and false negatives. Therefore it is important to have the urine properly cared for and sent out to a licensed clinical laboratory for confirmation, which is usually done by gas or liquid chromatography. Heavy metal screening can be done by most clinical laboratories, but a complete screening usually requires a specialty laboratory. The existence of heavy metals such as (but not limited to) lead and mercury impairs synaptic communication and will affect the timing, frequencies, amplitudes and incidence of focal events and seizures observed in the EEG. In acute situations metabolic signs of their existence can be detected by eyeball inspection on the EEG.[33] Likewise, exposure to solvent-based toxins can also influence the EEG.[34]

The presence of heavy metals or illicit drugs, undetected and untreated, may impair clinical effectiveness because they affect neuronal interactions. Neurofeedback treatment of crack cocaine users showed better abstinence rates than without neurofeedback, but not as high as with alcoholics and opiate addicts using the Peniston–Kulkowsky protocol.[35] Crack cocaine seems to have persistent deleterious effects on the EEG.[36,37] Alper's observation on the affect of cocaine on global measures of the EEG raises the question of whether or not training crack cocaine users with phase-reset neurofeedback, either as a lone neurofeedback protocol (coordinated with other treatment) or prior to or after the use of the Peniston–Kulkowsky protocol, might improve this limitation on success.

Pharmaceuticals may also be a hidden factor. The use of benzodiaz-epines may make the change in beta or high beta amplitudes difficult to alter. One little known hidden factor is Buspar or buspirone. In a study replicating the protocol of Peniston and Kulkowsky using polysubstance abusers,[38] an examination of two patients who should have improved with the protocol and did not revealed that they both were taking bus-pirone. Buspirone reduces the power of 7–9 Hz activity and thus was a limiting factor in the success of the protocol.[39] In a more recent study using LORETA, decreased alpha and theta were seen in the prefrontal and anterior limbic areas in the 8th hour of administration.[40] Clinicians using neurofeedback with patients on this substance might be well advised to discuss a medication change or discontinuation with the prescribing healthcare provider and the patient.

Hormones are neuronal messengers and regulators. This is mentioned in the case of an autistic spectrum adolescent (above) who was treated for a seizure disorder. Premenstrual factors have also been reported.[41]

Case of "Small but Wanna Be Good"

This is a case of a latency age male child who was diagnosed with oppo-sitional defiant disorder. He was experiencing difficulty at home and at school. He was taking growth hormone and Zoloft. He was undersized for his age. Major complaints were inattention, aggression, oppositionality, periods of rage, argumentative, distractible, compulsive and intense dislike of change. His parents were informed, and they agreed that neurofeedback with a child on growth hormone was experimental and that there was no way to predict the outcome, or whether there would be an interac-tion between the two – or if there was, what the extent of that interaction would be.

There was normal EC (eyes closed) posterior alpha dominance, but EO (eyes open) and listening showed dominance in theta, respectively along the midline, centrally and frontally. His summary qualitative EEG (qEEG) maps looked like this baseline compared to 50 sessions of training (Figures 4.2, 4.3, 4.4 and 4.5a,b):

Although we can see that substantial progress was made, the maps did not normalize and improvement was not sufficient. After careful tracking we

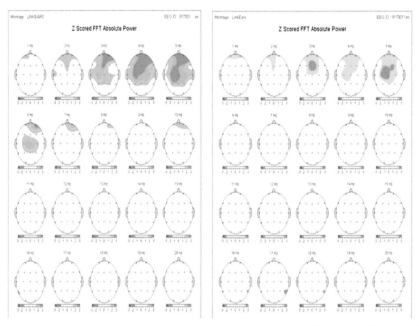

Figure 4.2 Pre-/post absolute power linked ears Z-score maps of the Case of Small But Wanna Be Good.

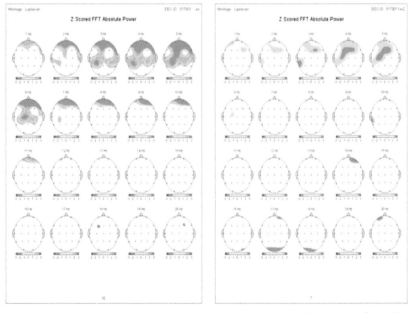

Figure 4.3 Laplacian Pre-/post absolute power Z-score maps of the Case of Small But Wanna Be Good.

Z-Scored FFT Absolute Power	EO1					Z-scored FFT Absolute Power	EO2					
	1 Hz	2 Hz	3 Hz	4 Hz	5 Hz		1 Hz	2 Hz	3 Hz	4 Hz	5 Hz	6 Hz
FP1	1.70	1.92	2.15	2.46	2.46	FP1	2.41	2.10	2.26	2.24	2.10	1.18
FP2	1.08	1.83	3.14	4.37	3.78	FP2	2.32	1.97	2.07	2.22	2.18	1.21
F3	-0.03	1.01	1.86	2.84	2.30	F3	-0.52	1.36	1.97	1.95	2.37	1.07
F4	0.25	0.60	1.26	2.56	2.20	F4	-0.91	0.97	2.12	2.07	2.34	0.97
C3	0.04	1.17	2.23	2.69	2.86	C3	-0.45	1.31	1.92	2.41	2.76	1.49
C4	0.04	0.74	1.56	2.42	2.36	C4	-0.89	0.86	1.85	1.66	2.13	1.05
P3	-0.28	1.10	1.65	1.90	2.16	P3	-0.57	-0.02	1.21	1.44	1.34	0.73
P4	0.23	1.08	1.52	1.62	1.85	P4	-1.36	0.40	1.31	0.86	1.36	0.46
O1	-0.78	-0.26	0.41	0.16	0.34	O1	0.01	0.69	0.77	0.36	0.45	0.28
O2	0.16	0.42	0.79	0.43	0.63	O2	-0.28	0.50	0.67	0.09	0.28	0.11
F7	0.15	1.06	1.31	1.48	1.40	F7	-0.65	0.53	0.86	1.25	1.17	0.52
F8	0.16	1.11	1.08	1.80	1.42	F8	1.08	0.93	0.96	0.92	0.76	0.54
T3	-0.48	1.69	1.77	1.77	1.46	T3	-0.05	0.98	1.47	1.51	1.40	0.84
T4	0.04	0.55	1.49	1.83	2.00	T4	-0.19	0.45	1.43	1.31	1.54	0.72
T5	-0.84	0.06	0.60	0.84	0.69	T5	-0.62	0.49	1.17	0.72	0.84	0.62
T6	-1.10	0.41	0.64	0.45	0.70	T6	-1.74	-0.34	0.30	-0.28	0.06	-0.33
Fz	1.05	1.79	2.62	3.30	2.53	Fz	0.01	2.09	2.90	2.41	2.45	0.96
Cz	0.61	1.39	1.89	2.42	2.58	Cz	-0.35	1.75	1.93	2.00	2.55	1.43
Pz	0.24	1.18	1.58	1.73	2.09	Pz	-0.43	1.04	1.48	1.65	2.02	1.10

Figure 4.4 Table of before and after actual Z-scores absolute power in the Case of Small But Wanna Be Good.

observed that although his attention improved, the aggressive episodes went in cycles. These cycles were accompanied by growth spurts or a change in the amount of growth hormone. A call was placed to the pharmaceutical company and the author spoke with a person identified as a nurse clinician familiar with this drug. She said that the company had received reports of explosiveness and irritability in a few cases.

Coherence appears to have improved in high beta, but the abnormal Z-scores shown in the post treatment coherence maps were still 6, 7 and 8 standard deviations from normal. Alpha coherence did not appear to improve at all. Other coherence improved (Figure 4.6).

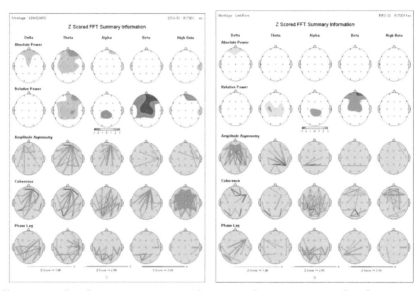

Figure 4.5a Baseline summary maps EO compared to 50 sessions of surface neuro-feedback training.

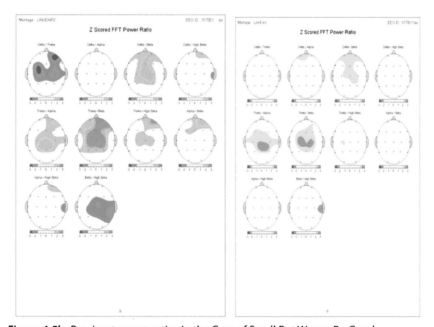

Figure 4.5b Pre-/post power ratios in the Case of Small But Wanna Be Good.

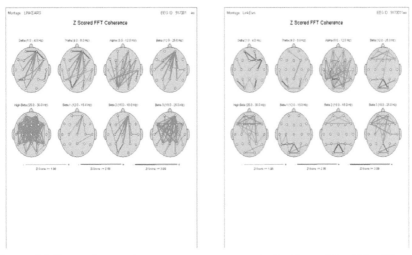

Figure 4.6 Pre- and postcoherence summary maps in the Case of Small But Wanna Be Good.

The patient made good progress and improved functionally in some ways. He had longer stretches of good behavior, and "green cards" – or at least no "red cards" – at school. Outbursts were shorter in duration. However, after each improvement the growth spurts and the growth hormone seemed to set him back. It appears that the growth hormone interacted with neurofeedback in a way that set a limit on success. It is unknown from this case whether this would be true in a child that did not already have signs of an irritable cortex or an Axis I diagnosis. However, because hormones are neuronal regulators and neurofeedback is a form of neuronal regulation, it is reasonable to conclude that there is some interaction. Unfortunately, in this case it was not beneficial for the patient. Phase-reset statistics were abnormal for this child, both before and after. Had we had the ability to train phase reset and use LORETA neurofeedback at that time, it is interesting to speculate whether the outcome would have been different.

Neurofeedback therapists are not equipped to diagnose endocrine disorders, but they need to be equipped to ask the right questions in the history, be open-minded, and consider this as a possibility based on a reasonable knowledge of human physiology and what is an appropriate developmental stage behavior in order to make a good referral to a collaborating medical professional. Although we cannot be experts in all of the forces in the field, we can be experts in identifying reasonable hypotheses based on scientific thinking, and proactive in bringing together a treatment team to help the patient.

Organic Causes Masked as Psychological

What, not just who, is sitting in your treatment chair? Are they in mask or costume?

Examples are the child who cannot sit still and squirms and scratches his buttocks: would you consider pin worms? The patient who is constantly tired, wakes up sluggish, gained weight and is feeling depressed, and complains of lack of motivation and failure to initiate actions he or she knows need to be taken: would you consider hypothyroidism? Or in the patient who is 45, male, and reports these symptoms, would you consider low testosterone?

How about an autistic spectrum patient diagnosed with a seizure disorder completing a successful year of neurofeedback without one incident of seizure suddenly becoming aggressive and unreasonable? Mother blames the neurofeedback therapist, because he was not like this before. Would you consider high testosterone?

Although we are not physicians, we need to be detectives to discern hidden factors that challenge the success of treatment. We should at least be sufficiently skilled to know when to make a referral for suspected organic illness.[42] There are clues to look for that should trigger our suspicion of a psychological masquerade. Taylor[43] provides some guidance in this area. Here are some clues he provides:

1. Is there a history of similar symptoms?
2. Is there a readily identifiable cause?
3. Is the patient over 55?
4. Does the patient have any chronic disease(s) or are there any in blood relatives, e.g., mother, father, grandparents, siblings?
5. Is there use of drugs or alcohol?
6. Does the person seem oriented?
7. Is recent or short-term memory impaired?
8. In conversation, does the person appear able to reason?
9. Is there a history of hitting of the head, head injury, "bell ringing", contact sports or motor vehicle accidents?
10. Does the person seem to be able to handle normal light, temperature, sound?
11. Is headache present? If so is this different, or the same as in the past?
12. Is the complaint involving vision or hearing?
13. Can the person find words, construct sentences and assemble ideas coherently to express himself or herself, or is there difficulty doing this? Does the person have difficulty naming common objects in your office?

14. When the patient walks, or during the interview, are there any abnormal body movements?

15. Is there a history of breathing or heart problems or hypertension?

16. Is speech normal in speed, sound, variation and intonation?

17. Is there a consistent or logical occupational and educational history? Is the educational history consistent with siblings, and the patient's occupational history?

18. Has there been one or more hospitalizations or visits to the emergency department? If so, why?

19. How is the patient dressed? Is there anything unusual about the way he or she is dressed, e.g., long sleeves, warm clothing worn on a hot day? or conversely shorts or a bathing suit in 30° weather?

20. What is the patient's sleeping pattern? Is the pattern a problem for the patient or anyone else?

21. Has the patient ever had the sense of losing time, or blanking out? Do others call his or her name and complain the patient is unresponsive?

22. Has the patient ever had moments or episodes where he or she had difficulty speaking or moving a limb? (Adapted from Taylor[43] p94).

Most of this information can be obtained using a good intake questionnaire, and observational data can be elicited by simple observation and normal conversation. If you are in doubt, Taylor[43] recommends asking the patient to draw a clock, draw a three-dimensional figure and write a sentence. You may also test the patient's short-term memory by asking him or her to recall three objects, at 5 or 10 minutes, that are common but unrelated (in different categories).

ADD/ADHD AS THE GREAT CONCEALER

Attention deficits may present as hidden disorders of other kinds that make persons appear as though they have ADD or ADHD – that is, people who are inattentive may be inattentive for a number of reasons. Or, they may present with comorbid disorders such as mood and/or learning disorders.

Case of X

This is a case of a 24-year-old Caucasian man who flew to Florida with his spouse for a consultation. He had had 20 sessions of infra-low frequency (ILF) on a Cygnet, and before and after Tests of Variables of Attention (TOVA) showed improvements in response time and response variability.

(ILF, also known as infra-slow oscillations [ISO], are oscillations <0.01 and usually 0.001 to 0.0001 or even lower, and are considered nonneuronal in origin,[44] perhaps as a result of a shortage of adenosine from adenosine triphosphate (ATP) of astrocytes. ISO are associated with different types of epileptic events.[45] ILF is usually done in sequential (bipolar) montages between T3 and T4 and other sites. TOVA is a neuropsychological continuous performance test of attention. See www.tovatest.com/about-the-t-o-v-a.)

The patient stated that he liked his provider. There was a previous psychological evaluation that indicated ADD, executive functioning difficulties, handwriting difficulties and auditory processing difficulties. Daily ILF sessions marked the most improvement, but improvement ceased when the sessions stopped. On the initial interview both the patient and his wife reported that he had moments of blanking out or being unresponsive to his name.

No qEEG was done prior to treatment and no baseline EEG assessment was done. Treatment was reported by the provider as a bipolar montage at T3–T4, with reinforcement at 0.0001 with a "dynamic threshold" set at 85%, which meant that the threshold was automatically adjusting so the patient received consistent 85% reinforcement. In the past 6 months the patient has appeared distractible, answers before hearing the whole question, has a hard time concentrating for long periods, seems as if he is always talking and interrupts others; he frequently loses things that are needed for work. He sustained two remote hits to the head without loss of consciousness. There is no medication at present.

The patient lists the following problems as severe or very severe:
- Attention deficits, distractible
- Auditory sequencing – being able to listen and put things in the correct order
- Organizing himself and planning for multistep projects
- Low motivation
  - Multitasking
  - Sequential planning
  And as moderate:
- Concentration
- Short-term memory

The findings on the qEEG, done as part of the consult, were a loss of delta more right than left, but mostly right central (C4) and diffuse loss of alpha, mostly alpha 1 (Figure 4.7). The second finding was pronounced hypocoherence in the frontal lobes (Figure 4.8).

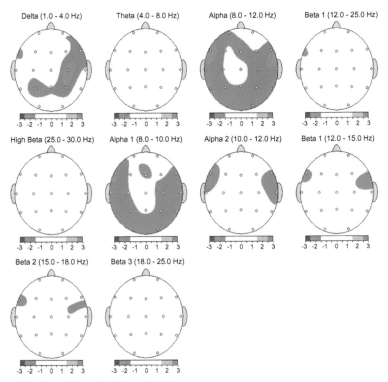

Figure 4.7 Case X loss of delta and alpha.

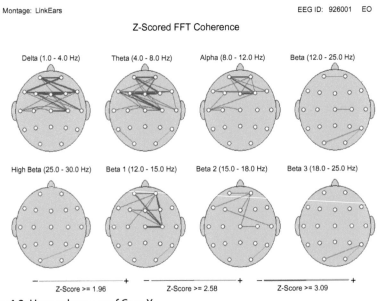

Figure 4.8 Hypocoherence of Case X.

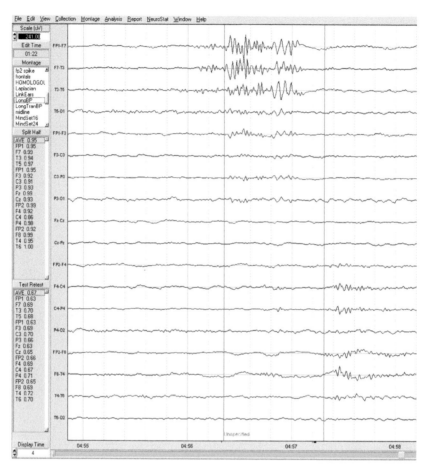

Figure 4.9 Case X post hyperventilation paroxysmal event in long bipolar montage.

The raw EEG showed phase reversals, sharp waves and paroxysmal activity. LORETA analysis of these focal events demonstrated source localization in the temporal lobes. Above and below there is an example of a paroxysmal event at about 4:56 post hyperventilation showing frontal temporal lead involvement. Note the gain is over 240 in Figure 4.9. Figure 4.10 shows the actual contrast of the event with the background.

Using LORETA time series analysis[46] in delta, source localization was in the middle temporal gyrus, BA 21 right (Figure 4.11).

Using LORETA time series in high beta, the results in Z-scores were even more pronounced. The areas involved in high beta were the left amygdala, left parahippocampal gyrus, right and left temporal lobes and

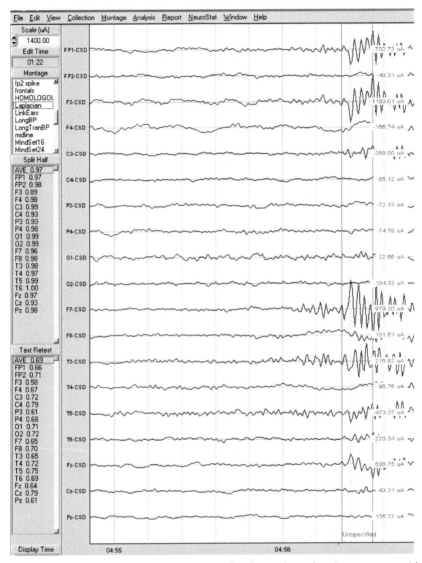

Figure 4.10 Post-hyperventilation event amplitude markers showing contrast with background in laplacian montage.

Brodman areas 20 and 22 on the left, the uncus and the left inferior frontal gyrus (Figures 4.12 and 4.13).

Finally, we see a sharp wave in the left front followed by a slow wave component (Figure 4.14).

The entire record was referred for review to a neurologist, who also examined X and determined that he should be treated with neurofeedback

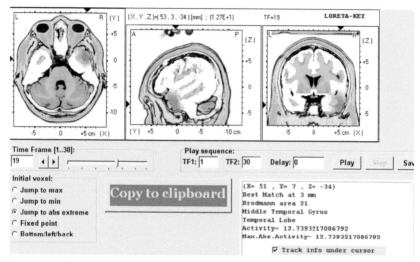

Figure 4.11 Case X delta source localization BA 21 middle temporal gyrus.

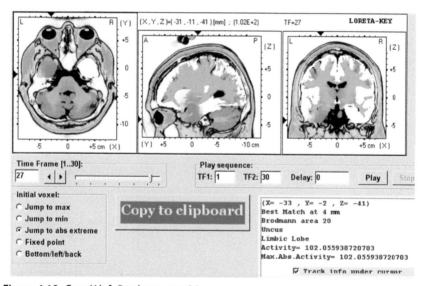

Figure 4.12 Case X left Brodman area 20.

and an anticonvulsant. The patient agreed to the medication but declined neurofeedback treatment, saying that the funds for neurofeedback treatment were now depleted after the 20 sessions of ILF training.

The hidden factors that thwarted success were therapist-controlled variables. The fact that changes were seen immediately following treatment but then faded is likely indicative of some placebo effect,

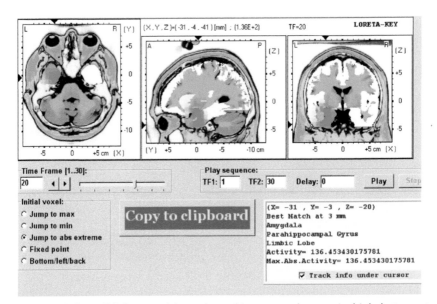

Figure 4.13 Case X left amygdala and parahippocampal gyrus in high beta post hyperventilation.

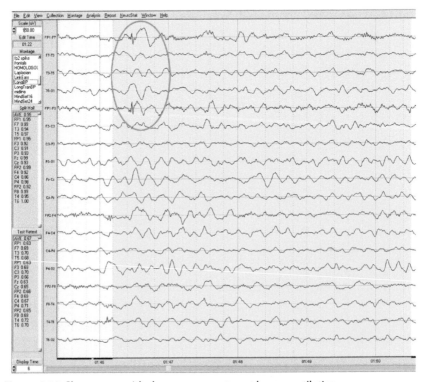

Figure 4.14 Sharp wave with slow component post hyperventilation.

and the fact that whatever was in fact changed or affected was not actually learned. The treatment was also inappropriate to the patient's difficulties, which were hidden from view because the provider did assess the EEG adequately – in fact they did no EEG assessment at all, believing that this was unnecessary. There were social driving forces favoring treatment, but technical factors that acted as restraining forces.

Factors that thwart success can remain hidden if we do not use the tools available to us to find them. Under such conditions, factors that can be driving forces, and help us to successfully complete treatment through proper assessment matched to a treatment plan, become restraining forces. Here the patient was unsuccessful in neurofeedback and was unable to take advantage of further neurofeedback treatment because the provider's belief system and training caused a depletion of funds. Thus the patient was treated pharmacologically. Further related material is covered below in the section Methodology as a Hidden Factor: Good Clinical Hygiene, which summarizes the therapist's contribution to the treatment field.

Nutrition

For our purposes nutrition means ensuring that adequate raw materials are delivered to the brain to permit proper functioning of the neurons (see Chapter 14 for a full discussion of this subject). This means that nutrients necessary for the ATP cycle, critical to the movement of ions in and out of neurons,[47] must be present.

Fatty acids play a crucial role in brain functioning, and their levels are not detectable by interview. We need to manufacture some of these acids, and therefore we must ingest sufficient amounts of the precursors and some other fats to ensure neuronal communication and change. The fatty acids most concerned with brain health are: arachidonic acid, alpha-linolenic acid, docosahexaenoic acid (DHA), gamma-linolenic acid, phosphatidylcholine and phosphatidylserine.[48] Some of the symptoms that we might treat with neurofeedback but which may be wholly or partly caused by fatty acid deficits or metabolism are aggression, memory difficulties, anorexia, anxiety, attention deficit, autistic-like symptoms, bipolar mood, chronic fatigue, migraine, parkinsonism, phobias, rage, reading disorders, schizophrenia, developmental delay, hyperactivity, brain injury, learning disability, depression, slow processing or reaction time.[48] Synapses are rich in DHA. Fatty acids are the main element in the construction of neuronal membranes and the myelin sheath that surrounds most neurons. The myelin, and hence the fats that help build it, is essential because the presence of myelin vastly speeds up the transmission of neuronal signals, permitting them to jump from node to node, rather like an express overpass on a superhighway.

The role of dietary consumption just prior to EEG acquisition and neurofeedback sessions should not be underestimated. Dietary consumption of products laden with caffeine can influence EEG and cognitive functioning.[49] Carbohydrate consumption has been noted to influence glucose curves, with the primary effect of an increased load in glucose leading to a subsequent decline in blood glucose and increase in delta and theta relative power in the temporal and parieto-occipital regions.[50]

THE FAMILY AS A HIDDEN FACTOR

Remember the child's game where a structure is built and everyone goes around the circle removing one piece at a time in the hope that the structure will still stand? The one who removes the strategic piece loses the game as the structure clatters to the floor.

No one is going to bring in little Johnny or Sally to "fix" him or her and then proceed to tell how and when they are going to sabotage what you are doing. No, it is hidden, and how the child holds the family (or the marriage) together is a secret. In situations like this the covert assignment is to relieve everyone's guilt by removing the crucial symptom of the child's brain, which may "conveniently" show up as an abnormality on qEEG. Often the child does have a real brain deregulation that fits happily into the secretly dysfunctional family, which appears quite normal thanks to this child. Or perhaps you wonder about the 20-something-year-old who cannot get launched: the parents have tried everything and he presents with depression and daytime sleeping. He presents wanting help to regulate his mood and sleep.

As neurofeedback therapists, we understand that there is a strong relationship between brain regulation and behavior. What is sometimes hidden from us is that the brain is also regulated by reality because it is constructed between the patient and those significant in his or her life. Families want strong input into treatment choices in the treatment of ADD and ADHD in their children, and according to parents the disorder has a strong impact not only on the child but on the family as well.[51] It might be useful to pause and note the images that the family brings into our treatment field of the child and the disorder: in their own words: "Boys are like that...He'll grow out of it...lot of energy...playful...inherited...

chemical imbalance…a disability…a little retarded…traumatized by the whole thing [marital separation]…physical abuse…crack cocaine…sexually molested"[51] (p4).

It is important to understand that the patient is more often than not the ambassador for the family. The family may be visible and present as part of the presenting system to be treated, or may simply be invisible, their safety and protection from change and disequilibrium held responsibly in the patient's psyche. The family is in fact mapped in the mind of the patient.[52]

The brain is an equal opportunity responder. It responds to psychotherapy,[53,54] because it learns from and responds to its repetitive environment. It will respond to the ministrations of operant conditioning,[55] whether they are in the therapy room or its own environment. In psychotherapy the brain responds to the change in symbols and dangers to affective ties, and the patient's position in the family and family relationships. The brain bridges what is learned in therapy back to the family and what is learned in the family back into psychotherapy.

In the same way that neurofeedback alters brain regulation, the brain is a bridge back into the family system. As often happens in psychotherapy, the family mounts a response to this new information, which may be perceived as a change, a threat, an accomplishment or a combination of any of these. Thus the patient rightly wonders, consciously or unconsciously, whether this will change his or her family. Families are systems and systems abhor disequilibrium, just as the brain does. So as the brain pushes back as we train it, so do family systems push back. There are restraining forces in all fields, but there are many variations on the patterns of those forces that make the job of the therapist a creative and challenging one requiring great range as well as technical skill. Although all patients are subject to these forces, those with the greatest vulnerability are those living in a defensive, chaotic or rigid system, or trying to negotiate the boundary from one developmental stage to another. So if neurofeedback is an agent of change in a family with a dysfunctional marriage, it is likely to involve arousal of the autonomic and central nervous system, which interact with other forces in the field (an interforce) to undermine success.[56,57]

A hidden factor in sabotaging success when treating children and adolescents (and unseparated or unindividuated young adults) is high expression of parental emotional expression. In a young man who presents with stuttering, Chapman gives good examples of high and low emotional expression by parents in coping with a child who stutters.[58] Many children will be accustomed to being yelled at, feel they are responsible, feel protective of their parents, be fearful of complaining about the parent, or feel hopeless about complaining about it and thus not present it as a problem. Yelling and being attacked may be their normal. Some children or adolescents will complain or report, so even the slightest hint of this would justify a curious inquiry into how the parent handles misbehavior, or obtaining a natural history of one or two incidents of conflict or discipline in the home. Usually parents are more comfortable (and the child more protected) when they discuss this with the therapist without the child present. High emotional arousal undermines therapy because the patient may not be able to put aside the arousal and his or her reaction to it, and be able to train. It is hard to focus on training, or believe in the magnitude of the reward of getting points by moving a racing car, when your most pressing problem is that you do not feel peaceful or safe at home. Just because the event is over it does not mean that the brain has finished processing what has happened. Both conscious and unconscious processes may be at work. Adult ego to adult ego communication, or nurturing parent-to-child communication, focused on problem-solving, sensible, calm discipline and boundaries that are consistent and fair, rather than inflammatory and threatening, are most supportive of neurofeedback. Critical parenting and high emotional arousal are restraining forces. They overarouse the limbic system and may easily become a distraction, a hidden factor undermining success.

The skill set of a neurofeedback therapist involves being able to think, plan and act systemically in treating the patient's family system. It is important to know where, when and with whom to enter the system. Understanding the language of the family, the culture (not necessarily ethnic culture), and even the generational heritage affects the effectiveness of intervention and the progress of the person. How does this family create its reality? What do the rigidities of the system defend? Family therapy may be needed, although you may not always get the opportunity to do this; however, the therapist must be able to guide the patient through the restraining forces and if necessary rearrange them, perhaps in strategic visits with other family members.

Case 1: Evan presents with the problem of drinking nightly when he comes home from work. He is diabetic and has been advised to stop drinking but continues to do so to the point of often being drunk. Six drinks a night, or a bottle of wine, is not unusual. His partner drinks, but not as much. Drinking and dinner are often followed by an angry confrontation – not over drinking, but over something immediate in the environment, e.g., doing the dishes, how the food was cooked, etc. This is followed by distance, and the pattern then repeats itself. They have a child in residential care. Evan presents wanting neurofeedback because his wife has heard that it could help with his temper. "My wife will tell you that I never stay long with one therapist." On the second visit they are seen together, and the wife indeed warns the therapist that he never sticks around long, but she hopes neuro-feedback will help. The therapist advises them both that this is not a short-term treatment. Their unconscious minds receive this information gleefully, knowing that no real change will occur. He refuses twice-weekly treatment and terminates after about five sessions. The therapist's real job was to rein-force their shared belief that they must be happy with the way things are, because change is impossible, so they both can continue to drink and avoid the painful issues that resulted in the child being in care.

Case 2: An adolescent presents with his mother for treatment of ADHD and makes a commitment to treatment. As he begins to improve, his grades become better and better and his behavior in the home improves, according to the mother. He is restrained in his joy at his own achievement. Not soon after the initial success, conflict increases between him and his mother, and neurofeedback progress becomes more difficult. He comes in angry and depressed and finds it difficult to concentrate. A series of single sessions is held with the mother on parenting skills and communication, and explaining how her interactions with her son support or can harm his progress, i.e., a driving or restraining force in treatment. After a series of individual sessions parallel with continued training of the teen, the therapist meets every 3–4 weeks with mom for reinforcement, and dad eventually comes in on his own. The teen's ADHD provided a perfect excuse for mom's poor communication skills, as well as dad's and dad's role in the family to stay just as they were. As the teen improved, mom was shamed and embarrassed and so undermined treatment. When helped with her problem (restraining force attenuated), she became a sup-porter, and the burden of protecting mom (restraining force) from her shame was removed (from the teen) and training was able to move for-ward. Here the child was the agent to get help for mom. Improved com-munication also helped the marital relationship, which was somewhat burdened with disagreement over child management issues (there were siblings as well), and the teen successfully completed his role in the family; the therapist rearranged the restraining and driving forces to permit the completion of treatment. The patient can be the ambassador or agent of a family covertly reaching out for help.[59]

From time to time we see requests on list serves from anxious parents inquiring whether neurofeedback will help their child with some psycho-physiological disorder.

Because neurofeedback is *voluntary*, it is necessary to gain both the conscious and the unconscious cooperation of the patient, which often means the conscious and unconscious alliance of significant others around him or her. If intervention directly in the system is not possible, owing to distance for example, other therapeutic maneuvers are needed. A catalog of these maneuvers is, however, beyond the scope of this chapter.

Historically Hidden Factors

Almost everyone reading this will be aware of the impact that head injury, even mild closed head injury, can have on individuals. Whereas most people recover from mild traumatic brain injury (TBI), they may do so – or their brain may do so – by making compensatory changes. Then, in the face of additional future stressors, there may be less resilience or reserve to call on to cope with the new neural stressors, all because of a long-forgotten injury that they may not even have been aware of at the time.

It is not unusual for an individual, or their family and friends, to not notice that they have continuing symptoms of a TBI because they may not connect the symptoms to the event that caused the injury, think they have recovered from the event, or may not even understand why they are having symptoms.[72] In fact, physicians are just as likely to miss the mild TBI as are the patient, family and friends. When the assignment of ICD-9 codes is examined in the emergency department directly following an injury, such code assignments have only a 45% sensitivity in identifying mild TBI.[60] Therefore, even trained emergency department physicians have a high rate of false positives and false negatives using the gold standard of physical examination of the patient. How much more accurate can we expect our patients to be? Thus the development of a careful interviewing technique to elicit a history of brain injury is essential to identifying a hidden force in the treatment field.

For any number of reasons, people are often reluctant and/or unable to talk about trauma, difficult or critical family experiences. A careful history with good interviewing technique taken with an appropriate historian is important to uncovering hidden historical facts that may in fact influence the presenting symptoms. If not unearthed, these become a hidden factor in treatment. For example, sexual abuse, even in healthy college women who might present for peak performance training, has been found to affect their inhibitory capacity during a vigilance task, math aptitude and to show memory impairments.[61] Sexual abuse also affects the coherence patterns of female survivors into adulthood.[62]

If history can affect the EEG, failure to properly assess the EEG may become a hidden factor in treatment, as we saw in the Case of X above. In other words, just as the person may present with hidden factors that a good history will elicit, so too does the brain present with hidden responses to historical patterns that might affect treatment. Their clinical significance can be determined only once they are identified. This can be true even in otherwise apparently well-functioning adults, as the Navalta and Black studies[61] above demonstrated. The therapist cannot know unless the EEG is directly assessed. Failure to do so may leave a force hidden. For this and other reasons, an assessment of the EEG is considered essential prior to treatment.[63] How one does so will depend on clinical training, skill and cost. Although qEEG is not yet considered essential as an assessment prior to treatment, as long as it follows established statistical principles it increases sensitivity,[64] i.e., the detection of EEG characteristics in a sample. With the exception of the detection of epilepsy, qEEG is more sensitive and accurate than eyeball examination of the EEG, especially when used with a properly validated database.[30] Databases should publish and adhere to certain standards of quality and uniformity in order to serve clinicians reliably.[65] A definitive description of the use of neurometric analytic tools and a database can be found in Thatcher.[30]

The Unconscious Mind as a Hidden Factor: the Patient

Not everything we sense necessarily comes into our conscious awareness, that is, to the extent that we take note, can witness it, sense it or communicate it to another.[66] We can call this an unconscious in a true analytic or neoanalytic sense, or we can take the view that reality is constructed in our minds,[67] that is, piecemeal, assembled by the bits of symbolic code we call the EEG,[6] but with the number of neural events occurring in over 1 billion neurons and a trillion connections, and neural events lasting from nanoseconds to milliseconds, what we would be aware of is already gone. It is not my intention to review all the literature on unperceived stimuli or operants in the environment. However, as therapists we often must deal with hidden emotions, and so what Tamietto and De Gelder write may give us some insight into the task-laden environment of neurofeedback training that "non-consciously perceived emotional stimuli elicit physiological responses that are indicative of autonomic arousal"[66] (p698) and elicit activity in subcortical structures such as the amygdala. Modern neuroscientists also theorize about unconscious thoughts,[68] consciousness itself and neuroscientific evidence of its impact.[69] The unconscious is related to event-related potentials[70] and to organizing inputs and outputs in hierarchies,[71] all of which are critical to learning.

Case of the Nervous Nephew

A pre-teen was making consistent progress in lowering theta over the midline using a referential montage to treat his attentional deficit when theta amplitude began to rise. When questioned, he denied that anything was bothering him. Later on, when properly engaged in conversation, he said that his aunt was travelling in from a distant country and would be staying in his house. He really did not like this aunt but felt powerless to do anything about it. When discussing this in the family, he was made to feel that there was no room for his objections, and he felt as though his privacy was being encroached upon. After this discussion, in the next session he did a little better. After his aunt departed, he did substantially better and successfully completed treatment.

Case of the Silent Observer

A latency aged child was undergoing neurofeedback for ADHD, and although he was attentive, cooperative and polite in session, and with no change in the inhibit thresholds, for no apparent reason he started to decline. Results seemed to indicate he was getting worse, not better, over about a 2-week period. He denied anything was different in his life, and this was confirmed by his mother. We sat and talked for a while, doing what appeared to be just social chatting as he described his play areas, neighborhood, friends, etc. As we were finishing our conversation, he turned away from me and said, "Oh you know, I forgot, but the man next door was murdered." "When?" I asked. "A couple of weeks ago. I dunno exactly." "Oh," I said (trying to maintain my nonreactive but supportive demeanor), "that doesn't happen too often." He replied, "Yeah, well, no, but I just remembered it. I'd forgot." No one had discussed this with him in his family. Things improved after that.

The Unconscious Mind as a Hidden Factor: the Therapist

Lest we think of ourselves as exempt from membership in the human race, there is ample evidence that therapists themselves have unconscious processes. Training does not inoculate us or prevent the operation of our unconscious, but if it is properly done it should teach us awareness and good management skills to minimize or eliminate its power – or at least how to use it creatively in the treatment of our patients. If our patients are having unconscious reactions, it is unlikely that we are immune.

One tool to help us manage this is to learn how to think and feel about how the interactional field between us and our patient could be an interpersonal role classification system of the treatment field. It might help us explore and gain an observing ego, an imaginary third person ally, in our relationship with the patient. I have provisionally named it the Biofeedback Field Treatment Grid (BFTG) (Figure 4.15).

These "types" are tools to help the clinician assess how he or she is contributing to the treatment of any one patient, as well as where the clinician stands, typically, or how the BFTG characterizes his or her long-term functioning in the treatment room. The BFTG may also assist not only supervisors, mentors and trainees in conceptualizing part of the treatment field but may also be useful in tracking their progress, developing a treatment style and identifying development goals (Figure 4.16).

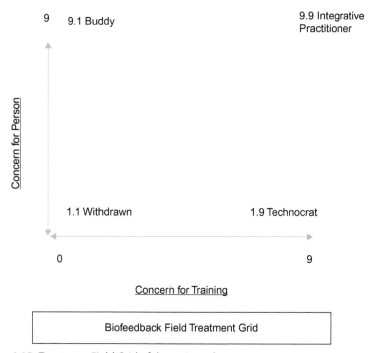

Figure 4.15 Treatment Field Grid of therapist style.

TYPES	DESCRIPTION	CHALLENGES	IN A NUTSHELL	SOME THINGS TO CONSIDER
1,1 Withdrawn	Unstructured, low technical competence, distant from client	Client may drop out, decrease motivation, violate research design, perceive therapist as uncaring, cold, distant and incompetent. Client may experience decreased safety and confidence in treatment. Client may fail to develop image of therapist as someone he or she wants to please. Client may act out to express frustration with unmet needs. Adverse reactions may go unnoticed, minor discomforts exaggerated by client, client may fail to share important events, feelings or changes. Treatment may lack appropriate or realistic goals. Therapist may have low ability to adapt in the face of treatment challenge. May fear invasion and/or abandonment. Mostly self-oriented, cares little for people or data. May mechanically apply protocol, oversimplify and miss complexity of treatment situation.	On vacation from people and things, temporarily or permanently.	Consultation or ongoing relationship with supervisor or mentor. Additional training. Assessing stressors acting on therapist. Character structure of therapist, i.e., trait vs. state. Sources of therapist's discomfort. Increased review of session treatment reports and trends.
1,9 Technocrat	High software and hardware competence, focuses on structure, rules of treatment, possibly rigid, may believe too much closeness will distort power or "purity" of treatment, i.e., specificity. Low concern for client, distant.	Patient may feel like a "number", views therapist as distant, may not share important events or feelings or changes in his or her life or reaction to treatment. May notice objective evidence of adverse reaction or decreased treatment efficacy but may not know how to approach patient to ask for information. May not know how to motivate client, client may not care if therapist is pleased or not. High competence in maintaining and fixing technical problems, low ability to adapt or solve problems of motivation or adapt training when life circumstances of patient changes. May genuinely enjoy learning, may also use competence as compensatory for fear of rejection. May adhere to treatment approach.	I'm smart and competent, even if you don't like me.	Supervision or mentoring to consider source of optimal interpersonal distance from client; reframe problem in what is in best interest of client, provide supportive nondefensive environment in supervision. Therapist self-inquiry as to own comfort zone, people vs. machines.

Figure 4.16 Summary of therapist's hidden contribution to treatment field.

9.1 Buddy	Warm, friendly, good interpersonal skills, poor technical skills. Highly likeable, so patients will want to please and maintain relationship. May compensate for poor technical skills by recruiting others to solve problems repetitively appropriate to his or her expected level of competence.	May breach boundaries with client or client family. May become stressed through overinvolvement or overidentification. Good relationships may not bring good results. May have difficulty with following structure and require increased day-to-day technical supervision. May fear rejection. May adhere to treatment approach based more on personality of mentor than science.	If patients like me and it is a pleasant environment. they will return and eventually achieve their goals. People are more important than computers and things. The software is so good it can almost take care of itself.	Increase training if needed. Carefully review session treatment reports and trends. Therapist may be sensitive to criticism. Explore belief system around scientific method, methodology, operant conditioning. Discuss boundary issues, red flags, procedures for coping.
9.9 Integrative Practitioner	High commitment to scientist practitioner model, scientific approach, tries to individualize research data (grouped) to patient's goals, high concern for patient, has ability for great range in interpersonal distance with patient, skills and ability to be very close and cope with sensitive issues, and distant when needed for separation or individuation; may think about patient systemically as well as intra-psychically but able to put client in context. Has well-developed observing ego.	Struggles with generalization vs. specificity. Struggles with issues of how actions affect the field or next generation of therapists, and/or can contribute to body of knowledge. Struggles with difference between "clean" laboratory treatment and "messy" real-life clinical circumstances. Others may be idiopathic. Open to investigating paradigm blind spots.	Patient care is the first consideration, which means safety and efficacy based on scientific principles. I endeavor to have a good relationship, a good outcome and being able to make a contribution to my field so others may learn from my success or failure.	Peer consultation, maintaining membership in scientific community, self care.

Figure 4.16 (Continued)

Transferential issues can cause us to act defensively, to over- or under-evaluate events, to misjudge what is important and what is less important, and even to entirely miss both critically obvious and nuanced events. The fine distinctions our frontal lobes help us to make can be affected by our own amygdala and hippocampus. There is enough here for a book of its own, but let us just leave this with the awareness that we too contribute to the hidden forces. This typology is offered in the hope that it will stimulate some curiosity in neurofeedback therapists and supervisors alike to courageously begin to collaboratively spelunk in this terrain.

METHODOLOGY AS A HIDDEN FACTOR: GOOD CLINICAL HYGIENE

Before Joseph Lister's intervention it was common for doctors to perform surgery in dirty, bloody coats. No one washed his or her hands before treating a wound, and there was no perceived need to wash one's hands before seeing a new patient. Hospital rooms were aired out daily, probably to relieve the stench as much as for the proclaimed reason of getting rid of "bad air," which might be the cause of illness. Where science lives not, superstition and magic take hold. Adapting Pasteur's discovery, Lister experimented with the idea that microbes could be causing illness and began using carbolic acid as an antiseptic, insisting on hand-washing and sterile operating theaters. Unsurprisingly, the rates of infection and mortality decreased. Just as importantly, methodology changed, which made physicians better observers, so that with adherence to good technique, results could be taught and replicated. The elements were close observation, measurement replication and scientific method, with knowledge being linked slowly to known science (as Lister did with Pasteur's findings) so that medicine could progress.

Using this kind of approach, and with the blessing of fast computers, we have learned more about the human brain in the last 20 years than in the whole of human history. Consequently, we must eschew magic and superstition and practice a modern version of good clinical hygiene. Otherwise, our obscured perceptions may lead to self-justification rather than scientific understanding. All too often, largely for historical reasons and the paucity of knowledge about neuroscience compared to today, we work backwards from our results, inductively to produce overarching rules or principles based on iterative trial-and-error learning.

I suggest that a careful reading of Seung, Kandel, Linden, Levasque and others provides a strong biological basis for good clinical hygiene. To recapitulate, neuronal change is a combination of newness and destruction, or pruning. In order for the new neuron to take root[21] "rewiring, reconnection, and re-weighting" are necessary.[21] We know that reinforcement plays a role in creation, growth and pruning of neurons. That was one of the points argued by Levasque, Beauregard and Monseur when they showed changes in the before and after fMRIs and related them, at least in part, to the dopamine system. Thus good clinical hygiene has a biological basis when we think of it as a set of procedures that maximize the probability that pleasure will support a new connectome, or improve the efficiency of the existing one.

There are some practical rules for good clinical hygiene that can be followed without fear of smothering therapeutic creativity.

1. Equipment should not be asked to perform beyond its rated specifications, nor claims be made therefrom.
2. Sensors should not be expected to measure beyond their ratings. Thus, for example, if measuring slow cortical potential (SCP), silver–silver chloride sensors should be used. Sensor metals should not be mixed during the same acquisition.

3. Gels and pastes must be cared for properly and protected against oxidation or degradation by minimizing exposure to the air or to excessive heat or cold. If damaged, they may not make a good connection to the scalp, or they may lose effectiveness and thus produce artifact or a poor signal.

4. The amplifier and wires must be shielded from electrical environmental artifact.

5. The patient should be isolated from any electrical hazard.

6. Therapists should instruct patients on how to minimize movement and muscle artifact.

7. Sampling rate must be appropriate to the frequencies being trained or studied. A minimum of 128 samples per second is usually required for EEG training.

8. Therapists should use equipment and software that permit viewing of the raw EEG, and they should be able to read and interpret the raw EEG during a session to the extent that they can distinguish between cerebral and noncerebral signals, and identify a record or event that may require referral to another healthcare provider.

9. Therapists should be able to answer the following questions:
    a. What was the EEG parameter like before my intervention?
    b. How does my intervention relate to the complaint anatomically and functionally?
    c. How is my intervention related to known science? If it is not, how could I explain the procedure?
    d. Does the risk of the procedure justify the expected benefit, and does the patient understand this and consent to it?
    e. Could I or someone else replicate my intervention? If so, with what reliability? If not, why not?
    f. Can I, if need be, reverse my intervention?
    g. What evidence is there for the validity of my intervention, content, concurrent, predictive or construct?
    h. When performing neurofeedback, am I following the laws of learning and operant conditioning?:
        i. Is the reward of sufficient magnitude?
        ii. Is the reward contingent?
        iii. Is the reward as close to the desired event as possible?
    i. Are there sufficient repetitions for learning to occur?

10. Do I have a therapeutic alliance with my patient?

11. Do I have someone more experienced or knowledgeable to back me up?

12. Am I reluctant to seek advice from supervisors or more experienced peers? If yes, why?

13. What possible alternative explanations are there for my results?

14. Do I follow the results of the training, show them to the patient when appropriate, and explain the results?

15. If other modalities are required, am I equipped to provide them, and if not, is there someone in the treatment constellation that can provide them for the patient?

16. Am I well trained to use the techniques I am using, and if not, do I have a mentor or supervisor?

17. Do I stay current with the knowledge base of the techniques I am using?

CONCLUSION

We are conscious, sentient and meaning-creating beings who are cortically responsive to operant conditioning and responsive, even at the genetic level of analysis, to the context in which treatment takes place. The brain is an equal opportunity responder, linking us to our environment, and therefore requires an approach that takes into consideration all the things to which the brain responds lest we plague ourselves with hidden limitations to our success. Specific use of operant conditioning using proper equipment by a qualified therapist is a necessary – but not sufficient – requirement for success. We must also understand and manage the contextual system of the patient to maximize learning, and thereby minimize limitations on our success. Therapist self-awareness, understanding the conscious and unconscious world of our patients, adherence to good scientific methodology, linking our treatment to scientific rationales, adhering to good clinical hygiene, properly using assessment tools – from low-tech, a good interview and history, to high-tech, a quantitative EEG and a well-validated database – and understanding the genetic and chemical neural environment will help push back the limits of success.

REFERENCES

1. Shellenberger R, Green J. *The Ghost in the Box*. Greeley, CO: Health Psychology Publications; 1986.
2. Green E, Green A. *Beyond Biofeedback*. Boca Raton, FL: Knoll Publishing; 1977.
3. Hammond D. Placebos and neurofeedback. *J Neurotherapy*. 2011:94–114.
4. Colloca L, Miller F. Harnessing the placebo effect: the need for translational research. *Philo Tran R Soc Lond B Biol Sci*. 2011;366:1922–1930.

5. Oken B. Placebo effects: clinical aspects and neurobiology. *Brain*. 2008:2812–2823.
6. Siegel D. *The Developing Mind*. New York, NY: Guilford; 1999.
7. Thatcher R, Biver C, North D. *EEG and Brain Connectivity: A Tutorial*. Retrieved from Applied Neuroscience: <http://www.appliedneuroscience.com/Brain%20Connectivity-A%20Tutorial.pdf>; 2009, December.
8. Sauseng P, Klimesch W. What does phase information of oscillatory brain activity tell us about cognitive processes? *Neurosci Biobehav Rev*. 2008. http://dx.doi.org/10.1016/j.neubiorev.2008.03.014.
9. Palva J, Palva S, Kaila K. Phase synchrony among neuronal oscillations in the human cortex. *J Neurosci*. 2005:3962–3972.
10. Trist E, Bamforth K. Some social and psychological consequences of the longwall method of coal getting. *Hum Relat*. 1951:6–24,37–38.
11. Rice A. *The Enterprise and Its Environment*. London, England: Tavistock Institute of Human Relations; 1963.
12. Lichtenstein PH. Dimensions of occupations: genetic and environmental influences. *J Biosoc Sci*. 1995:193–206.
13. Cardino A. Twin studies of schizophrenia. *Am J Med Genet*. 2000;97(1):12–17.
14. Segalowitz S, Schmidt L. Capturing the dynamic endophenotype: a developmental psychophysiological manifesto. In: Schmidt L, Segalowitz S, eds. *Developmental Psychophysiology*. New York, NY: Cambridge University Press; 2008.
15. Peniston E, Kulkowsky P. Alpha theta brainwave neurofeedback for Vietnam veterans with combat related post traumatic stress disorder. *Med Psychother*. 1991:47–60.
16. National Collaborating Centre for Mental Health Bisson J, Ehlers A, eds. *Post Traumatic Stress Disorder: The Management of PTSD in Adults and Children in Primary and Secondary Care*, vol. 26. London, England: Cromwell Press Ltd of Trowbridge, Wiltshire, England: Gaskell and the Royal College of Psychiatrists and the British Psychological Society; 2005.
17. Yehuda R, Bierer L. Transgenerational transmission of cortisol and PTSD risk. De Kloet E, Oitzel M, Vermetten E, eds. *Progress in Brain Research*, vol. 167; 2008121–135.
18. Linden D. *The Compass of Pleasure*. New York, NY: Viking; 2011.
19. Kandel E. *In Search of Memory*. New York, NY: W.W. Norton; 2006.
20. Stark R, Bauer E, Merz CJ, et al. ADHD behaviors are associated with brain activation in the reward system. *Neuropsychologia*. 2010:1–39. http://dx.doi.org/10.1016/j.neuropsychologia.2010.12.012
21. Seung S. *Connectome*. New York, NY: Houghton Mifflin; 2012.
22. Levesque J, Beauregard M, Mensour B. Effects of neurofeedback on neural substrates of selective attention in children with attention deficit/hyperactivity disorder: a functional magnetic resonance imaging study. *Neurosci Lett*. 2006:216–221.
23. Marshall P, Fox N. Electrophysiological measures in research on social and emotional development. In: Schmidt LA, ed. *Developmental Psychophysiology*. New York, NY: Cambridge University Press; 2008.
24. Tye C, Rijsdijk F, Grevon C, Kuntsi J, Asherson P, McLoughlin G. Shared genetic influences on ADHD symptoms and very low frequency EEG activity: a twin study. *J Child Psychol Psychiatry*. 2011:1–10.
25. Peterson S, Posner N. The attention system of the human brain: 20 years after. *Annu Rev Neurosci*. 2012:73–89.
26. Monastra V, Monastra D, George S. The effects of stimulant therapy, EEG biofeedback and parenting styles on the primary symptoms of attention-deficit/hyperactivity disorder. *Appl Psychophysiol Biofeedback*. 2002:231–249.
27. Pinker S. *How the Brain Works*. New York, NY: Norton; 2009.
28. Nelson C, de Haan M, Thomas K. *Neuroscience of Cognitive Development: The Role of Experience and the Developing Brain*. New York, NY: John Wiley; 2006.

29. Task Force on Nomenclature. *Home*. (International Society for Neurofeedback and Research) Retrieved July 5, 2012, from <www.isnr.org>: <http://www.isnr.org/neurofeedback-info/learn-more-about-neurofeedback.cfm>; 2008.

30. Thatcher R. *Handbook of Quantitative Electroencephalography and EEG Biofeedback*. St. Petersberg, FL: ANI Publishing Co.; 2012.

31. Dawson G, Bernier R. Development of social brain cirucuitry in autism. In: Coch DD, ed. *Human Behavior, Learning, and the Developing Brain*. New York, NY: Guilford; 2007.

32. Liegeois F, Morgan A, Vargha-Khadem F. Neurocognitive correlates of developmental verbal and orofracial dyspraxia. In: Coch DD, ed. *Human Behavior, Learning, and the Developing Brain*. New York, NY: Guilford Press; 2007.

33. Van Sweden B, Niedermeyer E. Toxic encephalopathies. In: Niedermeyer E, Lopes Da Silva L, eds. *Electroencephalography: Basic Principles, Clinical Applications, and Related Fields*. *4th ed*. Baltimore, MD: Williams & Wilkins; 1999:692–701.

34. Keski-Säntti P, Kovala T, Holm A, Hyvärinen HK, Sainio M. Quantitative EEG in occupational chronic solvent encephalopathy. *Hum Exp Toxicol*. 2008;27(4):315–320.

35. Burkett V, Cummins J, Dickson R, Skolnick M. An open open clinical trial utilizing real time EEG operant conditioning as an adjunctive therapy in the treatment of crack cocaine dependence. *J Neurotherapy*. 2005:27–47.

36. Alper K, Pritchep L, Kowalik S, Rosenthal M, John E. Persistent QEEG abnormality in crack cocaine users at six months abstinence. *Neuropsychopharmacology*. 1998:1–9.

37. Alper K. EEG and cocaine sensitization. *Neuropsychiatry Clin Neurosci*. 1999:209–211.

38. Gluck G. *The Peniston Kulkosky Protocol in a Poly Substance Abusing Population*. Hollywood, FL, Memorial Regional Hospital: Unpublished. 1996.

39. Kasamo KT. Effects of several 5HT1A agonists on hippocampal rhythmical slow activity in unanesthetized rats. *Neuropharmacol*. 1994:905–914.

40. Anderer PS-M. Effects of the 5HT1A partial agonist buspirone on regional brain electrical activity in man. *Psychiatry Res: Neuroimaging*. 2000:81–96.

41. Cantor DS, Strickland OL, Elmore D. *Pre-Menstrual Syndrome: Brain Functional Correlates to Dysphoria in PMS*. Presented at the National Academy of Neuropsychology, Orlando, Fl; November 2000.

42. Grace D, Christenson R. Recognizing psychologically masked illnesses: the need for collaborative relationships in mental health care. *J Clin Psychiatry*. 2007:433–436.

43. Taylor R. *Distinguishing Psychological from Organic Disorders. 2nd ed*. New York, NY: Springer; 2000.

44. Legarda S, McMahon D, Othmer S, Othmer S. Clinical neurofeedback: case studies, proposed mechanism and implications for pediatric neurology practice. *Journal of child neurology*. 2011 http://dx.doi.org/10.1177/0883073811405052

45. Lorincz M, Geall F, Bao Y, Crunelli V, Hughes S. ATP dependent infra slow (<.01) Oscillations in thalamic networks. *PLOSONE*. 2009:E4447. http://dx.doi.org/10.1371/journal.pone.0004447

46. Thatcher R. Neuroguide V2.7.1. Tampa, FL, USA. Retrieved from <www.applied-neuroscience.com>; 2011.

47. Thompson M, Thompson L. *The Neurofeedback Book*. Wheat Ridge, CO: Association for Applied Psychophysiology and Biofeedback; 2003.

48. Schmidt M. *Brain Building Nutrition. 2nd ed*. Berkeley: Frog Books; 2007.

49. Diukova A, Ware J, Smith JE, et al. Separating neural and vascular effects of caffeine using simultaneous EEG-fMRI: differential effects of caffeine on cognitive and sensorimotor brain responses. *Neuroimage*. 2012;62(1):239–249.

50. Fishbein D, Cantor DS, Thatcher RW. Ingestion of carbohydrates varying in complexity produce differential EEG responses. *Clin Electrophysiol*. 1990;vol. 21(1):5–11.

51. Davis C, Claudius M, Palinkas L, Wong J, Leslie L. Putting families in the center: family perspectives on decision making and ADHD and implications for ADHD care. *J Atten Disord*. 2011:1–10.

52. Slipp S. *Object Relations: A Dynamic Bridge Between Individual and Famiy Treatment*. New York, NY: Jason Aronson; 1984.
53. Roffman J, Marci C, Doughterty D, Rauch S, Glick D. Neuroimaging and the functional anatomy of psychotherapy. *Psychol Med*. 2005:1385–1398.
54. Dennis J, Schutter G, Knyazev G. Cross frequency coupling of brain oscillations in studying motivationo and emotion. *Motiv & Emot*. 2011. http://dx.doi.org/10.100 7/s.11031–011–9237–6
55. Sherlin L, Arns M, Lubar J, et al. Neurofeedback and basic learning theory. *J Neurofeedback*. 2011:292–304.
56. Gottman J. *Why Marriages Succeed or Fail*. New York, NY: Fireside; 1994.
57. Gottman J. *The Marriage Clinic*. New York: Norton; 1999.
58. Chapman AH. *The Games Children Play*. New York, NY: Berkeley Medallion Books; 1971.
59. Stierlin H. *Separating Parents and Adolescents*. New York, NY: Quadrangle/New York Times Book; 1974.
60. Bazarian J, Veazie P, Mmookerjee S, Lerner E. Accuracy of mild traumatic brain injury case ascertainment using ICD-9 Codes. *Acad Emerg Med*. 2006:1–8.
61. Navalta C, Polcari A, Webster D, Boghossian A, Tucker M. Effects of childhood sexual abuse on neuropsychological and cognitive function in college women. *J Neuropsychiatry Neurosci*. 2006:45–55.
62. Black L, Hudspeth W, Townsend A, Bodenheimer-Davis E. EEG connectivity patterns in childhood sexual abuse. *J Neurotherapy*. 2008:141–160.
63. Hammond D, Bodenheimer Davis G, Gluck G, et al. Standards of practice for neurofeedback: a position paper of the international society for neurofeedback research. *J Neurotherapy*. 2011:54–64.
64. Thatcher R, Walker R, Biver C, North D, Curtin R. Sensitivity and specificity of an EEG normative database. *J Neurotherapy*. 2003:87–121.
65. Thatcher R, Lubar J. History of scientific standards of normative databases. In: Budzinsky TB, ed. *Introduction to Quantitative EEG and Neurofeedback: Advanced Theory and Applications*. San Diego, CA: Academic Press; 2008.
66. Tamietto M, De Gelder B. Neural basis of the non conscious peception of emotional signals. *Nature reviews: Genetics*. 2010:697–709.
67. Gutterman J. *Solution Focused Counseling*. Alexandria, VA: American Counseling Association; 2006.
68. Dijksterhuis A, Nordgren LF. A theory of unconcious thought. *Perspectives Psychol Sci*. 2006:95–109.
69. Churchland P. *Brain Wise: Studies in Neurophilosophy*. Cambridge, MA: MIT Press; 2002.
70. New York Academy of Sciences. Some psychophysiological and pharmocological correlates of a developmental, cognition and motivational theory. In: Grossberg S, ed. *Ann NY Acad Sci*. New York, NY: New York Academy of Sciences; 1984:70–71.
71. Scarabino TA. *Atlas of Morphology and Functional Anatomy of the Brain*. Naples, FL: Springer; 2003.
72. U.S. Department of Health and Human Services, Center for Disease Control. (n.d.). *Facts About Concussion and Brain Injury*. Retrieved from CDC: <www.cdc.gov/concussion/pdf/Facts_about_Concussion_TBI-a.pdf>.

CHAPTER FIVE

Defining Developing Evidence-Based Medicine Databases Proving Treatment Efficacy

J. Lucas Koberda

The escalating costs of healthcare in the United States are not sustainable; therefore, our current government and insurance companies are open to any alternative treatment that could contribute to lowering this cost burden. Neurofeedback, which offers noninvasive and potentially cost-effective treatment, may become a favorable option in this competitive environment. Many patients who have failed in expensive and frequently invasive treatments and procedures respond to neurofeedback therapy. For example, patients who suffer from medication-resistant depression are subjected to electroconvulsive therapy (ECT). This type of treatment encompasses "shock" therapy, which involves an anesthesiologist and other ancillary support staff, making it relatively expensive. In addition, ECT works by evoking a generalized seizure and frequently leaves the patient with residual memory problems, most likely because of neuronal damage. Chronic pain is another example. Many patients undergo treatment in expensive pain management clinics, where an anesthesiologist under radiology guidance completes a procedure, frequently with mixed results. Sometimes these patients require multiple pain management visits and surgery for lower back pain, with no subsequent improvement. Quantitative electroencephalographic (qEEG) analysis with low-resolution electromagnetic tomography (LORETA) frequently shows a dysregulated insular cortex in these patients.[1] Therefore, neurofeedback targeting the dysregulated insular cortex observed in individuals suffering from chronic pain may become an attractive and cost-effective option. In my practice, I have had many patients who responded to neurofeedback therapy after undergoing multiple failed specialized treatments. Other neurofeedback clinics report similar results in other complex cases.[2–4] The cost of neurofeedback ranges between $100 and 150 per session. The newest neurofeedback modalities offer faster, more efficient and cost-effective

Clinical Neurotherapy.
Doi: http://dx.doi.org/10.1016/B978-0-12-396988-0.00005-2

127

results, where even a few sessions may give a substantial improvement in depression, chronic pain or other symptoms.[1] Therefore, it is crucial to document any positive neurofeedback treatment outcomes and not to rely only on word of mouth from patients who have experienced improvement of their symptoms. Also, more case-controlled or randomized studies need to be designed that will place neurofeedback higher in the rank of the evidence-based medicine (EBM) hierarchy.

Healthcare in the 21st century relies not only on individual medical skills, but also on the best information about the effectiveness of each intervention being accessible to practitioners, patients and policy makers alike. This approach is known as "evidence-based healthcare."

EBM has been defined as "the conscientious, explicit and judicious use of current best evidence in making decisions about the care of individual patients."[5,6] It seeks to assess the strength of the evidence on risks and benefits of treatments (including lack of treatment) and diagnostic tests.[7] This helps clinicians predict whether a treatment will do more good than harm.[8]

The purpose of EBM and practice guidelines is to provide a stronger scientific foundation for clinical work, to achieve consistency, efficiency, effectiveness, quality and safety in medical care. Besides escalating healthcare costs and inequality in healthcare access, major variations in accepted clinical practice are considered a third major issue facing contemporary US healthcare, because observers agree that at least some of the variation stems from overuse, underuse and misuse of medical care.[9]

The quality of evidence can be assessed based on the source type (from meta-analyses and systematic reviews of triple-blinded randomized placebo-controlled clinical trials with concealment of allocation and no attrition at the top end, down to conventional wisdom at the bottom), as well as other factors, including statistical validity, clinical relevance, currency and peer-review acceptance.[9]

EBM recognizes that many aspects of healthcare depend on individual factors such as quality- and value-of-life judgments, which are only partially subject to quantitative scientific methods. The application of EBM data therefore depends on patient circumstances and preferences, and medical treatment remains subject to input from personal, political, philosophical, ethical, economic and esthetic values.

Since the beginning of neurofeedback (also called EEG-biofeedback), there has been increasing interest in applying this therapy in clinical practice. Recent data obtained from the International Society for

Neurofeedback and Research (ISNR) lists more than 1050 members. It is speculated that the number of neurofeedback therapists is around 2000–3000 and growing. The words "biofeedback" and "electroencephalography" entered into the PubMed database identify more than 800 articles. Multiple neuropsychiatric conditions have been reported to benefit from neurofeedback treatment; however, the greatest number of papers (over 100) was devoted to the application of neurofeedback in behavioral disorders such as attention deficit disorder/attention deficit hyperactivity disorder. Most of the papers published are case or multiple case reports, with only a few randomized controlled studies.[10–19]

Shorter-term studies are commonly used in medical research as a form of clinical trial, or a means to test a particular hypothesis of clinical importance. Such studies typically follow two groups of patients for a period of time and compare an endpoint or outcome measure between the two.

Randomized controlled trials (RCTs) are a superior methodology in the hierarchy of evidence, because they limit the potential for bias by randomly assigning one patient pool to an intervention and another patient pool to nonintervention (or placebo). This minimizes the chance that the incidence of confounding variables will differ between the two groups.

An RCT or randomized comparative trial is a specific type of scientific experiment and the preferred design for a clinical trial. RCTs are often used to test the efficacy of various types of intervention within a patient population. RCTs may also provide an opportunity to gather useful information about adverse effects, such as drug reactions.

The key distinguishing feature of the usual RCT is that study subjects – after assessment of eligibility and recruitment but before the intervention to be studied begins – are randomly allocated to receive one of the alternative treatments under study. Random allocation in real trials is complex, but conceptually the process is like tossing a coin. After randomization, two (or more) groups of subjects are followed in exactly the same way, and the only differences between the care they receive, for example in terms of procedures, tests, outpatient visits, follow-up calls, etc., should be those intrinsic to the treatments being compared. The most important advantage of proper randomization is that it minimizes allocation bias, balancing both known and unknown prognostic factors, in the assignment of treatments.[20]

In 2001, a task force of the Association for Applied Psychophysiology and Biofeedback and the Society for Neuronal Regulation developed guidelines for the evaluation of the clinical efficacy of psychophysiological interventions,[21,22] which were subsequently approved by the boards of directors of both organizations. These Criteria for Levels of Evidence of Efficacy, described below, were used to assign efficacy levels for the vast number of conditions for which biofeedback has been used.

- **Level 1: Not empirically supported.** Supported only by anecdotal reports and/or case studies in non-peer-reviewed venues. Not empirically supported.
- **Level 2: Possibly efficacious.** At least one study of sufficient statistical power with well-identified outcome measures but lacking randomized assignment to a control condition internal to the study.
- **Level 3: Probably efficacious.** Multiple observational studies, clinical studies, wait-list controlled studies, and within-subject and intrasubject replication studies that demonstrate efficacy.
- **Level 4: Efficacious.**
  (a) In a comparison with a nontreatment control group, alternative treatment group or sham (placebo) control using randomized assignment, the investigational treatment is shown to be statistically significantly superior to the control condition, or the investigational treatment is equivalent to a treatment of established efficacy in a study with sufficient power to detect moderate differences; and
  (b) The studies have been conducted with a population treated for a specific problem, for whom inclusion criteria are delineated in a reliable, operationally defined manner; and
  (c) The study used valid and clearly specified outcome measures related to the problem being treated; and
  (d) The data are subjected to appropriate data analysis; and
  (e) The diagnostic and treatment variables and procedures are clearly defined in a manner that permits replication of the study by independent researchers; and
  (f) The superiority or equivalence of the investigational treatment has been shown in at least two independent research settings.
- **Level 5: Efficacious and specific.** Evidence for Level 5 efficacy meets all of the criteria for Level 4. In addition, the investigational treatment has been shown to be statistically superior to credible sham therapy, pill or alternative bona fide treatment in at least two independent research settings.

Neurofeedback is not a passive form of therapy, as in the case of the pharmaceutical industry, which uses medication as a mediator of the treatment effect.

Double-blinded research is generally held in high regard because subtle expectations on the part of both subjects and practitioners are supposedly eliminated. However, the double-blind and even the single-blind procedure frequently do not make sense in biofeedback because ongoing knowledge of changes in a physiological variable is central to the learning process. Eliminating expectations by double-blinding supposedly keeps things pure, but expectations may be the essence of the placebo effect, which is a very interesting self-healing phenomenon, not simply a confounding factor in experiments. In biofeedback at least, such an effect is something to be maximized and mastered, not eliminated.[23] Many rigorous standards are not easily applied to feedback therapies. There are inherent difficulties, for example, in creating a double-blind condition for a therapy that is founded on enhancing self-awareness of body and mind. For example, "sham feedback" (feedback that does not reflect the subject's actual physiological state) has been used as a control condition in biofeedback research. Yet perceptive individuals quickly notice that the sound or light feedback does not fit with their perceptions of their bodies: they are not blinded as the methodology requires.[23]

Most therapeutic success in clinical settings is measured by the patient's subjective response. A patient comes for a visit with a specific chief complaint and would like to see an improvement in this problem. In case of chronic pain, any subjective response can be graded using a scale of 1–10 or a percentage of pain improvement. For a particular patient the subjective response is of the most importance. However, for scientific reports the subjective response is usually not sufficient, and the objective response needs to be associated with a subjective improvement. One reason may be that the placebo effect frequently seems to "contaminate" the subjective impressions. Therefore, the objective response should be included in the design of any future studies hoping to improve the ranking of neurofeedback in EBM. Since the introduction of qEEG, many authors[16,24–28] have used the brain maps generated by this testing modality to show that neurofeedback induced an improvement in a dysregulated region of the brain. An improvement in a dysregulated area of the cortex can be even better seen on LORETA. For example, dysregulation of the insular cortex, which is frequently seen in individuals with chronic pain, can be assessed before and after neurofeedback. Demonstrating the resolution of this functional abnormality with neurofeedback may be an excellent way of showing the objective response to neurotherapy. I will demonstrate this by presenting a case from my practice illustrating a patient suffering from chronic pain associated with depression.

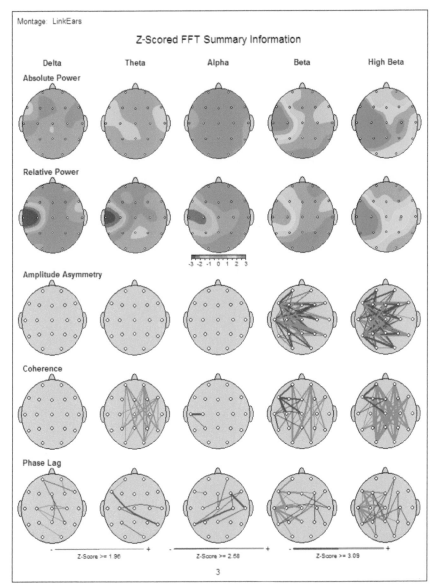

Figure 5.1 qEEG before neurofeedback in a 59-year-old man with chronic neuropathic pain: a marked increase in frontal and temporal beta power was recorded. qEEG compares the data to normal controls with color coding based on standard deviation (SD). Green color indicates regions where values of power were between 0 and 1 SD; yellow between 1 and 2 SD; red between 2 and 3 SD.

This was a 59-year-old physician who developed neuropathic pain in his groin after a urological procedure. The pain was reported as burning in character and lasting all day. The patient was treated with multiple anti-pain medications, including narcotics. He also was treated by pain management using multiple nerve blocks, with no significant improvement. Because of overlapping resistance to the antidepressant medications, he was treated with ECT, which contributed to his possible cognitive problems and did not result in any mood improvement. This patient was referred to me by a local psychiatrist for neurofeedback therapy because of refractoriness to conventional medical treatment for pain and depression. His initial qEEG maps showed marked elevation of temporal beta power (Figure 5.1). The LORETA showed an increase of theta and beta activity in the left insular cortex (Figure 5.2).

After just four sessions of Z-score LORETA neurofeedback, the patient reported major improvements in his symptoms: 80% of neuropathic pain reduction as well as marked improvement in his depression. Subsequent qEEG showed major reductions in temporal beta power, and

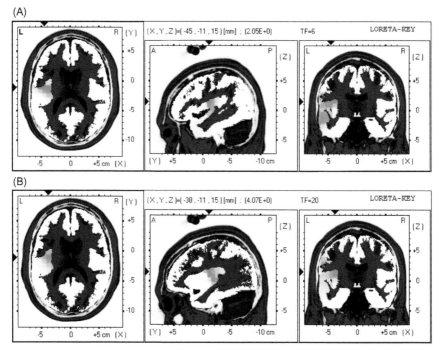

Figure 5.2 A and B. LORETA before neurofeedback in a 59-year-old patient with chronic neuropathic pain.

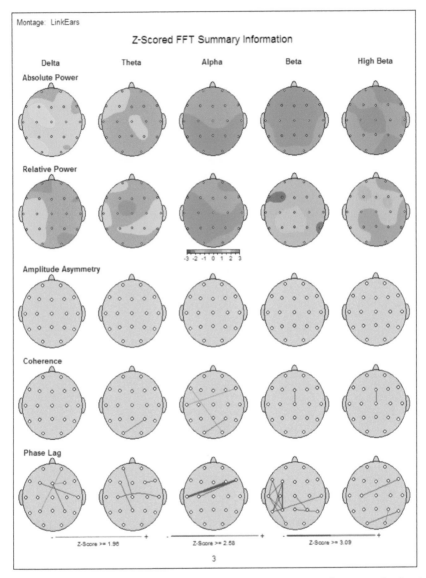

Figure 5.3 qEEG of a 59-year-old patient with chronic pain after neurofeedback showed resolution of previously elevated beta power.

LORETA demonstrated resolution of the left insular cortex theta and beta dysregulation (Figures 5.3 and 5.4).

This case report clearly illustrates neurofeedback–induced improvement in both the patient's subjective (reduction of pain and lessened depression) and objective (qEEG, LORETA) findings. Additional patient

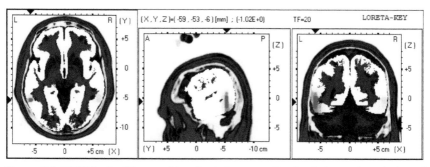

Figure 5.4 LORETA of a 59-year-old patient after neurofeedback showed resolution of dysregulation of the insular cortex.

randomization and the application of sham neurofeedback would be an appropriate next step (assuming future financial aid for further research will be granted) in order to increase the EBM ranking.

There is no doubt that neurofeedback treatment was cost-effective in this particular case. Therefore, a database of effective neurofeedback therapies will be the best tool for future negotiations with insurance companies.

In the case of therapy with patients having attention deficit disorder, the incorporation of attention scales before and after neurofeedback is always beneficial. For individuals complaining of cognitive problems, pre- and post-neurofeedback cognitive testing may suffice as good objective testing showing a potential improvement in a performance.

This will be illustrated by yet another case from my practice of a 27-year-old law student who completed law school, but experienced major problems with passing his bar examination because of memory problems and information-processing deficiency. He was treated with 10 sessions of Z-score LORETA neurofeedback and reported a subjective improvement in his cognitive skills. In order to see whether any objective enhancement of his memory and cognitive functions was achieved, computerized neuro-psychological testing (NeuroTrax, Inc., Bellaire, Texas) was conducted before and after neurofeedback therapy. Figure 5.5 shows seven different cognitive domains tested before and after neurofeedback, with marked improvement in both memory and speed of information processing.

In the case of more advanced technology, the correlation of findings on functional magnetic resonance imaging (fMRI) and neurofeedback-trained areas may be an excellent tool in demonstrating the objective improvement. In the case of fMRI, usually an increase in the blood oxygen level-dependent signal is detected in the region of interest during the neurofeedback training.[29,30] The increase in size of the gray and white

27 y.o.-Computerized neurocognitive testing before and after (neurofeedback)

	before	after
▪ Global CS:	89.7	105
▪ Memory:	43.4	91.5
▪ Executive Function:	109.4	105.1
▪ Attention:	91.8	103
▪ Info Processing Speed:	80.3	103.3
▪ Visual Spatial:	105	122
▪ Verbal Function:	96.2	102.3
▪ Motor Skills:	102	107.4

Figure 5.5 NeuroTrax showed marked improvements in global cognitive score, memory and information processing speed after just 10 sessions of Z-score LORETA neurofeedback.

matter attributed to neurofeedback was also reported at the most recent meeting of the ISNR.[31] This discovery illustrates an example of enhanced neuroplasticity induced by neurofeedback therapy, and of course serves as an elegant objective finding contributing to EBM.

Despite these obvious obstacles, every neurofeedback provider should try to maximize his or her efforts to produce the data that could enhance the EBM ranking of this treatment modality. Therefore, the following recommendations could be followed:

1. Any case of successful treatment of any condition not previously reported in the neurofeedback literature should be made available to the scientific world, so that more detailed research investigations may be developed in the future.
2. Any case report or case report series of successful neurofeedback therapy should include a detailed description of the neurofeedback protocol, including electrode localization, frequency and duration of treatment, as well as the number of sessions completed.
3. More studies should be designed to address optimal protocols for achieving the best results in particular medical conditions (for example,

in the case of depression, exact electrode localizations, number of sessions, duration of sessions and frequency).

4. If possible, randomized studies may be of additional benefit, assuming funding is available.

5. More studies using advanced technology (for instance fMRI) should be conducted in order to enrich the evidence of correlation of neurofeedback with neuronal stimulation and neuroplasticity.

6. Currently there are no available data to guide clinicians on the predictors of response to neurofeedback and on optimal treatment protocols. Therefore, further research needs to be conducted to define potential biomarkers that could identify patients who are potential responders and nonresponders to neurofeedback.

REFERENCES

1. Koberda JL, Moses A, Koberda P, Koberda L. Comparison of the Effectiveness of Z-Score Surface/LORETA19-Electrode Neurofeedback to Standard 1-Electrode Neurofeedback. Presented during the ISNR conference in Orlando, September 2012.
2. Thompson L, Thompson M, Reid A. Neurofeedback outcomes in clients with Asperger's syndrome. *Appl Psychophysiol Biofeedback*. 2010;35(1):63–81.
3. Walker JE. QEEG-guided neurofeedback for recurrent migraine headaches. *Clin EEG Neurosci*. 2011;42(1):59–61.
4. Ibric VL, Dragomirescu LG. Neurofeedback in pain management. In: Introduction to Quantitative EEG and Neurofeedback Advanced Theory and Application (T. H. Budzynska et al. eds), 2nd ed. Academic Press, San Diego; 2009.
5. Sackett DL, Rosenberg WM, Gray JA, Haynes RB, Richardson WS. Evidence based medicine: what it is and what it isn't. *BMJ*. 1996;312(7023):71–72. PMC 2349778. PMID 8555924.
6. Timmermans S, Mauck A. The promises and pitfalls of evidence-based medicine. *Health Aff (Millwood)*. 2005;24(1):18–28. http://dx.doi.org/10.1377/hlthaff.24.1.18
7. Elstein AS. On the origins and development of evidence-based medicine and medical decision making. *Inflamm Res*. 2004;53(suppl 2):S184–S189. http://dx.doi.org/10.1007/s00011–004–0357–2
8. Atkins D, Best D, Briss PA, et al. Grading quality of evidence and strength of recommendations. *BMJ*. 2004;328(7454):1490. http://dx.doi.org/10.1136/bmj.328.7454.1490
9. Cutler DM. *Your Money or Your Life: Strong Medicine for America's Healthcare System*. Oxford, England: Oxford University Press; 2004.
10. Duric NS, Assmus J, Gundersen D, Elgen IB. Neurofeedback for the treatment of children and adolescents with ADHD: a randomized and controlled clinical trial using parental reports. *BMC Psychiatry*. 2012;12:107.
11. Bakhshayesh AR, Hänsch S, Wyschkon A, Rezai MJ, Esser G. Neurofeedback in ADHD: a single-blind randomized controlled trial. *Eur Child Adolesc Psychiatry*. 2011;20(9):481–491. Epub 2011 Aug 13.
12. Gevensleben H, Holl B, Albrecht B, et al. Is neurofeedback an efficacious treatment for ADHD? A randomised controlled clinical trial. *J Child Psychol Psychiatry*. 2009;50(7):780–789.

13. Lansbergen MM, van Dongen-Boomsma M, Buitelaar JK, Slaats-Willemse D. ADHD and EEG-neurofeedback: a double-blind randomized placebo-controlled feasibility study. *J Neural Transm.* 2011;118(2):275–284. Epub 2010 Dec 17.

14. Kayiran S, Dursun E, Dursun N, Ermutlu N, Karamürsel S. Neurofeedback intervention in fibromyalgia syndrome; a randomized, controlled, rater blind clinical trial. *Appl Psychophysiol Biofeedback.* 2010;35(4):293–302.

15. Choi SW, Chi SE, Chung SY, Kim JW, Ahn CY, Kim HT. Is alpha wave neurofeedback effective with randomized clinical trials in depression? A pilot study. *Neuropsychobiology.* 2011;63(1):43–51. Epub 2010 Nov 9.

16. Breteler MH, Arns M, Peters S, Giepmans I, Verhoeven L. Improvements in spelling after QEEG-based neurofeedback in dyslexia: a randomized controlled treatment study. *Appl Psychophysiol Biofeedback.* 2010;35(1):5–11. Epub 2009 Aug 27.

17. Kouijzer ME, van Schie HT, Gerrits BJ, Buitelaar JK, de Moor JM. Is EEG-biofeedback an effective treatment in autism spectrum disorders? A randomized controlled trial. *Appl Psychophysiol Biofeedback.* 2013;38(1):17–28.

18. Arnold LE, Lofthouse N, Hersch S, et al. EEG neurofeedback for ADHD: double-blind sham-controlled randomized pilot feasibility trial. *J Atten Disord.* 2013;17(5):410–419.

19. Wangler S, Gevensleben H, Albrecht B, et al. Neurofeedback in children with ADHD: specific event-related potential findings of a randomized controlled trial. *Clin Neurophysiol.* 2011;122(5):942–950. Epub 2010 Sep 16.

20. Moher D, Hopewell S, Schulz KF, et al. CONSORT 2010 explanation and elaboration: updated guidelines for reporting parallel group randomized trials. *Br Med J.* 2010;340:c869. http://dx.doi.org/10.1136/bmj.c869 PMC 2844943. PMID 20332511.

21. Moss D, Gunkelman J. Task force report on methodology and empirically supported treatments: introduction and summary. *Biofeedback.* 2002;30(2):19–20.

22. Moss D, Gunkelman J. Task force report on methodology and empirically supported treatments: introduction and summary. *Appl Psychophysiol Biofeedback.* 2002;27(4):261–262.

23. Yucha C. Evidence-based practice in biofeedback and neurofeedback. University of Nevada Libraries; 2008.

24. Surmeli T, Ertem A, Eralp E, Kos IH. Schizophrenia and the efficacy of qEEG-guided neurofeedback treatment: a clinical case series. *Clin EEG Neurosci.* 2012;43(2):133–144. Epub 2012 Mar 27.

25. Arns M, Drinkenburg W, Leon Kenemans J. The effects of QEEG-informed neurofeedback in ADHD: an open-label pilot study. *Appl Psychophysiol Biofeedback.* 2012;37(3):171–180. http://dx.doi.org/10.1007/s10484-012-9191-4

26. Arani FD, Rostami R, Nostratabadi M. Effectiveness of neurofeedback training as a treatment for opioid-dependent patients. *Clin EEG Neurosci.* 2010;41(3):170–177.

27. Coben R, Myers TE. The relative efficacy of connectivity guided and symptom based EEG biofeedback for autistic disorders. *Appl Psychophysiol Biofeedback.* 2010;35(1):13–23. Epub 2009 Aug 1.

28. Monastra VJ, Monastra DM, George S. The effects of stimulant therapy, EEG biofeedback, and parenting style on the primary symptoms of attention-deficit/hyperactivity disorder. *Appl Psychophysiol Biofeedback.* 2002;27(4):231–249.

29. Zotev V, Krueger F, Phillips R, et al. Self-regulation of amygdala activation using real-time FMRI neurofeedback. *PLoS One.* 2011;6(9):e24522. Epub 2011 Sep 8.

30. Zhang G, Zhang H, Li X, Zhao X, Yao L, Long Z. Functional alteration of the DMN by learned regulation of the PCC using real-time fMRI. *IEEE Trans Neural Syst Rehabil Eng.* 2013;21(4):595–606.

31. Beauregard M. Neurofeedback Training Induces Changes in Grey and White Matter. Presented during the ISNR meeting-invited presentation. 2012.

CHAPTER SIX

Treating Attention Deficits and Impulse Control

Dagmar Timmers

INTRODUCTION

This chapter will cover the treatment of attention deficits and impulse control problems with neuromodulation techniques, and more specifically neurofeedback. The most common disorder of attention is attention deficit hyperactive disorder (ADHD). Although ADHD has been described as early as 1775[1] and is among one of the most researched disorders in medicine,[2] there is still much debate about what causes ADHD. The condition is still diagnosed using a list of behavioral symptoms,[3] although the larger part of research nowadays focuses on the underlying brain functions. Treatment of ADHD mostly relies on stimulant medication influencing particular circuits within the brain. Although the treatment effect of medication on ADHD symptoms is well established,[4] the neurobiological causes of ADHD are not yet fully understood. Studies using functional magnetic resonance imaging (fMRI) show effects of psychostimulants in the dorsal anterior part of the mid-cingulate cortex and dorsolateral prefrontal cortex.[5] The cingulate gyrus has, among other functions, an important role in the supervisory attention system. The prefrontal cortex, especially the dorsolateral part, is highly involved in working memory tasks by integrating different kinds of information. For example, the dorsolateral part of the prefrontal cortex is involved in more emotion-driven decision-making tasks, such as approach or withdrawal tasks.[6] In short, there is much evidence supporting the hypothesis that ADHD is a brain-related disorder, but also much debate on which areas and functions are unique to ADHD. In addition, medication does not effectively treat all patients diagnosed with ADHD. Studies show that prescribing methylphenidate (Ritalin) to healthy subjects increases interest in and motivation for the academic task at hand.[7] These findings led to statements by some experts claiming that ADHD might not be brain

Clinical Neurotherapy.
Doi: http://dx.doi.org/10.1016/B978-0-12-396988-0.00006-4

related at all, but instead be a result of a motivational or even parental skills problem. But most models of ADHD propose a certain set of brain regions that appear to be responsible for this behavioral problem.

Starting with a case report, this chapter will discuss common theories on ADHD. This is followed by a review of commonly used neuromodulation techniques, turning the focus more on the brain than on behavior. However, because the goal of neuromodulation should be to change the behavior of the patient, a neuropsychological framework is presented of how brain and behavior might be related. Also, different kinds of neuromodulation techniques are placed within this framework to help reach an understanding of how different methods of neuromodulation can treat the same disorder. Because behavioral change is the goal, the chapter will end with how changing the brain can lead to behavioral change.

A CASE REPORT OF NEUROFEEDBACK TREATMENT

A boy aged 14 was brought for neurofeedback treatment. Although he was diagnosed and treated by a child neurologist, he did not respond well to his medication. In addition to his attention problems, the boy suffered from impulsiveness and rage. The raw electroencephalogram (EEG) and quantitative EEG (qEEG) of this boy were reviewed, blinded to history and diagnosis, by a qEEG expert during a case example master class. When reviewing the raw EEG and upon seeing the clearly visible beta spindles, the expert responded with the remark: "This boy is like matches and dynamite within the same room, an explosive situation. He needs only a small spark to arouse in anger." This remark was based on the raw EEG and the boy's age alone. Although these kinds of diagnostic remarks based upon reviewing an EEG alone should be viewed with extreme caution, it illustrates nicely how brain and behavior can be linked.

Treatment was a great success. The starting point was parental counseling. After intensive parental counseling, the situation at home was more stable and the client more motivated for intensive neurofeedback treatment. Although he still had problems with sustaining attention and impulsivity, his behavior was less drastic and the interaction between client and parents was less negative. In this case, to really treat all his problems, neurofeedback was needed, because his behavioral problems originated from his ADHD related to his underlying beta spindles.

This case example is typical for ADHD patients receiving neurofeedback treatment, because this qEEG pattern is seen in an estimated 17%

of the ADHD population.[8] Most parents or patients applying for neuro-feedback treatment seek an alternative to medication, but for many different reasons. In this case medication and extensive parental counseling were not effective. Furthermore, the boy's qEEG demonstrated an EEG pattern that might not have been noticed by many electroencephalographers and qEEG specialists, but caught the eye of the qEEG expert involved. Without any background knowledge of this boy, he described just this type of behavior associated with ADHD, resistant to other treatments. But what information did his EEG contain that explained both the lack of medication treatment effect and the likely cause of his behavioral problems?

FROM BEHAVIOR TO BRAIN

Most models of the ADHD brain focus on prefrontal and subcortical areas. Russell Barkley, one of the leading experts in the field of ADHD, stated that suppression of desire-driven behavior is the unique problem in ADHD. Problems with attention skills are found in other disorders, but impulsiveness and hyperactivity are unique to ADHD, according to Barkley. Both symptoms can be driven by problems in response inhibition deriving from problems within the orbital frontal parts of the brain. He states that this might be the reason why symptoms often diminish in adulthood, that is, one learns to cope with postponed rewards.[9] EEG research supports the involvement of these brain areas but also suggests another factor. Because EEG measures brain activity in real time, the pioneers of EEG and neurofeedback found that lower activation of prefrontal areas of the cortex might be the cause of ADHD symptoms. Many research results indicate excessive frontal slow activity in the ADHD population, albeit less consistent in the more recent literature (about 30% of patients); for an overview and meta-analysis see:[10] Most EEG-driven neuromodulating techniques aim to reduce this excessive slow-wave activity.[11–13] Excessive slow-wave activity in general is seen as a manifestation of lower arousal within that area of the brain. A study based on combining behavioral data with findings from fMRI, genetics and lesion studies proposes a mechanistic model of lack of cognitive control in ADHD performed by Casey and colleagues.[14] In healthy children, irrelevant information is suppressed by the basal ganglia in order to maintain relevant information and conditions in the frontal cortex, so they can act upon this relevant information. This mechanism is compromised in children with ADHD, but also in other disorders such as Tourette's.[14]

Many more models have been proposed, and most include the frontal lobe in some fashion. Because humans have the largest frontal lobes of all primates, this area would be expected to be strongly involved in uniquely human cognitive functioning. ADHD patients show problems in working memory tasks, focusing and sustaining attention, impulse control and executive functioning. Most of these functions are mediated largely by the prefrontal cortex. The prefrontal cortex has a high degree of connectivity with other parts of the cortex and with subcortical areas, receiving input information from all primary cortex regions, such as the primary visual or auditory cortex. The primary and premotor areas are part of the frontal lobes and are highly connected with the basal ganglia and cerebellum for executing complex motor skills. Because the anterior part of the cingulate is part of the frontal lobe, regulating emotional behavior is also partly a function of that lobe. The anterior part of the cingulate gyrus also is considered a part of the limbic system, which includes the thalamus, hippocampus and amygdala. In short, the frontal lobe is interconnected with almost all the major structures of the brain.

Because the frontal lobes do not contain any primary cortex (except the primary motor cortex at its posteriormost part), damage to the more prefrontal areas may have less overt impact on functioning than damage to, for instance, the occipital lobe, which can result in cortical blindness. This is best and most cruelly demonstrated in the procedure of frontal lobotomy.[15] It is this high connectivity of the frontal lobe that makes it difficult to pinpoint ADHD to a particular brain injury or damage to a specific brain area. However, it has been found that in ADHD patients frontal injuries show high correlations with behavioral and cognitive problems.[16] The cognitive impairments that characterize both ADHD and frontal lobe injury are most prominent in the domain of executive functioning. The term "executive function" covers a wide variety of functions all working together to create complex decision-making and the execution of more complex tasks. In Lezak's[16] definition, executive functioning has four components: volition, planning, purposive action and effective performance, and results in purposeful behavior. Thus, the result of executive functioning is more than the sum of its parts. ADHD is sometimes defined as a disorder in executive functioning. Because ADHD cannot be consistently linked to a particular area of the brain, why call it attention deficit disorder and not something like executive function disorder? One answer is that executive functioning problems also are symptoms in many very different types of brain disorders, ranging from depression to Alzheimer's and Parkinson's diseases.

Furthermore, the positive effects of ADHD medication are largely a result of the arousal of the brain (although by different methods, as discussed next).

MEDICATION IN ADHD: TREATMENT THROUGH DOPAMINE AND NOREPINEPHRINE

Psychostimulant medication such as methylphenidate "normalizes" excessive slow-wave patterns in in 80% of children with ADHD,[17] but nonstimulating medication is also used in the treatment of ADHD. For example, atomoxetine is used for nonresponders to psychostimulants. Atomoxetine works by preventing presynaptic reuptake of norepinephrine within the synapses of the brain. Although both norepinephrine and dopamine fall within the category of catecholamine neurotransmitters, they have different effects within the brain. Because medication regulates the level of arousal within the brain and is used in treatment of approximately 80% of ADHD children, it is important to try to understand how medication alters the brain. Medication research indicates that positive effects of methylphenidate in children with ADHD involve changes in the function of the frontal lobe.[18] Methylphenidate achieves its functional result by influencing the dopaminergic projections and binding to the same receptors as amphetamines. Dopamine is also involved in executive functioning by projections from the basal ganglia to frontal areas of the brain, and through its role in motor planning and execution of movement (although the relationship of the latter to the executive functions is not clear). Applying a precursor of dopamine in the form of L-dopa has positive result in the executive functioning problems of Parkinson's disease patients,[15] but this result was not found in ADHD patients even though the brain can synthesize both dopamine and norepinephrine from L-dopa.[56]

Other medications such as atomoxetine are not regarded as psychostimulants because they do not bind to amphetamine receptors and work by influencing norepinephrine levels in the brain by selectively inhibiting norepinephrine reuptake.[19] Norepinephrine reduces the inhibitory effect of the locus ceruleus (LC) in the brainstem. The LC influences cortical excitability and is involved in regulating the sleep–wake cycle and initiating and maintaining neuronal activation of the forebrain. The rate of firing activity within the cells of the LC is directly related to the amount of vigilance or arousal of the brain: rate of fire is lowest in the deep sleep part of the sleep cycle and highest during awake states. Although stress does have some effect on the amount of activity in the LC, the amount of firing is related more to the overall salience aspects of the stimuli and less to the aversive or attractive aspects. Norepinephrine projects to the forebrain and thalamic regions. These regions react to norepinephrine by a increasing the state of arousal. This higher state of arousal within these areas of the brain in turn influences ability to sustain attention for a long period of time.[20]

Both neurotransmitters belong to the catecholamine amino acid group and are synthesized from the same basic amino acid: tyrosine. This amino acid is the basic material for L-dopa, from which dopamine is synthesized, which, in turn, can be transformed into norepinephrine; adrenaline can be synthesized from norepinephrine.[15]

An animal study performed by Andrews and Lavin[21] showed surprising effects of methylphenidate at the single cell level within the rat brain. They showed in single cell recordings that methylphenidate raises cortical excitability, not through the D1 dopamine receptors, but through alpha-2 norepinephrinergic receptors. These results suggest that the medication effect of methylphenidate might be similar to the effect of atomoxetine, which also influences the norepinephrine systems within the brain.[21] Thus, both medications may work in the same way: by influencing the noradrenergic systems rather than two different related systems. One thing is clear: no matter exactly how, medication alters the arousal of the brain, and as such can be seen as a neuromodulation technique, albeit not a focal treatment but a systemic one.

NONMEDICATION NEUROMODULATION AS A TREATMENT METHOD FOR ADHD: DIFFERENT APPROACHES TO THE SAME DISORDER

Most nonmedication neuromodulation techniques use EEG biofeedback (also called neurofeedback) as a method of operation. These methods are more recent developments, and the dynamics are not yet fully established. Therefore, the methods emphasized in this section involve applying EEG as a measurement tool and treatment technique.

Pioneering Work in EEG Neurofeedback Training Protocols and Current Status

Vigilance is best measured using EEG, and much of the research on this topic comes from EEG data. But the EEG signal can be processed in many different ways, which also leads to many different forms of modulation technique. One of the earliest modulation techniques involved increasing or reducing certain predefined frequency bands often linked to arousal (e.g., the theta/beta power ratio). Most of the earlier work in neurofeedback, and some more recent research, was based on the principle of training these predefined frequency bands at certain scalp locations. In general, a lower arousal state is linked to higher amplitudes in the lower frequency bands (e.g., delta and theta), and a higher arousal state is linked to higher amplitudes in the beta band. Because the goal is to influence the arousal of the brain as a whole, electrodes are generally placed centrally, at central locations C3, C4, Cz or FCz.[22] Electrode placement and the frequency bands to target often depend upon which neurofeedback pioneer's work is followed.

Theta/Beta Training

Joel Lubar first described the theta/beta ratio as an objective measure to discriminate children with learning disabilities and ADHD from normal controls.[23] His work was the basis for subsequent research on and the clinical use of theta/beta ratio neurofeedback. Monastra,[24] in a large multicentre study with 482 children, found 88% accuracy in identifying ADHD children based on theta/beta ratio scores measured at electrode site Cz alone. In a large treatment effect study (n = 100) comparing theta/beta ratio neurofeedback to stimulant medication, Monastra[25] found large clinical effects (effect size (ES) = 2.22) on attention (ES = 2,22), and hyperactivity (ES = 1,22). It is important to keep in mind the fact that in this study children were preselected for having a high theta/beta ratio before receiving neurofeedback treatment.[25]

Theta/beta training protocols target elevated theta power in children with ADHD. High theta generally is linked to a less aroused state[26] and a more inner directed focus of attention. Also, high theta can be linked to a more creative state of mind.[12] A helpful analogue to explain theta is one known to most readers: if you read a book before you go to sleep, at a certain moment in time you may find yourself turning a page but realizing you do not know what you just read. This generally relates to increased theta activity and low arousal. Although you are still awake (aroused), your attention is no longer focused outside. Children with ADHD experience this quite commonly. So, theta/beta training with them consists of reducing theta activity while rewarding increases in beta. An increase of power at beta frequencies reflects higher arousal and is generally the signal of an alert brain doing nothing in particular.[26]

SMR Training

Barry Sterman's[27] pioneering work generally focused on sensorimotor rhythm (SMR) training. This targets the central motor strip using central scalp electrode sites to train the SMR frequency band (12–15 Hz). In his studies he found that the SMR occurs when one is in a alert state of mind but without any movement, as shown in his famous EEG research with cats. SMR neurofeedback has a positive effect on the regulation of attention and tends to reduce motor activity, because the SMR occurs only when one is still.[12] SMR neurofeedback is commonly used in epilepsy, because it has been demonstrated to reduce seizure activity.[27] The SMR is regulated by a thalamocortical loop.[12] Regulation of attention is a function of certain areas in the thalamus, and therefore increasing SMR generally leads to a decrease in theta, which in turn is correlated with an increase in arousal.[28] Thus, SMR training is used in some cases of ADHD. When applying SMR feedback, localization of electrode placement is critical. The SMR is functionally bound to the primary motor and sensory cortices, found centrally within the brain at the most posterior part of the frontal lobe. In order to correctly measure SMR, the electrodes must be placed over these areas. Furthermore, the SMR has a unique pattern to it. Although it has a specific frequency band (12–15 Hz), simply uptraining this frequency is not the most effective method. The SMR comes and goes in a spindle-like pattern, and the longer these spindles persist, the better. So, apart from uptraining the amplitude of the frequency band, one might also reward the patient when he can produce the frequency for increasingly longer periods (rewarding based on a duration above the threshold). This kind of SMR feedback is known as discrete SMR training, because you reward each discrete spindle. In their studies concerning SMR feedback, Lubar and Sterman[28] suggest that "real" SMR occurs 10–20 times per minute in healthy persons and might be as low as five times per minute in ADHD children. Therefore, they have suggested a 0.25–0.5 s duration of the SMR signal as a target for reward.

Note, however, that the amplitude of an SMR signal can be low, around 5 μV. Because many children with ADHD show so little SMR, a training protocol requiring 0.5 s SMR duration 25% of the time might require a very low threshold setting in the neurofeedback software, resulting in a very poor signal-to-noise ratio. In order to deal with this problem in SMR training, one might begin with a shorter duration of SMR (e.g., 250 ms) and increase this as the child improves during feedback. In operant conditioning terminology this process is known as "shaping,"[28] and has been applied with great success in most, if not all, types of neurofeedback training.[29]

Siegfried Othmer took a somewhat different approach toward neurofeedback. In his opinion, neurofeedback trains the brain to become more dynamic as a whole. His early approach focused on a specific set of treatment protocols. If a patient had a low arousal level, increasing power in the 13–18 Hz frequency range at C3 was recommended. A high arousal level would be approached with SMR training (12–15 Hz) at site C4. When the patient showed signs of unstable arousal (meaning he or she had difficulty maintaining a certain level of arousal), a bipolar setup of SMR training at C3/C4 or T3/T4 often was advised. In all protocols close monitoring of a patient's symptoms was considered important. Protocols were expected to lead to changes in arousal levels, which would help the patient to become more balanced. Protocol changes and decisions on which protocol to use and when were based on both clinical judgment and introspection by the patient concerning his or her symptoms. Frequency bands were altered within very small bandwidths, sometimes going up in steps as small as 0.25 Hz in order to fine-tune the patient's "best" specific training frequency.[28,30] Using this general approach, Othmer and many of his associates report having successfully treated large numbers of cases of ADHD, with the largest study published by Kaiser and Othmer[31] on a sample of 530 patients. Today, however, Othmer generally advocates what he refers to as infra-low-frequency training for a variety of clinical conditions. Because there is no controlled research on this method, it is hard to estimate its clinical efficacy.

Michael and Lynda Thompson are other neurofeedback pioneers who remain very active in the field. They frequently combine SMR training with theta/beta ratio training and/or with alpha/theta training. The latter aims to help the patient enter and maintain a relaxed state of mind without slipping into drowsiness. It involves rewarding increased power at frequencies near where the alpha and theta band frequencies intersect. The comprehensive training protocols they advocate also involve a focus on learning to control one's self-awareness. They use a combination of neurofeedback and peripheral biofeedback techniques along with metacognitive strategies to teach patients to cope with different situations that might, for instance, induce stress. An extensive overview of their training protocols can be found in their book.[12]

Although all the protocols mentioned above were used in early published research claiming effective treatment for ADHD, many of the studies were lacking in aspects of research design, and none included placebo controls. However, as will be discussed in the next section, support for these methods continues to come, using better research design and qEEG.

qEEG-Based and Phenotype-Based Protocols

qEEG analysis of the EEG signal provides a whole new insight in the analysis of EEG. In qEEG, features of a patient's individual EEG are quantified using the method of fast Fourier transformation (FFT). For example, average power in microvolts (µV)in the alpha frequency band produced by an individual over a 5-minute sampling period could be calculated (measured; quantified), and then compared to the same measure in a normative (reference) database collected from a large number of persons' EEGs. By comparing an individual's "score" on any of a large number of EEG features to the average score on the corresponding feature in the normative database, the degree of deviation from normal can be determined. The deviation commonly is expressed in terms of standard deviations (SDs) from the average and presented as "Z-scores," where, for example, a Z-score of −1 means the individual's score on a given EEG feature was 1 SD below the average (or mean) of persons of the same age in the normative reference group. Thus, qEEG makes neurofeedback research and training protocol decisions more data driven. Relevant to this, a large meta-analysis of qEEG research showed that most children with ADHD do, in fact, show an increase of power in slower frequencies (between 4 and 8 Hz) frontally;[32] however, this is not as consistently reported in more recent studies,[10] which is most likely explained by reduced duration of sleep in healthy children these days. However, excess theta or a deviating theta/beta ratio is consistently found in a subgroup of 25–30% of patients and is a relevant finding related to a more favorable treatment outcome of stimulant medication or neurofeedback.[33] These findings support the arousal theory and the symptom-based neurofeedback protocols discussed earlier for this subgroup.

Because both executive functioning and attention focusing are mediated largely by the prefrontal cortex, training this area within these frequency bands makes sense. Reducing theta and increasing beta activity should enhance vigilance and thereby reduce cognitive and behavioral problems. This reasoning, now supported further by qEEG research, sometimes leads neurotherapists to claim that a prior qEEG analysis is not necessary with ADHD patients, and the "up beta/down theta"-type protocol fits all. Although decreased arousal is a common finding in the ADHD population, this finding is not linear the relation is not purely causal. As will be discussed later, *higher* arousal levels might also lead to problems with attention. Therefore, stating that ADHD is purely correlated to lower arousal with higher amplitudes of theta is an oversimplification, as we now know from applying sophisticated techniques such as qEEG. An important subgroup of ADHD, found by comparing qEEG findings with databases, involves other frequencies, notably an increase in the beta frequency most often seen as beta spindles.[8] In these cases simply downtraining theta and uptraining beta can be counterproductive and could result in a seizure. This is an example of why prior qEEG measurement is preferred, rather than simply applying general rules to all.

Although qEEG enables a more scientific approach to EEG analysis and protocol development than do general protocols, some precautions should also be taken into account. Many qEEG reports and training protocols use predefined frequency bands as a measurement and output tool, and this could lead to some misleading interpretations. Because the FFT procedure is done by computers, these predefined frequency bands often become a major part of the score reports generated using normative databases, and hence influence the planning of treatment protocols. Work done by Arns and colleagues[8] involving in-depth visual inspection of the raw EEG concluded that it is possible that a slow alpha peak frequency (as defined as <8 Hz, measured on Pz with eyes closed) might be falsely included in the theta frequency band when one uses predefined frequency bands. This could lead to a false finding of increased theta, and the consequent reporting of a larger subgroup with abnormal theta within the ADHD population.[8] This finding is based upon a new way to analyze the EEG involving what are called phenotypes, and which will be discussed below.[34]

EEG Phenotypes

A more comprehensive method of evaluating EEG includes examining both raw EEG and qEEG data and looking for so-called phenotypes within the EEG. Phenotypes were first described by Johnstone et al.[34] in 2005. Because EEG is a stable biological trait, they defined a set of EEG phenotypes as larger categories within all the variations of individual EEGs. These phenotypes cannot be linked to any particular disorder, so they may not be used as diagnostic criteria. They do, however, define certain subgroups of stable EEG patterns and can therefore be used, for instance, to help decide which medications are likely to yield the best treatment outcome according to the phenotype of the individual EEG.[34]

Phenotypes and ADHD

Arns and colleagues[8] phenotyped a small sample of EEG reports of both healthy (n = 49) and ADHD children (n = 49) and found a certain subsection of phenotypes within their dataset, i.e., they found that the "frontal slow" and the "slow alpha peak" frequency phenotypes occurred more often in ADHD, albeit not significantly compared to normal. The "low-voltage EEG" was significantly more prevalent in ADHD. They did not find a correlation between behavioral symptoms (e.g., attention deficit disorder versus ADHD) and EEG phenotypes. They did find a differential response to psychostimulant medication for the frontal slow and frontal alpha phenotypes, whereas the slow alpha peak frequency subgroup did not respond at all to stimulant medication. The latter had been found earlier by Johnstone et al.[34] in their phenotype study of 2005. This suggests that it is important to take one's individual alpha peak frequency into account when calculating theta/beta ratio or excessive theta. Also, they found that almost 16% of their ADHD subjects fell within the beta spindle phenotype (excessive beta).[25] This clearly demonstrates the clinical relevance of phenotyping and considering qEEG data, instead of simply applying theta/beta ratio training to all ADHD children. As noted earlier, the latter can be counterproductive if the patient has a beta spindle phenotype.

Combining Vigilance Theory and Phenotypes

Hegerl and colleagues in their studies[35] propose a model based on findings of unstable vigilance regulation in both patients with ADHD and mania. Vigilance (or arousal) should change over a longer period of time with the eyes closed, because the patient will tend to drift into sleep. Unstable vigilance regulation means that the patient drops very quickly into the lower vigilance stages (e.g., frontal theta or frontal alpha) and/or switches very rapidly between vigilance stages.[35] Arns and colleagues[29] further propose that some of the core symptoms of ADHD (mainly inattention) are a direct consequence of unstable vigilance regulation, and that hyperactive and sensation-seeking behaviors might be forms of self-regulating or vigilance autostabilization behavior.

Arns and colleagues[22,29] propose a method of making training protocol decisions for individual patients based on this model of vigilance, the phenotype model presented earlier, qEEG findings and the large meta-analytic study conducted in 2009. They suggest a set of five common protocols to choose from based on this combination: (1) frontocentral theta/beta training; (2) frontocentral alpha/beta training; (3) beta downtraining; (4) low-voltage EEG training; and (5) SMR training. In this protocol set many of the earlier findings are incorporated, such as the theta/beta ratio and SMR protocols for both frontal theta/beta and frontocentral alpha. It can be seen, however, that other approaches are used in individual cases, e.g., beta downtraining is included (beta spindles phenotype), as is targeting of the low-voltage EEG phenotype. These last two are included because it has been noted that the beta spindles and low-voltage phenotypes often occur in ADHD patients. Patients are also sometimes treated with SMR training (at sites C3 or C4), and/or with eyes closed alpha uptraining at site Pz. The beta-down protocol is included because this is considered the best protocol for the beta spindle phenotype. Early results from research and clinical experience suggest that this is a promising type of protocol decision-making. In an open label study published in 2012, an ES of 1.8 (n = 21) was found when protocol decisions were made based on these criteria.[29] Most treatment protocols used in this pilot study incorporated to some degree the methods discussed for theta/beta training and SMR protocols as discussed by Lubar and Sterman.[28]

The ES is one of the largest ever published and is comparable to that published by Monastra et al.,[24] who preselected patients based on elevated theta/beta ratios, demonstrating that personalizing neurofeedback to the qEEG potentially doubles the ES for inattention. This large ES is considered likely a result of the fact that protocol decisions were based on individual qEEG and raw EEG findings.

Live Z-Score Neurofeedback

The availability of Z-scores obtained from comparing an individual's qEEG data to a normative database has led to a whole new approach to neurofeedback training, often referred to as "real-time Z-score neurofeedback". Protocol decision-making, especially with regard to sites to be trained, is based on qEEG findings, but microvoltage thresholds are not set by the therapist. Instead, feedback is given to the patient when his or her EEG signal reflecting a selected EEG feature or multiple features (e.g., power in the 8–12 Hz frequency band) is within ±1 (or 1.5, 2, etc.) SD of normal, based on real-time comparisons with average scores in a normative database. In short, a specific set of frequencies (or even all frequencies) and/or other qEEG features, such as coherence, are either up- or downtrained to approximate the "normal" score(s), the goal being to normalize the features being trained, i.e., to keep them within ±0.5 or 1 SD of normal. There is less clinical judgment involved, because the training goals are preset as the average Z-score levels for a client's age. All frequencies should be trained to follow the "normal" amplitudes reported in the database.

Training with live Z-score neurofeedback means that feedback can be provided over a much larger array of frequencies, training not just one specific frequency but several (or even all) relevant frequencies. The brain appears capable of processing such vast amounts of information, thereby potentially enabling more time-efficient training. No large-scale effect studies using Z-score training with ADHD have so far been published, but a review of case studies done in 2010 suggests significant changes in qEEG findings after relatively few sessions of live Z-score training.[36] Furthermore, no studies have been published comparing "traditional neurofeedback" to this approach, making it difficult to evaluate the clinical efficacy.

Although this method looks promising, there is a potential drawback. Using live Z-score training, one might rely too heavily upon computations that were *averaged* over time, yet based on a dynamic signal. Although Z-score training improves objectivity and comparison between different types of training, one might miss important data within the raw signal. As with the theta/beta ratio example mentioned earlier, these kinds of EEG signal averages must be viewed by an experienced neurofeedback trainer in combination with the raw signal.[37]

Slow Cortical Potential Neurofeedback

Another area of considerable interest in the neurofeedback field involves slow cortical potentials (SCPs). As the name suggests, these slow components of the EEG are not so much frequencies as *shifts* in the brain's electrical potential or baseline. The normal resting potential, measured between the inside and the outside of a neuron within the pyramidal cell membrane of the brain, is around $-70\,\mu V$. Firing of a neuron is the result of a small chemical chain reaction leading to a decrease in this voltage all the way up to a positive charge within the neuron, also known as an action potential.[15] This fast shift of potential also generates the EEG. In order to produce this fast depolarization of the neuron, the brain maintains this normal negative resting potential at all times. It is interesting that increasing or reducing the potential difference between the inside and outside of a neuron can influence the reaction time needed by the neuron to reach its firing potential.[15,26] This forms the basic mechanism underlying SCP neurofeedback. That is, the shift to a more negative resting potential value – or hyperpolarization – prepares the neuron for a more rapid fire response, whereas a shift to a lesser negative value – depolarization – reduces the neuron's firing response. These shifts in resting potential occur naturally within the brain and are known as SCPs.[26]

SCP neurofeedback focuses on learning to control these SCPs. More work on SCP neurofeedback has been done by Ute Strehl and colleagues at the University of Tübingen and Hartmut Heinrich at the University of Erlangen, both from Germany. In short, SCP neurofeedback teaches the patient to deliberately "switch" his or her brain on and off. The method of training and feedback is different from frequency-based neurofeedback. In single trials, the patient is asked to shift his baseline potential to either a more negative or a more positive value, according to what is asked on a computer screen. The goal is learning to self-regulate these SCPs. A shift to a more negative value will reduce the excitation threshold. Because SCP neurofeedback uses frequencies in the DC range <1 Hz special attention must be paid to the amplifier used. Most regular amplifiers filter out these very low frequencies in order to reduce artifacts in the EEG (such as eye movements) and are thus called AC amplifiers. More detailed information on both apparatus and training protocols can be found in publications by Strehl and colleagues.[38,39] SCP neurofeedback might not simply influence the brain's resting potential. Because they depend on the event of active decision making by the patient ("I want to switch my brain on"), these trained SCPs are a form of event-related potential (ERP).

When patients learn to actively control their SCPs, the SCPs can also be called contingent negative variations (CNVs) or *Bereitschaftspotential*, a specific SCP pattern that has been found to be linked to certain cognitive tasks. These CNVs behave differently in children with ADHD and are associated with difficulty in anticipating stimuli. The latter may result in some of the behavioral problems common to ADHD.[40] This will be discussed in a later section.

The results of SCP neurofeedback in ADHD are promising. In a large study (n = 59), Gevensleben and colleagues[41] compared a combination of SCP and theta/beta neurofeedback to a computerized attention skill training program. After a total of 36 counterbalanced neurofeedback sessions, the neurofeedback group displayed a greater improvement in both parent and teacher behavior rating scales than did the attention skill training group.

GENERAL COMMENTS CONCERNING RESEARCH ON NEUROMODULATION TECHNIQUES WITH ADHD

As stated before, when we consider the behavioral symptoms of ADHD and want to change those behaviors by modulating areas of the brain involved in producing them, we tap into a complex system of brain areas that is not yet fully understood. One might ask whether modulat-ing something that is not fully understood is even possible. How does one know what one is doing if one does understand the underlying organ? And some may claim that, although neuromodulation might be a prom-ising technique for the future, for now we should leave the brain to neuroanatomists to figure out how it works before proceeding. This is a common argument opposing neuromodulation techniques. Certainly, cau-tion must be exercised when using neuromodulation techniques, and we must keep in mind that many consider these procedures to be experimen-tal. On the other hand, most neuromodulation techniques have been used to treat ADHD-type symptoms and other disorders for over 50 years, with very few reports of significant negative side effects.

The fact that with many neuromodulation procedures we aim to treat a specific portion of a brain network has both drawbacks and advantages. A network may be seen as analogous to a spider's web: touch one area and fibers in all other areas will vibrate. Networks within the brain can be viewed in a similar way, that is, influencing one certain part may cause all other parts to be affected as well. Thus using neuromodulation techniques such as neurofeedback for ADHD may target one specific area but can influence many different systems via the targeted network.

Although many studies using different techniques claim effectiveness for neurofeedback with ADHD, they vary greatly in quality. However, the results of a few high-quality studies have been published, and some, including some with placebo controls, are currently in progress. As the work of researchers such as Arns, Gevensleben, Heinrich, Monastra and Strehl, cited earlier, shows, neurofeedback training has a high probability of having positive clinical effect. The large meta-analytic study by Arns and colleagues in 2009[22] shows that certain sets of neurofeedback proto-cols are effective in the treatment of ADHD. They concluded that a level-5 efficacy can be claimed based on the large number of studies (n = 1149) included in their study, using APA guidelines. They found neurofeedback to be effective for both attention and impulsivity. Furthermore, they found an effect (albeit smaller) on symptoms of hyperactivity. All studies included in this meta-analysis used one or a combination of three training proto-cols: theta/beta, SMR or SCP neurofeedback, all applied to central loca-tions. Therefore, the use of one or more of these protocols is advised in order to claim level 5 efficacy.[22]

Some related placebo-controlled studies are currently in progress. A first feasibility study of one of these[42] found no difference between a pla-cebo group and an active group, but it was suggested that this might have been the result of a drawback of double-blind placebo-type research with neurofeedback. In order to reach double-blind criteria, auto-thresholding was used in both placebo and active conditions. This may have resulted in no significant learning effect in the active condition,[42] because with auto-thresholding (where a therapist may not be closely monitoring) it is possible for persons with minimal motivation to receive feedback even when making little or no progress toward the training target. More importantly, recent double-blind studies have used 'nonconventional' neurofeedback protocols that have not previously been investigated, e.g., two-channel neurofeedback training of SMR activity at F3 and F4.[42] Therefore, these studies have not investigated the above-mentioned well-investigated protocols, e.g., SMR, theta/beta or SCP neurofeedback at central locations.

FROM BRAIN TO BEHAVIOR

In this section, several issues regarding ADHD as it relates to brain function will be discussed, along with some generally accepted diagnostic and treatment considerations. There is still much to learn about ADHD, in relation to both brain functioning and treatment. In the author's opinion, and as emphasized in the introduction, ADHD should be viewed as a brain disorder, and diagnosis should not be made solely upon behavioral observations. However, we still lack consistent clinical neuromeasurement findings. Different measurements often implicate different brain structures as dysfunctional in persons diagnosed with ADHD. As for treatments, there are about as many opinions on which is best as there are different treatments. It may be, however, that these different measurement results, treatments and models underlying treatment are not really that different. Perhaps they all tap into the same attention system, but at different levels. Regarding neurofeedback, the question is sometimes asked whether it involves an active learning process, demanding focused attention and motivation, or is more of a subconscious process not requiring awareness. Some neurofeedback experts claim that successful neurofeedback does not require conscious awareness and that patients do not need to learn to voluntarily manipulate EEG patterns.[36] However, some methods, such as SCP training, very much involve active manipulation of one's EEG patterns.[38] In their treatment protocols the Thompsons[12] combine treatment procedures that may not necessarily require conscious awareness, with learning of certain meta-cognition skills, thus applying both active learning and potentially unconscious self-regulation methods.

Some things have remained quite consistent over the years with regard to the ADHD/neurotherapy connection. For example, most neurotherapists and neurotherapy researchers use a continuous performance task (CPT) as a measure of attention (although the term concentration might be more accurate) during diagnostic procedures, and as before- and after-treatment indicators of success or lack thereof. Although such measures have their limitations, they remain one of the most useful. Also, most training protocols for neurofeedback include some sort of means of reducing theta power in their method of operation. These protocols all seem to influence arousal, which would be commensurate with the vigilance model proposed by Arns and colleagues (referenced earlier). SCP training seems to differ from the other methods, but, as noted earlier, this might not be the case.

The different types of training protocols can fit into a more general model of attention. As the name implies, problems with attention are prominent in persons classified as ADHD. Therefore, in the next section we take a closer look at what exactly is to be treated in ADHD.

A Framework of Attention

Attention is a core deficit in ADHD. But, as we speak about attention, this single word tends to suggest that we are referring to a single function. A common definition of attention is maintaining focus for a longer period of time, which is the sense in which it is most often used when diagnosing ADHD and assessing treatment outcomes, but attention also involves functions such as the selection of information and wakefulness. So it is important to define more broadly what is meant by the term "attention".

Attention is a name for a group of functions, some regulated by the autonomic nervous system, and some by conscious decision-making by the person attending. This leads to the model proposed in Figure 6.1.[43]

In this framework, attention is divided into six different functions, in which the lower half is more or less regulated by a bottom–up (autonomous) process, while the upper three forms involve top–down decision-making by the person paying attention (an important part of executive functioning). Different forms of attention are regulated by different parts and systems within the brain. A brief discussion of these forms of attention follows.

Arousal

Located at the lower part of the model, arousal or vigilance is a bottom-up system (autonomous) of attention, regulated by the reticular activation system in the brain stem. It is located in several different parts of the

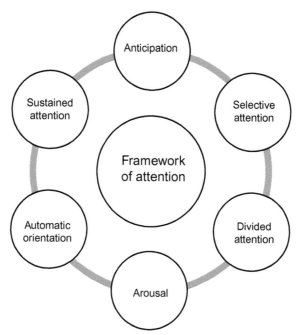

Figure 6.1 Framework of attention.

brain stem, including the LC and has projections via the thalamus to the cortex.[15]

When one is asleep, arousal, as commonly defined, does not exist. Generally, the higher the arousal level becomes, the more alert one becomes. Drowsiness is a low arousal state, whereas stress and anxiety are associated with the high end of the scale. Arousal has a parabolic relationship with performance and achievement. When one is not aroused, as when asleep, one is not "achieving" in the usual sense of that term. Low arousal leads generally to lower achievement. For instance, performance will become lower when one is fatigued or otherwise drowsy. On the other hand, high arousal, as during fear or stress, also leads to lesser achievement, especially with more complex tasks. So, there is an optimal level of arousal for achievement that is somewhere in the middle between these extremes. Problems in regulation of arousal leading to either excessively high or low arousal result in low performance in executive functioning as noted in Figure 6.2. Research by Yerkes and Dodson[30] that led to the Yerkes–Dodson law of attention of optimal arousal made a further distinction. They found that the optimal level of arousal is task-related: a

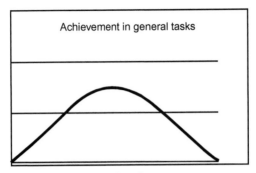

Figure 6.2 General curve – attention and performance.

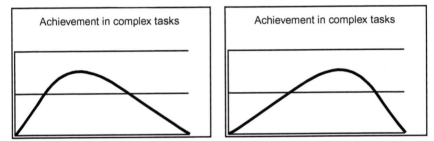

Figure 6.3 Yerkes–Dodson law of attention – performance and optimal arousal.

complex task is performed better in a slightly lower level of arousal, whereas a higher level of arousal facilitates a better performance in simple tasks. Both curves are displayed in Figure 6.3.

Orientation and divided attention, which are both found at the same level in the model, are primarily automated processes but allow for a degree of conscious regulation. The orientation of attention is best known from the work of Posner regarding cueing tasks. In these tasks, subjects keep their eyes focused on the center of a screen. A stimulus is shown left or right from the point of focus, and the subject has to react to the stimulus. Next, two different kind of cues are introduced, a congruent cue that predicts the location of stimuli in advance or an incongruent cue that points in the opposite direction to the site where the stimulus will appear. Posner demonstrated that congruent cueing, although it precedes the stimulus by <300 ms (and thus is not likely to be a conscious process), enhances reaction time, and incongruent cues slow reaction time significantly, even more than neutral cueing.[15] As noted earlier, some forms of attention, including orientation, can involve both automatic and conscious control. The superior parietal lobe is involved in the conscious orientation aspect of attention,[44] also known as covert attention, whereas the automatic orientation response is regulated by the pulvinar thalamus.[45]

The automatic form of orientation happens only if the cue is followed within 300 ms by a relevant stimulus. If a relevant stimulus does not appear within these 300 ms, the cued area is actively inhibited. This process is known as inhibition of return.[15] This covert attention after automated cueing is different from conscious guidance of covert attention in anticipation of an upcoming stimulus, which can be sustained for more than 300 ms. This form of attention is discussed in the section regarding anticipation.

Divided attention is best shown in automated tasks such as driving a car while talking to the person next to you. The ability to perform two tasks simultaneously is only possible when one of the tasks is overlearned and thus fully automated. For instance, the skills required for driving are stored in procedural memory and therefore require no consciousness processing. However, the *acquisition* of these skills starts with a large cognitive component requiring sustained and focused attention. Areas involved importantly in the acquisition of skills are the lateral prefrontal cortex and the parietal lobe. Once the skill is learned, the cognitive component declines and the skill becomes an automated process executed without awareness, but monitored by regions in the frontal lobe for fault detection and error correction.[46] Both skill acquisition and error detection are very often impaired in patients with ADHD.[2] A common test of error detection involves the so-called "go/no-go" task. Patients with ADHD are generally known to perform poorly on these kinds of tasks. A study by O'Connell and colleagues[47] showed decreased involvement of the anterior part of the cingulate gyrus in ADHD patients, leading to less error detection on the task. They suggest that this might be a result of a motivational insensitivity to performance errors, because the anterior cingulate gyrus is involved in emotion-driven information processing.[47] These findings are in line with Barkley's proposition that problems in response inhibition deriving from problems in the orbital frontal regions of the brain are unique symptoms of ADHD.[1]

Sustained and Selective Attention

The next levels of attention include sustained attention and selective attention. Freedom from distractibility is a key component of selective attention, which can be defined as the ability to block out irrelevant stimuli while attending to relevant stimuli. The ability to concentrate on a specific task involves a combination of both skills. Both distractibility and inability to sustain attention are core components of ADHD, although both also are closely related to other forms of attention. Freedom from distractibility is a filtering process, often seen as a top-down process. Friedman-Hill and colleagues[48] investigated the hypothesis that the lack of freedom from distractibility in children with ADHD is caused by an inefficient top-down filtering process. They used an attention filtering paradigm in which discrimination difficulty and degree of distractor salience could be manipulated. They expected that children with ADHD would perform less well in more difficult conditions, because of a larger loading on top-down processing of the stimuli, but found the opposite: response time increased in the ADHD subjects in the easier condition, and there was no difference in response time between healthy and ADHD subjects in the more difficult condition. They came to the conclusion that children with ADHD fail to efficiently engage in top-down filtering.[48] These findings match those of some vigilance researchers suggesting that low vigilance is a core component in ADHD,[49] and with the Yerkes–Dodson law of performance and arousal, which states that somewhat lower than average arousal favors more complex tasks.[30]

Sustained attention is defined as the capability to focus on a particular task for rather long periods of time. A commonly used technique to measure sustained attention is a CPT in which patients are asked to respond to certain stimuli, such as a series of the number 1 presented for a prolonged period on a computer screen. It has been found that as the stimuli appear, the brain produces a task-specific ERP, referred to as P3. Although the exact properties and meaning of P3 are not yet fully understood, much research suggests that it is linked to task-relevant information processing. The emergence of the P3 peak is linked to the moment basic stimulus evaluation is done. Therefore, latency of the P3 peak provides information on the time it took to process the basic properties of the event, up to the point of decision-making as to whether action is to be taken, i.e., "go", or not taken – "no-go". The amplitude of P3 is closely related to the intensity of processing the stimulus.[50] In an overview, Tannock[18] summarizes P3 studies in ADHD, and all indicate a smaller P3 amplitude in children with ADHD in both visual and auditory modalities. It was found that task performance is linearly linked to P3 amplitude.[18] There is also evidence of longer P3 latencies, suggesting that stimulus evaluation takes longer in children with ADHD.[51] Similar results with prolonged P3 latencies have been shown in clinical trials. Ozdag and colleagues[51] evaluated the effect of methylphenidate on auditory oddball ERPs on 23 drug-free boys with combined-type ADHD, based on DSM-IV criteria. Ozdag suggests that ADHD is associated with abnormalities in signal detection (inattention), discrimination and information processing. His results indicate, as he emphasizes, that methylphenidate normalizes impaired information processing but has less effect on the receiving of information. These results suggest an information processing deficit in children with ADHD in which the speed and efficiency of stimulus evaluation is impaired, thereby creating a smaller-amplitude P3 and influencing its latency.[51]

Anticipation

Anticipation is found at the top of the model because it involves active, conscious decision-making. Anticipating something means that one knows it is coming and prepares for it. This preparation for upcoming stimuli can be seen on the EEG as an SCP waveform referred to as CNV. Although CNV can be observed in various brain regions in conjunction with the anticipation of different stimuli, the best-known CNV is the readiness potential (RP), which can be seen over the primary motor cortex just before one moves a finger, for example. The brain prepares for the neural activation subsequently needed for this movement by preparing the neurons for firing. To produce this action potential there is a negative shift in the electrical potential within the neurons of the brain. When certain stimuli are anticipated, there is also a temporary shift in potential to a more negative state.

Experiments with CNV involve set-ups in which a warning stimulus (S1) precedes a relevant stimulus (S2), which in turn triggers a response (R). Damen and Brunia[52] first demonstrated the existence of a negative wave preceding the S2 in a nonmotor task, providing evidence for the fact that the late part of the CNV wave not only consists of the RP, but also embodies the preparation of other functional parts of the brain. Further research into these CNV waveforms suggests that they originate from a corticocortical network from pulvinar to parietal lobe.[53,54] Some of the findings regarding brain activity and CNV show remarkable similarities with the findings of brain areas active in covert attention tasks that are cued, as, for example, in the research of Posner and Fan discussed in the section concerning orientation.[44] However, there is an important difference: cueing shows a facilitating effect for only a short time (<300 ms). When the target stimulus appears after 300 ms, the effect of cuing is different, i.e., the target is processed more slowly. There is a clear explanation for this effect: if a cue would cause attention to focus on a single stimulus for several seconds, naturally occurring cues would use all of one's attention capacities. Cueing is very common, because any unexpected event can act as a cue.[15] Anticipation is a more active process that involves directing attention to a stimulus that one knows is coming. However, the purpose of both processes, automatic orienting attention and anticipation, is the same: speeding up the attention process in order to process stimuli more efficiently.

METHODS OF NEUROFEEDBACK AND THE FRAMEWORK OF ATTENTION

As different as the various methods of neurofeedback for ADHD seem at first glance, it may be that they all affect brain networks and functions, but ones that vary in degree of relevance to the different levels in the attention model presented here. Arousal-based methods can be placed in the lower and more autonomous part of the model. Arousal is important in all forms of attention: without arousal, "attention," in the sense commonly used, is not possible. However, although one can be awake and aroused, arousal must be flexible and adapt to task-specific needs. Neurofeedback methods such as reducing theta or normalizing many features of one's brain electrical activity through Z-score training may have positive effects on this less conscious system, enabling flexible regulation of arousal at a fundamental level.

Beta spindles are seen in about 16% of ADHD cases,[9] and these tend to respond poorly to stimulant medication.[33] Furthermore, patients with beta spindles are often found to be impulsive, especially when the spindles are found in frontal or central sites and may originate from the anterior part of the cingulate gyrus. The latter area is known to be involved in emotion-based decision-making.[15] Therefore, it seems logical that arousal regulation may not be as relevant in such cases, and that neurofeedback training to reduce the presence of beta spindles at such sites could be especially helpful in reducing their (task-dependent) impulsive behaviors and excessive emotion-based decision-making. Of special relevance to this, a relatively new method referred to as low-resolution electromagnetic tomography (LORETA) neurofeedback holds promise as a means of directly training the cingulate gyrus. It will be described in some detail below.

SMR training involves a state of optimal alertness, without movement, in order to let SMR appear. This state of mind reduces theta activity because it involves a higher (optimal) alertness. Learning to maintain this state of mind does require a degree of focused attention in the learning phase, but once learned it can become a more automated response to certain tasks, such as mathematics. Although in the author's opinion all neurofeedback involves a skill learning phase and thus a level of focused attention, both beta spindle and SMR training involves more task-dependent skill learning, in contrast to increasing self-regulation of arousal as in, for instance, theta/beta training. Theta/beta training seems to treat more trait-like symptoms, whereas beta spindles and SMR seem to be more state-dependent training methods. In line with the clinical work of the Thompsons (discussed in their comprehensive manuals), state-dependent neurofeedback training requires a more active application of the skills learned in training in particular situations such as school or work.[12] This application of skills has much in common with the application of both focused and selective attention, and thus requires a greater degree of awareness because it seems to treat the higher levels of attention in the model.

In some contrast to neurofeedback methods, which may not require awareness by the patient and may have most impact on the more automatic levels of attention, SCP training is a skill learning technique which requires a very conscious process of anticipating stimuli. Thus, SCP training can be linked to the uppermost (and fully aware) parts of the attention model: anticipation. Although anticipation at a cellular level is an autonomic process, knowing when to anticipate involves a learning paradigm in which one learns to anticipate a relevant upcoming event based on pattern learning in the past. In SCP training the patient is very actively involved in learning the skill, evaluating its learning curve and applying it without direct feedback in transfer sessions.[38] As noted earlier, some research suggests that anticipation processes may be one of the core deficits underlying ADHD. But in order to anticipate, one has to recognize patterns. And, for this one has to pay attention to external stimuli, process those stimuli quickly and act accordingly. Because this process involves all levels of attention to some degree, all types of neurofeedback may influence it. However, SCP training may be especially useful for developing the more conscious aspects of anticipation.

A study involving theta/beta training alone, SCP training alone, methylphenidate alone or both treatments simultaneously is relevant here.[52]

Results have shown that no one treatment alone was as effective in treating ADHD as a combination of interventions. Methylphenidate alone positively influenced the P3. But the combination of SCP training and methylphenidate yielded the best results, superior to SCP training, theta/beta training or methylphenidate alone. The authors argue that both the relationship between CNV function in attention, and the relationship between P3 and arousal, could be critical in treatment of ADHD.

In a way, the neurofeedback methods used in treating ADHD discussed here may not be that much different. Although their methods of operation might differ significantly, they all may tap into a network of attention, albeit at different levels of awareness. Furthermore, they all have one thing in common: the patient's symptoms usually diminish, and hence the learning process, whether conscious or subconscious, is positively reinforced. This in turn helps maintain the attention-related skills learned even after neurofeedback training ceases.

In the future, it may prove possible to modify deeper cortical and subcortical areas of the attention network, such as the anterior cingulate. As mentioned in the introduction, Barkley has stated that emotional decision-making is a unique factor in ADHD; and dysregulation of the anterior cingulate, which is involved in mediation of aspects of emotionality, is often found in ADHD patients. A relatively new and interesting method of neuromodulation, LORETA neurofeedback, purports to enable direct training of such deeper brain areas. Because the origins of EEG are the pyramidal neurons of the cortex, much of any EEG signal detected at scalp electrodes contains information about the upper surface of the brain but does not provide information about its exact location of origin. Techniques such as MRI and computed tomography can look further within the brain at subcortical structures, but lose the time-dynamic information provided by the EEG. To solve this EEG limitation, a technique known as source localization can be applied to the EEG signal, which functions much the same as triangulation measurements of a mobile phone signal to pinpoint its location. This type of localization initially was very rough and sensitive to artifacts but has been greatly refined in recent years. Pasqual-Marqui introduced LORETA software for source localization of specific EEG components. The program is freely distributed by the Key Institute for Brain-Mind research in Zurich, Switzerland.[55,56] Although some believe it is not yet ready for clinical use, this method of source localization is being applied to EEG data and neurofeedback, with increasing numbers of clinical reports of its effectiveness. Scientific research concerning effectiveness of LORETA neurofeedback is still limited, but there are a few ongoing studies.

FROM BRAIN TO BEHAVIOR

Although sometimes taken for granted, the positive reinforcement involved in neurotherapy is very important. As shown in the case example at the beginning of the chapter, positive behavioral change because of neurofeedback may not occur, or be obvious, during the early stages of training. Change is difficult for humans in general: we tend to stick with certain behaviors, even if they are not as effective as we might think or wish. With neurofeedback we attempt to influence the brain in order to change behavior. But changing behavior involves more than changing the origin of the behavior – in this case the brain – alone. So, when using neurofeedback with a patient, one must keep in mind that the goal is to change behavior, and behavior can depend on many factors, including, for example, one's surroundings. This was clearly illustrated in the case of a teenage client seen by the author. When first seen for counseling, he was hyperactive and moved constantly during consultation. I proposed either medication or neurofeedback therapy as treatment, because of his apparently extreme need for motor activity to self-regulate attention. After about 10 sessions he managed to maintain a normal and still posture for a prolonged period of time (>5 minutes). However, as soon as the neurofeedback sessions were paused, he would resume hyperactivity. While confronting him about this, and pointing out that the goal was to learn to maintain a still posture without the aid of neurofeedback, he asked, "Why?" When told that it might help him in school, because he was considered a disturbance to teachers and classmates, he replied firmly and without any hesitation that his classmates liked his movement and considered it funny rather than disturbing. He noted that teachers might find it disturbing, but his grades were "good enough," and he was not spending an hour of treatment twice a week for over 20 weeks of his precious time after school to please his teachers. Furthermore, he explained, his hyperactivity was part of him, part of how he presented himself to others, and it gained him a lot of status among friends. So, the positive reward of his friends far exceeded any loss of reinforcement from his teachers. A decision was made to quit neurofeedback, although the results had been clear.

Transfer of training is important and is possible only if positive reward also is provided in real-life situations apart from the neurofeedback setting.

Because transfer is a desired goal, a neurotherapist should expect it and discuss it with patients. In the author's opinion, successful neurofeedback training always involves a conscious learning part, although in the end part of it should become automatic and part of it should become a skill that can be applied when required in real life. Otherwise, the therapist may see a very clear result in the neurofeedback setting, but none in real life.

In conclusion, neurofeedback is a promising nonmedication technique of neuromodulation, the various different forms of which appear to tap into different levels of the attention systems within the brain. However, just as different parts of the brain interact with each other in a complex network to reach a higher goal than the sum of their parts, behaviors are the result of more than brain functioning alone. It is considered always necessary to take interaction between humans, their environments and their conscious decision-making into account when treating any executive function such as attention and impulse control by any form of neuromodulation.

REFERENCES

1. Barkley RA, Peters H. The earliest reference to ADHD in the medical literature? Melchior Adam Weikard's Description in 1775 of "attention deficit". *J Atten Disord.* 2012:1–8.
2. Polanczyk G, de Lima MS, Horta BL, Biederman J, Rohde LA. The worldwide prevalence of ADHD: a systematic review and metaregression analysis. *Am J Psychiatry.* 2007:942–948.
3. American Psychiatric Association. *Diagnostic and Statistical Manual of Mental Diseases (DSM-IV).* 4th ed. Washington, DC: American Psychiatric Publishing; 1994.
4. Schachar R, Tannock R. Childhood hyperactivity and psychostimulants. *Rev Extended Treat Stud.* 1993;3:81–97.
5. Bush G, Spencer TJ, Holmes J, et al. Functional magnetic resonance imaging of methylphenidate and placebo in attention-deficit/hyperactivity disorder during the mutisource interference task. *Arch Gen Psychiatry.* 2008;65(1):102–114.
6. Fitzgerald MJT, Folan-Curran J. *Clinical Neuroanatomy and Related Neuroscience.* Edinburgh, London, New York, Oxford, Philadelphia, St Louis Sydney, Toronto: W. B. Saunders; 2002.
7. Volkow ND, Wang GJ, Fowler JS, et al. Evidence that methylphenidate enhances the saliency of a mathematical task by increasing dopamine in the human brain. *Am J Psychiatry.* 2004;161:1173–1180.
8. Arns M, Gunkelman J, Breteler M, Spronk D. EEG phenotypes predict treatment outcome to stimulants in children with ADHD. *J Integr Neurosci.* 2008;7(3):421–438.
9. Barkley A. *Taking Charge of ADHD.* New York, NY: Guilford Press; 2000.
10. Arns M, Conners CK, Kraemer HC. A decade of EEG theta/beta ratio research in ADHD: a meta-analysis. *J Atten Disord.* 2012:1–10.
11. Lubar JF, Swartwoord MO, Swartwood JN, O'Donnel PH. Evaluation of the effectiveness of EEG neurofeedback training for ADHD in a clinical setting as measured by changes in T.O.V.A scores, behavioral ratings and WISC-R performance. *Appl Psychophysiol Biofeedback.* 1995;20(1):83–99.

12. Thompson L, Thompson M. *The Neurofeedback Book*. Wheat Ridge Colorado: The Association for Applied Psychophysiology and Biofeedback; 2003.

13. Ogrim G, Kropotov J, Hestad K. The qEEG theta/beta ratio in ADHD and normal controls: sensitivity, specificity and behavioral correlates. *Psychiatry Res.* 2012; 198(3):482–488.

14. Casey BJ, Tottenham N, Fossella J. Clinical, imaging, lesion and genetic approaches toward a model of cognitive control. *Dev Psychobiol.* 2002;40(3):237–254.

15. Gazzinga MS, Ivry RB, Mangun GR. *Cognitive Neuroscience*. New York, NY: W.W. Norton; 1998.

16. Lezak MD. *Neuropsychological Assessment*. Oxford, England: Oxford University Press; 1995.

17. Chabot RJ, Orgill AA, Crawford G, Harris MJ, Serfontein G. Behavioral and electro-physiologic predictors of treatment response to stimulants in children with attention disorders. *J Child Neurol.* 1999;14(6):343–351.

18. Tannock R. Attention deficit hyperactivity disorders: advances in cognitive, neurobiological and genetic research. *J Child Psychol Psychiatry.* 1998;35:65–99.

19. Bymaster FP, Katner JS, Nelson DL, et al. Atomoxetine increases extracellular levels of norepinefrine. *Synapse.* 2002;5(3):140–149.

20. Berridge CW, Waterhouse BD. The locus coeruleus–noradrenergic system: modulation of behavioral state and state dependent cognitive processes. *Brain Res Rev.* 2003;42:33–84.

21. Andrews GD, Lavin A. Methylphenidate increases cortical excitability via activation of alpha-2 noradrenergic receptors. *Neuropsychopharmacology.* 2006;31:594–601.

22. Arns M, de Ridder S, Strehl U, Breteler M, Coenen A. Efficacy of neurofeedback treatment in ADHD: The effects on inattention, impulsivity and hyperactivity: a meta-analysis. *Clin EEG Neurosci.* 2009;40(3):180–189.

23. Lubar JF. Discourse on the development of EEG diagnostics and biofeedback for attention-deficit/hyperactivity disorders. *Appl Psychophysiol Biofeedback.* 1991;16(3):201–225.

24. Monastra VJ, Lubar JF, Linden M, et al. Assessing attention deficit hyperactivity disorder via quantitative electroencephalography: an initial validation study. *Neuropsychology.* 1999;13(3):424–433.

25. Arns M. EEG en neurofysiologie van ADHD. Subtypen, EEG-fenotypen EEG-vigilantie model. *Handvoek neurofeedback bij ADHD*. Amsterdam: Uitgeverij SWP; 2010:105–131.

26. Niedermeyer E, Lopes Da Silva FH. *Electroencephalography: Basic Principles, Clinical Applications, and Related Fields*. Philadelphia, PA: Lippincott, Williams & Wilkins; 2005.

27. Sterman MB, Macdonald LR, Stone RK. Biofeedback training of the sensorimotor electroencephalogram rhythm in man: effects on epilepsy. *Epilepsia.* 1974;15(3):395–416.

28. Bergh VDW. *Neurofeedback en toestandregulatie bij ADHD*. Lede: Lorré Engeineering; 2007.

29. Arns MM, Drinkenburg WHIM, Kenemans JL. The effects of qEEG-informed neurofeedback in ADHD: an open label pilot study. *Appl Psychophysiol Biofeedback.* 2012;37:171–180.

30. Reitsma B, Fekkes J. Symptoom gebaseerde neurofeedback. In: Arns M, ed. *Handboek bij Neurofeedback bij ADHD*. Amsterdam: Uitgeverij SWP; 2010:132–154.

31. Kaiser DA, Othmer S. Effect of neurofeedback on variables of attention in a large multi-center trial. *J Neurother.* 2000;4:5–15.

32. Boutros N, Fraenkel L, Feingold A. A four step approach for developing diagnostic tests in psychiatry: EEG in ADHD as a testcase. *J Neuropsychiatry Clin Neurosci.* 2005;17(4):455–464.

33. Arns M, Kenemans JL. Neurofeedback in ADHD and insomnia: Vigilance stabilization through sleep spindles and circadian networks. *Neurosci Biobehav Rev*. 2012. Available at: <http://www.sciencedirect.com/science/article/pii/S014976341200173X>.
34. Johnstone J, Gunkelman J, Junt J. Clinical database development: Characterization of EEG phenotypes. *Clin EEG Neurosci*. 2005;36:99–107.
35. Hegerl U, Himmerich H, Engmann B, Hensch T. Mania and attention-deficit/hyperactivity disorder: common symptomatology, common pathophysiology and common treatment? *Curr Opin Psychiatry*. 2010;23(1):1–7.
36. Collura TF, Guan JMM, Tarrant J, Bailey J, Starr F. EEG biofeedback case studies using Live Z-score training and a normative database. *J Neurother*. 2010;14(1):22–46.
37. Johnstone J, Lunt J. Use of quantitative EEG to predict therapeutic outcome in neuropsychiatric disorders. In: Coben R, Evans JR, eds. *Neurofeedback and Neuromodulation Techniques and Applications*. London, England: Academic Press; 2011:3–20.
38. Strehl U, Leins U, Goth G, Klinger C, Birbaumer N. Physiological regulation of slow cortical potentials: a new treatment for children with ADHD. *Pediatrics*. 2006;118(5):173–179.
39. Wyckoff S, Strehl U. Feedback of slow cortical potentials: basics, application and evidence. In: Coben R, Evans JR, eds. *Neurofeedback and Neuromodulation Techniques and Applications*. London, England: Academic Press; 2011: 205–222.
40. Doehnert M, Brandeis D, Schneider G, Drechsler R, Steinhauser AC. A neurophysiological marker of impaired preparation in an 11-year follow-up study of attention-deficit/hyperactivity disorder (ADHD). *J Child Psychol Psychiatry*. 2013;54(3):260–270.
41. Gevensleben H, Holl B, Albrecht B, et al. Is neurofeedback an efficacious treatment for ADHD? A randomized controlled clinical trial. *J Child Psychol Psychiatry*. 2009;50(7):780–789.
42. Lansbergen MM, Dongen-Boomsma VM, Buitelaar JK, Slaats-Willemse D. ADHD and EEG-neurofeedback: a double-blind randomized placebo-controlled feasibility study. *J Neurotransmission*. 2011;118(2):275–284.
43. Timmers DA. Neuropsychologie en ADHD. *Handboek Neurofeedback bij ADHD*. Amsterdam: SWP; 2010:71–92.
44. Corbetta M, Kincade JM, Ollinger JM, McAvoy MP, Shulman GL. Voluntary orienting is dissociated from target detection in human posterior parietal cortex. *Nat Neurosci*. 2000:292–297.
45. Posner MI, Fan J. Attention as an organ system. In: Pomerantz JR, ed. *Topics in Integrative Neuroscience: From Cells to Cognition*. Cambridge: Cambridge University Press; 2008:31–61.
46. Anderson JR. *Learning and Memory*. Hoboken, NJ: John Wiley & Sons; 2000.
47. O'Connell RG, Bellgrove MA, Dockree PM, et al. The neural correlates of deficient error awareness in attention-deficit hyperactivity disorder (ADHD). *Neuropsychologia*. 2009;47:1149–1159.
48. Friedman-Hill SR, Wagman MR, Gex SE, Pine DS, Leibenluft E, Ungerleider LG. What does distractibility in ADHD reveal about mechanisms for top-down attentional control? *Cognition*. 2010;115(1):93–103.
49. Sander C, Arns M, Olbrich S, Hegerl U. EEG-vigilance and response to stimulants in paediatric patients with attention deficit/hyperactivity disorder. *Clin Neurophysiol*. 2010;121(9):1511–1518.
50. Kok A. On the utility of P3 amplitude as a measure of processing capacity. *Psychophysiology*. 2001;38:557–577.
51. Ozdag YO, Ulas UH, Hamamcioglu K, Vural O. Effect of methylphenidate on auditory event related potentials in boys with attention defect hyperactivity disorder. *Int J Pediatr Otorhinolaryngol*. 2004;68:1267–1272.

52. Damen EJP, Brunia CHM. Slow brain potentials related to movement and visual KR in a response tiing task. *Biol Psychol.* 1985;20:195–201.
53. Brunia CHM, van Boxtel GJM. Wait and see. *Int J Psychophysiol.* 2001;43:59–75.
54. Brunia CHM, van Boxtel GJM. Anticipatory attention to verbal and non verbal stimuli is reflected in a modality specific SPN. *Experimental Brain Res.* 2004;156:231–239.
55. Pasqual-Marqui RD. LORETA. Available at: <www.uzh.ch/keyinst/loreta.html>.
56. Pasqual-Marqui RD, Michel CM, Lehmann D. Low resolution electromagnetic tomography: a new method for localizing electrical activity in the brain. *Int J Psychophysiol.* 1994;18:49–65.
57. Wilens TE, Spencer TJ, Biederman J. Pharmacotherapy of adult ADHD. In: Nadeau KG, ed. *A Comprehensive Guide to Attention Deficit Disorder in Adults.* New York, NY: Brunner/Mazel; 1995:168.

FURTHER READING

Congedo M, Lubar JF, Joffe D. Low-resolution electromagnetic tomography neurofeedback. *Trans Neural Syst Rehabil Eng.* 2004;12(4):387–397.
Jongsma MLA, Eichele T, Rijn VCM, et al. Tracking pattern learning with single trial event related potentials. *Clin Neurophysiol.* 2006;117:1957–1973.
Jonkman LJ, LAnsbergen M, Stauder JEA. Developmental differences in behavioral and event related brain responses associated with response preparation and inhibition in a go/no go task. *Psychophysiology.* 2003;40:752–761.
Heinrich H, Gevensleben H, Strehl U. Annotation: neurofeedback, train your brain to train behavior. *J Child Psychol Psychiatry.* 2007;48:3–16.
Sangel RB, Sangel JM. Attention-deficit/hyperactivity disorder: use of cognitive evoked potential (P3) to predict treatment response. *Clinical Neurophysiology.* 2006;117:1996–2006.

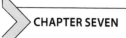

CHAPTER SEVEN

Treating Mood Disorders

Emily Stevens

According to the National Comorbidity Survey-Replication, the prevalence rate for mood disorders is 9.5% for Americans[1] and the fourth leading cause of disability in the world.[2] Depression is currently predicted to be the second largest disorder globally by 2020, according to the World Health Organization.[3] Major depression is characterized as a serious and severe psychiatric disorder that can recur in severity over a person's lifetime. Full remission is the ideal goal of treatment, but most patients fail to achieve this and only obtain partial remission, leading them to seek treatment throughout their lifetime. When patients do not reach complete remission after an acute episode, they are at a high risk for relapse, with continued and possibly more severe episodes.[4,5] The numbers of individuals of all ages with symptoms of a mood disorder are increasing, and women are 50% more likely to be depressed than men.[1] Antidepressant medications have become the first line of treatment and what is considered standard of care by most physicians and insurance companies. Broadhead[6] and associates estimated that 90% of patients with depression can be treated successfully, yet 50% are undiagnosed, misdiagnosed, undertreated or never treated. As the number of patients taking antidepressant medications has increased, so has the number of people who cannot tolerate the medications, have had poor to no response to medication or have had severe medication side effects.[7] Studies also support a powerful placebo effect that is equal to or very close to the actual response to medication in patients treated with antidepressants.[8–10] As a result, the need for safe, nonmedication approaches to treatment is on the rise. In this chapter, we will explore an array of treatments for mood disorders, including neurofeedback, auditory–visual stimulation, cranial electrotherapy stimulation (CES) and transcranial magnetic stimulation (TMS).

Since the mid-1980s considerable research has focused on the role of the frontal lobes and cortical asymmetry related to depression in brain functioning.

Clinical Neurotherapy.
Doi: http://dx.doi.org/10.1016/B978-0-12-396988-0.00007-6

The use of electroencephalographic (EEG) technology has increased the ability of clinicians to identify such neurological correlates and markers in patients with different disorders. Increased relative frontal alpha is associated with dysthymia and major depressive disorder (MDD),[11–13] and the onset of depression in patients with damage to the left frontal lobe. Henriques and Davidson[14] first hypothesized that frontal alpha asymmetry was an indicator and marker for vulnerability to depression in all ages. In 1992 Dawson and colleagues[15,16] published data that supported an EEG biological marker for depression that was noted in both the EEG of a mother who had a documented history of depression and the EEG profile of her infant with no documented symptomatology, owing to age.

Throughout the mid-1990s Davidson[17] continued to publish data noting increased frontal asymmetry in patients who were depressed. In 2000, Kentgen and colleagues[18] published a study looking at increased frontal alpha asymmetry in adolescents diagnosed with MDD and found that the same profile that had been identified in adults could be seen in adolescents. This information has provided not only a well-established neurological marker for depression in the EEG, but also a framework for clinicians to explore various approaches to brain stimulation to improve functioning.

NEUROFEEDBACK FOR DEPRESSION

As a result of these data, clinical practitioners trained in neurofeedback or EEG biofeedback began to develop protocols to improve alpha asymmetry and reduce symptoms of depression. Neurofeedback has been shown to be successful in modifying brain function in a number of disorders, which supports its exploration in treatment for depression. Various types of equipment have been used for this approach to treatment, with promising outcomes. Saxby and Peniston[19] published a study focusing on alpha/theta brainwave training as an effective treatment for alcoholics with depressive symptoms. This experimental study of 14 alcoholics in an outpatient setting focused on a treatment group of participants who presented with a history of both alcoholism and depression. The study was based on the Peniston–Kulkowsky[20,21] protocol which uses five sessions of temperature training, guided visualization, and 20 40-minute sessions of alpha/theta brainwave biofeedback. The results supported a 92% effectiveness rate in the use of neurofeedback to treat alcoholics with comorbid depression. A 21-month follow-up revealed sustained treatment effects and no relapse in 13 of the 14 participants. The one participant who relapsed returned for follow-up "booster" neurofeedback sessions and was able to remain abstinent for another 13 months of follow-up.

Baehr and colleagues[22] first reported on their work treating depression with an alpha asymmetry protocol where they reviewed six case study outcomes. The patients were seen twice a week and received a half hour of neurofeedback and a half hour of psychotherapy. F3 and F4 electrode sites were used, with a focus on activating the left frontal cortex and reducing alpha in the same region. Their protocol (ALAY – Alpha Asymmetry F4 – F3/F3 + F4 with reference at Cz) was first developed by Rosenfeld[23] and utilized by Rosenfeld and colleagues in multiple clinical case studies. Results for Baehr and colleagues revealed that four out of six patients indicated a positive outcome, with neurofeedback being identified as a "promising alternative adjunctive treatment for mood disorders." Follow-up on these patients demonstrated improved symptomatology and neurophysiology from 1 to 5 years.

In an effort to further explore the Rosenfeld alpha asymmetry protocol, Choi and colleagues[24] set up the first experimental neurofeedback alpha asymmetry protocol study. This study continued to look at the EEG research that correlates depression with hypoactivation in the left prefrontal cortex and variations in electrical frequency bands associated with depression. The study examined the effects of neurofeedback training when increasing the relative activity in the right prefrontal cortex with patients suffering from depression, as well as emotional, behavioral and cognitive problems. This experimental study included two randomized groups of patients: one neurofeedback group and one psychotherapy placebo group to control for treatment effect. The neurofeedback group received 10 sessions (twice a week) for 5 weeks and the psychotherapy group received psychological assessment and interpretation throughout the 5 weeks. After the 5 weeks of neurofeedback were completed, the patients continued on with a 1-month trial (twice per week) of self-training sessions replicating the mental state they experienced during neurofeedback, and the psychotherapy group was referred to other therapists during this time period for conventional therapy sessions. The results supported a positive training effect in the prefrontal cortex alpha band with neurofeedback, decreased symptoms of depression and enhanced executive functioning. Fifty percent of the neurofeedback subjects showed significant changes that were not reflected in the psychotherapy group. The experimental design of this study supports a causal relationship between the EEG alpha asymmetry profile and the symptoms of depression, and when treated with neurofeedback utilizing the Rosenfeld alpha asymmetry, protocol symptoms of depression can be decreased.

Hammond[25] explored a different protocol in his case study. Placing electrodes at Fp1 and F3, he inhibited slow alpha/theta and rewarded beta 15–18 Hz for 20–22 minutes, and then changed the reward band to 12–15 Hz for 8–10 minutes. In 2005, Hammond reported on nine patients he had taken through this protocol and seven who had completed the study. The average number of sessions was 20.75 at 30 minutes each. The results showed that 77.8% of the patients made a significant improvement. Hammond[26,27] reported ongoing success using this protocol with follow-ups from 6 to 24 months and an average 80% success rate.

Raymond and colleagues[28] also explored the effects of alpha/theta training for management of mood. Instead of focusing on rewarding beta as Hammond had, the study went back and reviewed the effects of deep state relaxation on personality and mood enhancement. There is no clear understanding of why alpha/theta training has shown to be so effective, but it appears to have a positive effect on feeling and sense of wellbeing. The participants in this study included 12 second-year medical students who were assessed with the Personality Syndrome Questionnaire-80 and the Profile of Mood States. All subjects chosen scored 30% higher on the withdrawal scale than their peers. The participants received 10 sessions of alpha/theta training over a 5-week period. The results showed no improvement in personality but did reveal improvement in mood. This study included a real feedback group and a mock feedback group with the real group showing significantly more improvement in mood. The subjects noted that they felt more energized after their neurofeedback sessions and overall more positive.

Dias and van Deusen[29] proposed a new protocol based on a comprehensive review of the literature for depression. The paper presents three parameters that are used to provide the neurofeedback training. The first is to increase alpha (9–14 Hz) asymmetry to the right side, increase the beta/theta ratio on the left prefrontal cortex and reduce beta (23–38 Hz) over the entire prefrontal cortex to reduce/manage anxiety. This protocol addresses the asymmetry issues associated with depression, the motivational issues often associated with depression, and the reduction of anxiety that might occur by increasing beta in the left frontal lobe for some clients. The initial case study that was used with this protocol is limited, but revealed positive improvement and supports the need for further research.

Another trend in the field is to combine the research that supports reducing alpha in the left frontal for depression and increasing beta to support improved executive functioning as a treatment protocol for depression. Currently, the most common approach to treating depression with neurofeedback is to develop a protocol that corresponds with the quantitative EEG (qEEG), if one is available, i.e., to treat the identified areas of the EEG where abnormal functioning was indicated. This may still include the protocols listed above but can include other protocols to complete the treatment relevant to the qEEG and symptomatology.

Z-score neurofeedback, low-resolution electromagnetic tomagraphic analysis neurofeedback and real-time functional magnetic resonance imaging (fMRI)-based neurofeedback are the newest areas of focus in the neurofeedback and brain-based regulation arena that are showing positive outcomes on a case-by-case basis. fMRI neurofeedback is growing rapidly, with the first studies being published and several under way.

Johnston and colleagues[30] published one of the first studies in 2010 utilizing real-time fMRI to train patients in neurofeedback to self-regulate emotion networks. First fMRI was used to identify areas reactive to positive and negative emotional stimuli, and then neurofeedback was used to train participants to upregulate the areas associated with reactions to negative stimuli. Thirteen volunteers were assessed utilizing fMRI, Profile of Mood States and Positive and Negative Affect Scale. The brain area identified as having the highest response to negative stimuli was identified in each subject as the target area for neurofeedback. Subjects were able to upregulate the emotion areas identified within 20 sessions of fMRI neurofeedback. The results of mood on the psychological assessments revealed increased mood disturbance after neurofeedback when increasing activation to the emotion areas with the highest response to negative stimuli. This study supported with proper feedback the ability to use fMRI to train individuals to self-regulate emotion areas in the brain.

In 2012, Linden and colleagues[31] published the next compelling study using fMRI-based neurofeedback to train patients with depression in self-regulation and self-control of emotion-related brain areas associated with depression. This study included eight neurofeedback participants and eight imagery control participants. Groups were matched by demographic characteristics, clinical parameters and severity of unipolar depressive symptoms. The localized areas of the brain targeted included areas responsive to positively valenced visual stimuli adapted by the team from the International Affective Picture System.[32,33] Results of the study showed that participants in the fMRI-based neurofeedback group successfully learned to upregulate the neurological target area in four sessions compared to the control group. Neurofeedback was identified as a significant aspect and component to the outcomes in this study, as shown by the lack of improvement in the control group.

After reviewing previous studies, Johnston and colleagues[34] decided to study the effects of fMRI and neurofeedback to increase positive mood and emotion. Thirty-one subjects were chosen from university staff and students to participate. This study included 17 subjects in the active neurofeedback experimental group and 10 in the control group. Using the same psychological assessments as the Johnston (2010) study, participants were screened before and after every neurofeedback session. Subjects were assessed utilizing fMRI to identify the highest activation response to positive pictures versus neutral and then trained to upregulate the area with highest response to positive stimuli. The results revealed the experimental group was able to upregulate their target areas with positive emotional stimuli, while the control group showed no change to the target areas during the sessions. However, the psychological assessment of mood did not show any significant change or improvement in positive mood in either group and only a slightly improved depression score in the experimental group. This study reinforced the outcome found in previous studies supporting that subjects can upregulate different areas of the brain utilizing fMRI neurofeedback. However, the benefits of real time fMRI neurofeedback need further evaluation to determine efficacy of treatment and reduction of symptomology or improvement of mood. The technology clearly demonstrates an individual's ability to upregulate emotion areas of the brain, but minimal changes in mood have been reported in the studies.

These studies continue to build the bridge between the importance of neuroimaging techniques in mental health and their future potential role in treatment.

AUDITORY–VISUAL STIMULATION

Auditory–visual stimulation has an extensive history of use and research. The foci of these studies range from depression, anxiety, seasonal affective disorder (SAD), hypertension, migraines and premenstrual syndrome to stress management. The majority of the studies involve a self-assessment of symptomatology and change in severity. This has worked against this technology and its broader use, yet over 100 studies showing before-and-after improvements of symptomatology argue for its use and the continued need for research.

Light stimulation was first documented as being used clinically with psychiatric patients in the early 1900s to produce a calming effect, by watching a flashing light produced by a wheel spinning in front of a lamp at a constant speed. Adrian and Matthews[35] first documented that the flashing light changed patients' brainwave activity. Over time, interest in this continued to grow in the arena of psychiatry and neuroscience. James Toman[36] performed a number of simple studies on the effects of flicker or photic stimulation on the flicker potentials of the brain. He studied and recorded the percentage of time that alpha was produced with the eyes closed, and the effects that entrainment or stimulation could have on an individual's natural brainwave levels. Toman was able to confirm previous work, which showed that people with strong alpha rhythms had a poor range of entrainment, and those with few or no alpha rhythms could be entrained to a wider range of frequencies. He also observed that the cerebral frequency of stimulation seemed to maintain itself for a period of time after the end of flicker stimulation, and hypothesized that this was a result of the mutual interaction of neurons. For many years research continued in the areas of both photic and auditory/binaural stimulation concerning its effects on pain management, anesthesia and calming hysterical patients. Cady and Shealy[37] studied the effects of 30-minute sessions of 10 Hz photic stimulation, taking regular measurements of blood serotonin, endorphin, melatonin and norepinephrine levels. They identified a drop in the daytime level of melatonin and substantial increases in levels of endorphin, serotonin and norepinephrine. Shealy's group theorized that an increase in beta-endorphins is associated with a sense of wellbeing, happiness and decreased pain. The increase in norepinephrine and serotonin and the decrease in melatonin suggested an increase in alertness and awareness. They also noted that people had a more positive relaxation response from photic stimulation than from using self-hypnosis, CES or "Hemi-Sync" tapes from the Monroe Institute.

However, changes in biochemistry are only a part of a wide spectrum of psychobiological effects reportedly produced by auditory–visual entrainment (AVE). It has been well established since the 1940s, for example, that various types of brain technology, ranging from lights flickering at various rates and frequencies to binaural beats at various rates, produce rapid and profound changes in brainwave frequencies when used to stimulate the brain.[36,38–40] The use of tools for brainwave "entrainment" or "driving" has enabled therapists to produce increased brainwave activity in desired ranges associated with different disorders, and reduction of symptom complaints without requiring the client to do anything other than relax passively throughout the session. Training goals usually included improvements in functioning and reductions in negative symptomatologies, such as pain.

Research has also shown that if a person's brain does not seem to entrain to the frequencies being presented, it does not mean that the individual will not benefit. Some studies show that photic stimulation increases cerebral blood flow and the production of neurotransmitters, regardless of whether or not it changes the baseline brainwave frequencies, with each aspect playing a different part in the overall AVE experience.[41,42] AVE has been used to improve academic performance[43] and clinically to reduce chronic pain,[44] treat migraines,[45] learning disabilities and attention deficit hyperactivity disorder (ADHD),[46] SAD,[47] depression[48] and more.

Kumano and colleagues[49] published one of the first case studies using photic stimulation on a patient who was hospitalized for depression. The client was given a set of 16 and 18 treatment sessions divided between two separate inpatient admissions. The protocol used photic stimulation in the alpha range. Results reported included improvements in general mood state, alpha rhythm increase, cardiac parasympathetic suppression, and increased skin conductance. An interesting aspect to this study is that one would not expect to see such significant improvement with alpha enhancement when, as noted earlier, increased left frontal alpha has been found to be a signature for depression. Limitations to this study are that baseline qEEG data were not provided regarding whether or not this individual had a classic depression profile, and the possible role of medications on the outcome was not considered, but it did begin to open the door for more published research in this area.

Berg and Siever[47] published a study using AVE for SAD using placebo and 20 Hz AVE treatment with 74 patients. In this study 58 patients received 2 weeks of the placebo and then 2 weeks of the 20 Hz AVE; the remaining 16 patients were in a control group and did not receive any treatment. The study used the Beck Depression Inventory and the Anxiety Sensitivity Index as before and after measures, as well as a personal diary that kept track of sleep time, sociability, eating, appetite, carbohydrate intake, cravings and energy. The results indicated a 36% reduction in depression symptoms in the placebo phase and a 100% reduction of symptoms in the treatment phase for the AVE group. Of the treatment group, it was reported that 84% became clinically nondepressed according to their scores. According to the study, the control group's symptoms increased on both the depression and the anxiety scales. They also reported that clients' journals revealed improvements in social/family/work life, energy, and reduced carbohydrate cravings and overeating. The results supported that 20 Hz AVE had positive outcomes in patients with depression. One of the limitations of that study is that it involved self-report and observation only, with no baseline neurological measures to suggest why those clients may have responded to this frequency, and no "post" measures to assess for neurological changes.

Cantor and Stevens[48] assessed the impact of AVE on patients with treatment-resistant depression. Sixteen patients with refractory depression (i.e., not responding to medication) ranging in age from 20 to 67 years were randomly assigned to two treatment groups. Subjects were assessed using Beck's Depression Inventory II (BDI-II) as well as qEEG assessments at baseline, at cross-over of treatments and after treatment. All were required to have a score of 15 or higher on the BDI-II to qualify for the study, as well as to move to the next stage and have a qEEG evaluation. All participants were required to have increased relative frontal alpha or increased relative frontal beta on a neurometric qEEG evaluation at baseline to qualify to participate in the study. This was based on other studies indicating such deviations in depression samples.[50,51] No patients were on medication during the study. The study compared a "sham" procedure to 14 Hz AVE. One group received 20 sessions of the sham procedure for the first 4 weeks and then received the active treatment, with qEEG data obtained at the beginning, following sham treatment, and then after AVE. The second group received 20 sessions of AVE in the first 4 weeks and then no treatment over the last 4 weeks to measure for sustainability. They also had qEEG evaluations at matching time points. In this study, significant improvements in both depressive symptoms and qEEG Z-score measures were noted during the AVE treatment period. Participants experienced an average 70% decrease in depressive symptoms as well as improved features within their individual EEGs. Although there were significant changes in the qEEGs, they were not uniform across all patients and varied from person to person. The group that received no treatment for 4 weeks following the 14 Hz AVE did maintain reduced symptoms of depression as well as improved neurological changes. In some cases the EEG continued to improve after no treatment, supporting the view that when the brain is given the opportunity to improve and reorganize, it often will.

More studies are needed to further validate this treatment modality, and the protocols leading to improved outcome.

CRANIAL ELECTROSTIMULATION

CES, also called cranial electrotherapy stimulation, is a noninvasive brain-based treatment being used for anxiety, insomnia, depression and many other disorders. This form of electromedicine is used to treat physical pain-related conditions and psychological symptoms with varying levels of electrical current stimulation. The stimulation is provided via electrodes or an electrode pen to the area identified to assist with the symptomatology. For chronic pain the electrode pads or pen are placed at the site where the patient is experiencing the pain, and for psychological disorders electrodes are often placed on the head or earlobes, where the individual feels a light tingling during the stimulation. This technology is easily adapted between clinical office use and home use by the client. Varying with the specific frequencies used for the stimulation, it reportedly produces a neurological response in the brain and other components of the nervous system that reduces pain, anxiety, hypervigilance, depression and more. There are currently over 150 published articles on the use of CES to treat an array of disorders, and symptoms with positive treatment outcomes.[52,53] Many frequencies from 0.5 Hz to 100 Hz have been used in the studies, with different frequencies being used to target different symptoms. The most current CES technology uses <1 mA of low-frequency (0.5 Hz) biphasic current applied with electrodes attached to the patient's earlobes, or on the head directly behind the ears. Treatment typically lasts anywhere from 20 to 60 minutes and can be done daily as needed. Patients can sit and relax, watch TV or even work on the computer while using CES. CES has been shown to increase electrical brainwave patterns in the alpha range (8–12 Hz), creating a calming, euphoric and soothing effect. Many clients report feeling a calm focus as a part of this treatment, increasing their ability to perform versus becoming overstressed and mentally shutting down. Kennerly[54] reported a decrease in beta frequency brain waves after treatment: these are often associated with anxiety and hypervigilance. He also noted deeper areas of activation, indicating that CES also affects subcortical areas of the brain. Patients report feeling a light tingling from the electrodes and report feeling effects of the stimulation within 2–5 minutes. Patients' reports on how long they feel the effects last vary considerably, with some reporting hours and others

1–2 days. There are currently minimal reports of any side effects, and no lasting adverse side effects have been reported. Many devices have been developed for CES, all reporting similar outcomes, but depending on the frequencies used. There are 25 published studies on the use of CES to treat depression.[55,56] They go back as far as the 1950s and include an array of treatment designs, with some patients on and off medications and some with previous medication failures. Gilula and Kirsch[57] published a literature review of multiple studies of CES for depression and highlighted those comparing CES to antidepressant medications. They reviewed data from 26 CES studies that included a placebo treatment group, and 52 medication studies that compared the efficacy of various antidepressants to placebo treatments. The standard protocol used in the studies of CES for depression included 20–60 minutes of CES daily for 3 weeks, with the intensity level at the comfort level of the participant, and then continued every other day or as needed. In the studies electrodes moistened with conductive solution were attached to the ears. Participants were encouraged to relax during treatment, but lying down or resting was not required. A total of 21 (81%) of the 26 CES depression studies reported improvements in depression symptomatology. According to study authors, the five studies that showed minimal or no improvement were early studies from the 1970s using equipment that is no longer used or available. Most participants reported having less anxiety, feeling less distressed, and having improved sleep, an improved sense of wellbeing and improved focus on tasks and learning activities. The review indicated that CES was three times more effective than medication when the effectiveness of each was compared to placebo. The average treatment effectiveness of placebo compared to antidepressant medications was 21.17%, whereas CES effectiveness compared to placebo was 63%. No significant side effects of CES are reported in the studies reviewed, and it can be used with or without medications. This is in contrast to the studies on antidepressants, which report multiple potential serious side effects ranging from increased suicidality in children and adolescents to liver metabolism issues and more. There are no reports of participants reporting dependence on the technology or increased suicidality. This meta-analysis comparison supports CES as a viable noninvasive brain-based therapy that is safe and effective for the treatment of depression, with or without medication. The study results support a need for more long-term studies measuring the efficacy, after 3–4 weeks, of CES to assess sustained effect on depression, and/or the need for adjunctive psychotherapy to produce long-term change. As a treatment it is cost-effective and easy to administer in the clinic and to observe effects and response, and is easily transferred to home use. However, in a very medication-focused western culture, some clients are convinced that medication is the best option and thus are resistant to the use of this technology. The other challenge that most clinicians are faced with includes the current standard of care, which considers medication as the first approach, and only if that does not work considers other safe alternatives. This leads to a situation where many clinicians continue to focus on the use of medications to treat depression, rather than reviewing, learning about or considering any nonmedication treatment options for their patients.

TRANSCRANIAL MAGNETIC STIMULATION

With an estimated 20–40% of depression patients not responding to medication, it is important to continue to search for alternative treatment interventions. Another such is TMS.[58] This is a noninvasive technique that provides electrical stimulation to the cerebral cortex in a specific area using a magnetic field. The stimulation occurs via an insulated coil placed above the scalp that is able to bypass the scalp and skull, thereby providing stimulation directly to the brain. This technique includes both single-pulse TMS and repetitive TMS. This procedure began to be explored after continued documentation and review of research showing patients with depression having reduced activity in the left prefrontal cortex. TMS is a procedure that is provided as an outpatient service, with minimal side effects and no cognitive impairment, such as is often documented after electroconvulsive therapy (ECT). The most common complaints include headaches and neck muscle tension. The sessions last 30–60 minutes and take place several times a week for a total of 20–30 sessions. The stimulation occurs at <1 Hz as well as at greater frequencies, depending on the chosen protocol and the disorder being treated. Many studies have explored the efficacy of this treatment, with varying results, often depending on the specific protocol. After a thorough review of protocols and previous single-center controlled studies showing mixed results, O'Reardon and colleagues[59] set up a double-blind, multisite study with 301 medication-free patients who had a history of negative response to antidepressant medication. The study was conducted at 23 sites in the United States, Australia and Canada, with participants ranging in age from 18 to 70 years. Patients were treated five times a week with 10 pulses/second stimulation for 3000 pulses/session over the left dorsolateral

prefrontal cortex for 4–6 weeks. TMS was shown to be safe and well tolerated when administered with this protocol, with minimal side effects and
no seizures reported. This study included both an active TMS and a sham
treatment group, with the TMS active group showing superior results to the
sham group by week 4, and increased improvement by week 6. The findings support that TMS administered for depression according to this protocol is safe and effective for MDD, and should be considered more often
in treatment-resistant patients. This study was the final documentation used
by the Food and Drug Administration (FDA) to support the use of TMS
for treatment-resistant depression. As a result, the FDA deemed that MDD
patients could receive TMS after one failed trial of antidepressants. Despite
FDA approval, insurance companies remain reluctant to reimburse for
TMS and still see antidepressant medication as the first line of defense in
treating MDD.

Dumas and colleagues[60] published a study looking not only at improvements in symptomatology in patients with MDD using TMS, but also at
health-related quality of life (HRQoL). Fifteen patients, 18 years and
older, diagnosed with MDD and a poor antidepressant treatment history, were selected to receive 20 low-frequency repetitive TMS (six 60-s
trains at 1 Hz) to the right dorsolateratal prefrontal cortex over a 4-week
period. The Role-Physical problems dimension they assessed showed a
statistically significant improvement, and before-and-after SPECT scans
showed a decrease in perfusion in the precuneus, an area involved in self-
processing and first-person perspective. The researchers correlated a direct
relationship between repetitive TMS and improvement in HRQoL with
the decrease in perfusion in the precuneus. This study indicated that low-
frequency repetitive TMS can improve HRQoL in patients with MDD.

Several other studies have investigated the role of TMS as an adjunct to
treatment in patients who are still experiencing symptoms despite being
medicated. Charnsil and colleagues[61] looked at the impact of 10 sessions
of repetitive TMS on patients in partial remission as an adjunct to treatment with medication. Patients were then followed up for 12 months
to determine the long-term effects. Nine patients were included in this
small study, and all had received medication for 8 weeks with no remission. Each patient received 10 sessions of TMS applied to the left dorsolateral prefrontal cortex while continuing their medication throughout.
Each Monday through Friday a daily session included 25 stimulation trains
at 10 Hz for 5 seconds, for a total of 10 sessions over a 2-week period.
The results revealed a positive outcome, with decreased symptomatology

and continued duration of the positive effects of treatment for up to 12 months. This research supports that TMS may be a viable adjunct to treatment for clients on medication but still experiencing symptoms.

Studies on TMS continue to increase, not only for MDD but for many other disorders, such as Parkinson's disease, bipolar disorder, anxiety and ADHD. TMS appears to be a promising noninvasive treatment that will increase in clinical use over the next several years. A key will be for insurance companies to begin to recognize this and other noninvasive brain-based therapies for reimbursement, which will increase their use substantially.

VAGAL NERVE STIMULATION

Vagal nerve stimulation (VNS) began to be considered as a possible treatment for depression when patients who were being treated for seizure disorders were reporting improvements in mood and affect as a result of the treatment. Later, clinicians began to look at it specifically for patients who had not responded to medications and/or ECT, and had clinically severe symptoms, with limited options for further treatment. It began being used in the early 1990s in Europe and the United States. VNS requires a brief outpatient surgery under local or general anesthesia, where a physician implants a small stimulation generator into the patient's left chest wall, and the lead from the generator is then connected to the vagus nerve. The generator is then activated by the physician with a "wand" to begin to create a set of stimulation settings to assist in reducing symptomatology. Side effects are minimal, but it usually takes a few months for patients to feel the full impact of relief. This would not be recommended for a patient having an acute episode of depression that is debilitating or indicative of harm to self or others, which requires immediate treatment. VNS is considered an adjunct to treatment and recommended only after all other options have been considered and tried.

In an open trial by Rush and colleagues,[62] 30 patients with major depression or bipolar disorder who had a minimum of two medication failures were treated with VNS. The patients received 10 weeks of stimulation along with medication. They showed a response rate of 40% and a remission rate of 17%. A second study completed in 2001, with 30 more patients, showed a positive response rate of 30% and remission rate of 15% over a 12-week period.[63]

The largest study using this treatment included 235 patients who received either VNS or a placebo/sham treatment. In this study, patients were at the highest level of treatment resistance, with multiple medication failures and failure to respond to ECT as well. Both groups received treatment over 12 weeks, and minimal difference was found between the two. There was only a 15% positive response rate and 10% remission rate; however, researchers noted that some true effects occurred over time, with a positive response increasing between 27% and 34%. Suicide attempts reportedly decreased, along with diminished levels of suicidal ideation.[64,65]

Overall, the efficacy and cost-effectiveness of this treatment need more study, especially when it is considered that the average cost for the stimulation generator is $40,000. It does appear to be effective in patients with MDD and bipolar disorder as an adjunct to medication management, and should be worth considering, especially after all other treatment modalities have failed or had minimal effect.

CONCLUSION

With the increased rate of mood disorders being diagnosed, there is enough clinical support to continue to explore the use of the various brain-based therapies discussed in this chapter in both children and adults. Considering such things as medication side effects and the lack of knowledge about the long-term impact of psychotropics (especially in children), these therapies may currently hold the best chance of producing long-term change in persons suffering from depression with and without medication. Upon review of the data from studies using the various brain-based therapies reviewed here, it is disappointing that the medical profession is not more willing to embrace neurofeedback, auditory visual stimulation, CES and TMS as potential viable treatments for patients with depression. With minimal side effects and the majority being cost-effective, it would seem that patients' long-term best interests would override a need to continue to use medications, especially for those experiencing little or no improvement. Currently many patients are prescribed not just one medication, but, when that medication is not yielding acceptable results or has negative side effects, others are added. Thus, many patients present clinically with as many as three, four or more psychotropic medications.

For motivated clients, neurofeedback is a viable option that can bring positive results over multiple sessions, but it does require the client to be involved in the process. It also requires ongoing sessions in a clinician's office setting for best practice and maximum results. Current research also supports that individualizing treatment with qEEG often affords the best outcomes, because the protocols are individualized for maximum results.

However, for many years protocols were developed, utilized and published that have shown consistent positive outcomes in studies without using qEEG as a determining factor for selecting protocols.

For clients who want quick relief in the moment, CES is a viable alternative that can be used in the clinical setting, or at the client's home, with maximal results occurring when used daily and consistently. This often requires some use of a home unit to accomplish. A benefit of this technology is that clients report symptom relief within 5 minutes. Another benefit of CES is that it requires minimal client involvement other than attaching the device to the ears and completing the session. AVE is another viable alternative that can be used both in the clinical setting and at home. It also requires minimal client involvement, other than to sit quietly throughout the session. The technology does the work for the client, with minimal side effects, but may take several sessions to achieve maximum relief or change. In contrast to CES, this technology does require multiple sessions to begin to achieve symptom reduction. TMS requires a medical provider at all times, and is not a device for home use. It also requires very little effort on the client's part other than regular trips to the clinicians office, and, compared to neurofeedback, CES and AVE are the most costly per session. VNS continues to be considered a last resort for treatment-resistant patients and is an invasive technique requiring surgery and multiple ongoing appointments with a provider. Of all of the techniques, VNS is the most costly, with probably the fewest published positive results compared to the other modalities. In summary, it is the author's opinion that in cases of mild to moderate depression that is not debilitating to the client, neurofeedback, CES and AVE are worthy of consideration. For more severe and treatment-resistant clients, TMS may be worth considering over ECT and prior to VNS.

REFERENCES

1. Kessler RC, Chiu WT, Demler O, Walters EE. Prevalence, severity, and comorbidity of twelve-month DSM-IV disorders in the National Comorbidity Survey Replication (NCS-R). *Arch Gen Psychiatry.* 2005;62(6):617–627.
2. Kessler RC, Burglund PB, Demler O, et al. The epidemiology of major depressive disorder: results from the national comorbidity survey replication (NCS-R). *JAMA.* 2003;289:3095–3105.
3. Blazer DG, Kessler RC, McGonagle KA, Swartz MS. The prevalence and distribution of major depression in a national community sample: The national comorbidity survey. *Am J Psy.* 1994;151(7):979–986.
4. McClintock SM, Husain MM, Wisniewski SR, et al. Residual symptoms in depressed patients who respond by 50% but do not remit to antidepressant medication. *J Clin Psychopharmacol.* 2011;31:180–186.

5. Judd LL, Paulus MJ, Schettler PJ, et al. Does incomplete recovery from first life-time major depressive episode herald a chronic course of illness? *Am J Psychiatry.* 2000;157:1501–1504.

6. Broadhead WE, Blazer DG, George LK, Tse CK. Depression, disability days, and days lost from work in a prospective epidemiological survey. *JAMA.* 1990;264(19):2524–2528.

7. Glenmullen J. *Prozac Backlash.* New York, NY: Simon & Schuster; 2000.

8. Antonuccio DO, Danton WG, DeNelsky GY, Greenberg RP, Gordon JS. Raising questions about antidepressants. *Psychother Psychosom.* 1999;68:3–14.

9. Kirsch I, Scoboria A, Moore TJ. Antidepressants and placebos: secrets, revelations, and unanswered questions. *Prev Treat.* 2002:5. Article 33.

10. Kirsch I, Sapirstein G. Listening to Prozac but hearing placebo: a meta-analysis of antidepressant medication. *Prev Treat.* 1998:1. Article 2.

11. John ER, Prichep LS, Friedman J, Eastman P. Neurometrics: computer assisted differ-ential diagnosis of brain dysfuntions. *Science.* 1988;293:162–169.

12. John ER, Prichep LS, Winterer G, Herrmann WM, diMichele F, Halper J. Electrophysiological subtypes of psychotic states. *Acta Psychiatr Scand.* 2007;116(1):17–35.

13. Robinson RG, Kubos KL, Starr LB, Rao K, Price TR. Mood disorders in stroke patients: importance of location of lesion. *Brain.* 1984:81–93.

14. Henriques JB, Davidson RJ. Left frontal hypoactivation in depression. *J Abnorm Psychol.* 1991;100:534–535.

15. Dawson G, Grofer Klinger L, Panagiotides H, Hill D, Spieker S. Frontal lobe activ-ity and affective behavior of infants of mothers with depressed symptoms. *Child Dev.* 1992;63:725–737.

16. Dawson G, Grofer Klinger L, Panagiotides H, Spieker S, Frey K. Infants of mothers with depressed symptoms: electroencephalographic and behavioral findings related to attachment status. *Dev Psychopathol.* 1992;4:67–80.

17. Davidson RJ. Cerebral assymetry, emotion and affective style. In: Davidson RJ, Hugdahl K. *Brain Asymmetry.* Cambridge, MA: MIT Press; 1995:369–388.

18. Kentgen LM, Tenke CE, Pine DS, Fong R, Klein RG, Bruder GE. Electroencephalographic asymmetries in adolescents with major depression: influence of comorbity with anxiety disorders. *J Abnorm Psychol.* 2000;109(4):797–802.

19. Saxby E, Peniston EG. Alpha-theta brainwave neurofeedback training: an effective treatment for male and female alcoholics with depressive symptoms. *J Clin Psychol.* 1995;51(5):685–693.

20. Peniston EG, Kulkowsky PJ. Alpha-theta brainwave training and beta-endorphin lev-els in alcoholics. *Alcohol Clin Exp Res.* 1989;13:271–279.

21. Peniston EG, Kulkosky PJ. Alpha-theta brainwave neurofeedback for vietnam veterans with combat related post traumatic stress disorder. *Med Psychother.* 1991;4:1–4.

22. Baehr E, Rosenfeld JP, Baehr R, Earnest C. Clinical use of an alpha asymmetry neu-rofeedback protocol in the treatment of mood disorders. In: Evans J, Abarbanel A, eds. *Introduction to Quantitative EEG and Neurofeedback.* San Diego: Academic Press; 1999:181–201.

23. Rosenfeld JP. EEG biofeedback of frontal alpha asymmetry in affective disorders. *Biofeedback.* 1997;25(1):8–25.

24. Choi SW, Chi SE, Chung SY, Kim JW, Ahn CY, Kim HT. Is alpha wave neuro-feedback effective with randomized clinical trials in depression? A pilot study. *Neuropsychobiology.* 2011;63:43–51.

25. Hammond DC. Neurofeedback treatment of depression with the Roshi. *J Neurotherapy.* 2000;4(2):45–56.

26. Hammond DC. Neurofeedback treatment of depression and anxiety. *J Adult Dev.* 2005;12:131–136.

27. Hammond DC. Neurofeedback with anxiety and affective disorders. In: Hirshberg LM, Chiu S, Frazier JA, eds. *Emerging Interventions Child and Adolescent Psychiatric Clinics of North America*; 2005:105–123.Vol. 14 (1).

28. Raymond J,Varney C, Parkinson LA, Gruzelier JH.The effects of alpha/theta neurofeedback on personality and mood. *Cogn Brain Res.* 2005;23:287–292.

29. Dias AM, van Deusen A.A new neurofeedback protocol for depression. *Span J Psychol.* 2011;14(1):374–384.

30. Johnston SJ, Boehm SG, Healy D, Goebel R, Linden DEJ. Neurofeedback: a promising tool for the self-regulation of emotion networks. *Neuroimage.* 2010;49:1066–1072.

31. Linden DE, Habes I, Johnston SJ, et al. Real-time self-regulation of emotion networks in patients with depression. *PLoS One.* 2012;7(6):e38115. http://dx.doi.org/10.1371/journal.pone.0038115 Epub 2012 Jun 4.

32. Lang PJ, Bradley MM, Guthbert BN. *International Affective Picture System (IAPS): Technical Manual and Affective Ratings.* Gainesville, FL: University of Florida, Center for Research in Psychophysiology; 1999.

33. Johnston SJ, Boehm SG, Healy D, Goebel R, Linden DE. Neurofeedback: a promising tool for the self-regulation of emotion networks. *Neuroimage.* 2010;49:1066–1072.

34. Johnston S, Linden DEJ, Healy D, Goebel R, Habes I, Boehm SG. Upregulation of emotion areas through neurofeedback with a focus on positive mood. *Cogn Affect Behav Neurosci.* 2011;11:44–51.

35. Adrian ED, Matthews BH.The Berger rhythm: potential changes from the occipital lobes of men. *Brain.* 1934;57:355–385.

36. Toman J. Flicker potentials and the alpha rhythm in man. *J Neurophysiol.* 1941;4:51–61.

37. Cady RK, Shealy N. *Neurochemical Responses to Cranial Electrical Stimulation and Photo-Stimulation via Brain Wave Synchronization.* Springfield, MO: Study performed by the Shealy Institute of Comprehensive Health Care; 1990.

38. Kroger WS, Schnieder SA. An electronic aid for hypnotic induction: a preliminary report. *Int J Clin Exp Hypn.* 1959;7:93–98.

39. Chatrian G, Petersen M, Lazarte J. Responses to clicks from the human brain: some depth electrographic observation. *Electroencephalogr Clin Neurophysiol.* 1960;12:479–487.

40. Sadove MS. Hypnosis in anesthesiology. *Ill Med J.* 1963;124:39–42.

41. Fox P, Raichle M. Stimulus rate determines regional blood flow in striate cortex. *Ann Neurol.* 1985;17(3):303–305.

42. Fox P, Raichle M, Mintun M, Dence C. Nonoxidative glucose consumption during focal physiologic neural activity. *Science.* 1988;241:462–464.

43. Frederick J, Lubar J, Rasey H, Brim S, Blackburn J. Effects of 18.5 Hz audiovisual stimulation on EEG amplitude at the vertex. *J Neurotherapy.* 1999;3:23–27.

44. Gagnon C, Boersma F.The use of repetitive audio-visual entrainment in the management of chronic pain. *Med Hypnoanalysis J.* 1992;7:462–468.

45. Anderson D. The treatment of migraine with variable frequency photic stimulation. *Headache.* 1989;29:154–155.

46. Carter J, Russell H.A pilot investigation of audio and visual entrainment of brainwave activity in learning disabled boys. *Texas Researcher.* 1993;4:65–72.

47. Berg K, Siever D. A controlled comparison of audio-visual entrainment for treating seasonal affective disorder. *J Neurotherapy: Investigations in Neuromodulation, Neurofeedback and Appl Neurosci.* 2009;13(3):166–175.

48. Cantor D, Stevens E. QEEG correlates of auditory-visual entrainment treatment efficacy of refractory depression. *J Neurotherapy.* 2009;13:100–108.

49. Kumano H, Horie H, Shidara T, et al.Treatment of a depressive disorder patient with EEG driven photic stimulation. *Biofeedback Self Reg.* 1996;21(4):323–334.

50. John ER, Prichep LS, Friedman J, Eastman P. Neurometrics: computer assisted differential diagnosis of brain dysfunctions. *Science*. 1988;293:162–169.
51. John ER, Prichep LS, Winterer G, Herrmann WM, diMichele F, Halper J. Electrophysiological subtypes of psychotic states. *Acta Psychiatr Scand*. 2007;116(1):17–35.
52. Kirsch DL. Why electromedicine? *Pract Pain Manage*. 2006;6(5):52–54.
53. Kirsch DL, Marksberry JA. Advances in cranial electrotherapy stimulation. *Pract Pain Manage*. 2011;11(3):77–81.
54. Kennerly, R. Changes in quantitative EEG and low resolution tomography following cranial electrotherapy stimulation. Unpublished doctoral dissertation, University of North Texas; 2006.
55. Kirsch DL, Gilula M. Cranial electrotherapy stimulation in the treatment of depression, Part 1. *Pract Pain Manage*. 2007;7(4):33–41.
56. Kirsch DL, Gilula M. Cranial electrotherapy stimulation in the treatment of depression, Part 2. *Pract Pain Manage*. 2007;7(5):32–40.
57. Gilula MF, Kirsch DL. Cranial electrotherapy stimulation review: a safer alternative to psychopharmaceuticals in the treatment of depression. *J Neurotherapy: Investigations in Neuromodulation, Neurofeedback and Appl Neurosci*. 2005;9(2):7–26.
58. Greden JF. The burden of recurrent depression: causes, consequences and future prospects. *J Clin Psychiatry*. 2001;22:5–9.
59. O'Reardon JP, Solvason HB, Janicak PG, et al. Efficacy and safety of transcranial magnetic stimulation in the acute treatment of major depression: A multisite randomized controlled trial. *Biol Psychiatry*. 2007;62(11):1208–1216.
60. Dumas R, Richieri R, Guedj E, Auquier P, Lancon C, Boyer L. Improvement of health related quality of life in depression after transcranial magnetic stimulation in a naturalistic trial is associated with decreased perfusion in precuneus. *Health Qual Life Outcomes*. 2012;10:87.
61. Charnsil C, Suttajit S, Boonyanaruthee V, Leelarphat S. Twelve–month, prospective, open label study of repititive magnetic stimulation for major depressive disorder in partial remission. *Neuropsychiatr Dis Treat*. 2012;8:393–397.
62. Rush AJ, George MS, Sackeim HA, et al. Vagus nerve stimulation (VNS) for treatment-resistant depressions: a multicenter study. *Biol Psychiatry*. 2000;47:276–286.
63. Sackeim HA, Rush AJ, George MS, et al. Vagus nerve stimulation (VNS) for treatment resistant depression: efficacy, side effects, and predictors of outcome. *Neuropsychopharmacology*. 2001;25:713–728.
64. Rush AJ, Marangell LB, Sackeim HA, et al. Vagus nerve stimulation for treatment-resistant depression: a randomized, controlled acute phase trial. *Biol Psychiatry*. 2005;58:347–354.
65. Rush AJ, Sackeim HA, Marangell LB, et al. Effects of 12 months of vagus nerve stimulation in treatment-resistant depression: a naturalistic study. *Biol Psychiatry*. 2005;58:355–363.

CHAPTER EIGHT

Diagnosing and Treating Closed Head Injury

Exposing and Defeating the Mild Huge Monster

Carlos A. Novo-Olivas

INTRODUCTION

Head injury, or traumatic brain injury (TBI), is a very heterogeneous entity, with no standardized diagnostic system – in fact, with no established and official definition (see below). The two major causes of trauma are falls and automobile accidents, although other violent events have increased substantially in the last decade.[1] Most patients are children (<5 years), young men (15–35 years) and the elderly (>70 years). The severity of TBI depends on multiple factors, and classification has a long and complex history. It is still under debate, as are the consequences of the traumatic event in the short and the long term.[2] An important project on this essential issue, Common Data Element (TBI CDE),[3] is being led by the National Institute of Neurological Disorders and Stroke, with support from the Brain Injury Association of America, the Defense and Veterans Brain Injury Center, and the National Institute of Disability and Rehabilitation Research. Through the Demographics and Clinical Assessment Working Group of the International and Interagency Initiative, the TBI CDE has formed an expert group that proposes the following definition: "TBI is defined as an alteration in brain function, or other evidence of brain pathology, caused by an external force".[4] An update can be found at the TBI CDE webpage and in Adelson et al.[5] An important paper by Ruff et al.[6] is also recommended.

Despite decades of research, TBI is still one of the leading causes of death and disability worldwide, and, in some populations, both geographically and age-wise, it is the leading one. In the last century, the field of TBI has

Clinical Neurotherapy.
Doi: http://dx.doi.org/10.1016/B978-0-12-396988-0.00008-8

been evolving and great advances have been made, especially with regard to intensive care, resulting in improved rates of survival. The numbers of mild and moderate disabilities have gradually increased in the last 30 years, and there are no pharmaceutical options to mitigate those consequences.[7] With some exceptions, cognitive and psychological approaches have little or no efficacy.[8–10] Excellent reviews and meta-analyses of cognitive training can be found elsewhere.[11,12] There is no efficacious therapy per se, so an integrative approach often is recommended. However, which therapies are the best to incorporate remains debatable. The Department of Veterans" Affairs of the Department of Defense, through the Management of Concussion/MTBI Working Group, has published clinical guidelines for the management of mild traumatic brain injury (MTBI);[13] other reviews and guidelines on the matter are also recommended.[14,15] For more than 40 years, operant conditioning using electroencephalography (EEG), also called neurofeedback, has been used to treat resistant epilepsy, attention deficit disorder, learning disabilities, autism, depression, anxiety disorders, the sequelae of acquired brain injury (traumatic and vascular), and other disorders and symptoms.[16–19] An overview of research especially relevant to MTBI is presented below. It is proposed that, although further research is badly needed, neurofeedback should be part of the integrative treatment for these patients.

EPIDEMIOLOGY

While you were reading the above, almost 50 people died from head trauma worldwide – almost 6 million a year.[20] In the United States in the last two decades around 1.5 million people were treated in emergency departments (EDs) for TBI each year; 80% of them were released from the ED. The incidence of MTBI is around 300–500/100,000 per year. The number of persons who have suffered a TBI and not sought medical attention in a hospital setting, or did not seek attention at all, is unknown, but could be as high as 50% more than the officially reported number (near 3 million). It has been estimated that 5–6 million people in the United States have long-term disabilities resulting from TBI,[21–24] and it is well established that MTBI is a risk factor for chronic degenerative disorders, such as Alzheimer and Parkinson's disease.[25,26]

The literature on the sequelae of MTBI is enormous, complex and contradictory. Some authors report that, of those suffering MTBI, around 20% (up to 70% or as low as 5%) will experience symptoms of post-concussion syndrome (PCS) for more than a year, the most common

symptoms being fatigue, affective disorders, irritability, vertigo, attention and memory deficits, low verbal fluency, chronic pain (especially
headache), anxiety disorders and sleep disturbances.[27–38] Very often these
after-effects are not considered significant, or are regarded as "psychological", meaning not real, or at least nonbiological, which seems illogi-
cal and ontologically wrong. The different criteria for diagnosis (DSM-IV
and ICD-10) of PCS make it impossible to have acceptable epidemiologic
data. A large study reported that only 56% of the patients from more than
2500 cases with MTBI had no symptoms 3 months after the injury;[39]
on the other hand, an elegant meta-analysis concluded that: "…to date
six meta-analytic reviews, including the present one, found no evidence
of a significant difference between the MTBI groups and the control
groups."[40] There is an urgent need for integrative prospective studies in
the general population to clarify the impact of MTBI and the variables
that may contribute to PCS.

PATHOPHYSIOLOGY

The forces (direct trauma and/or acceleration–deceleration and
rotational) producing the primary injury could last as little as 100 ms, but
the secondary processes that follow can occur in the next hours, days and
even months. It is known that the linear acceleration forces affect especially the cortex and the meninges, while the rotational forces have their
major impact on the axons (diffuse axonal injury), and the longer the
duration of injury, the more damage produced. There is some damage to
deep structures that could be explained by stereotactic theory, which considers the spherical shape of the cranial vault as well as the vibrations produced at the moment of the injury and their ability to generate secondary
pressure waves. These waves travel and focus energy on the middle of the
encephalic mass (deep cortical and subcortical structures). The trauma
also has a systemic influence (adrenaline rush, hypoxia, arterial hypoten-
sion, hyperglycemia), which can effect the whole brain (seizures, cortical
spreading depression, loss of autoregulation), and can act at the cellular
level (release of excitatory amino acids, increase of inflammatory molecules, influx of calcium ions, cytoskeletal degradation and apoptosis). Each
of these contributes to the primary and secondary processes of the brain
injury at different scales and times.[41–43] The pathophysiological mechanisms are complex and not the focus of this chapter but can be reviewed
elsewhere.[44–46]

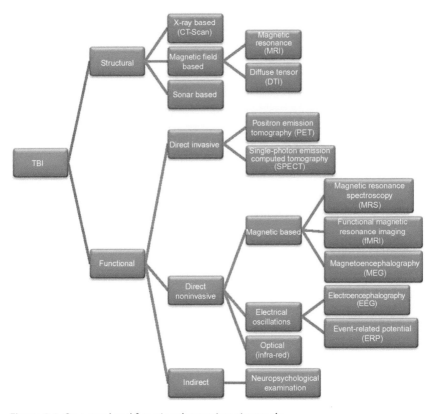

Figure 8.1 Structural and functional neuroimaging tools.

DIAGNOSTIC TOOLS

The tools used for the diagnosis of TBI are illustrated in Figure 8.1.

In this chapter the utility of EEG in the diagnosis of MTBI and PCS will be reviewed. For a more complete review of this topic, the reader is referred to the special issue of *Brain Imaging and Behavior* from June 2012,[47] and to another reference,[48] where neuropathological, neuroimaging and neuropsychological findings and their correlations are thoroughly covered.

ELECTROENCEPHALOGRAPHY (EEG)

The ability to measure brain electrical activity took a revolutionary step when Hans Berger and his engineers made the first modern electrical amplifier of brain electrical activity. A few years before, in 1924, when still using a galvanometer, he planned to create a better apparatus. He stated, "I have cherished over 20 years that the device would develop into some kind of cerebroscope."[49] The EEG captures the electrical changes produced by billions of synapses of the pyramidal neurons of the cortex. A way to imagine this is by taking a stadium (cranium) full of people (neurons) as a metaphor (dangerous, but necessary) and trying to imagine that we want to learn what is going on inside the stadium just by hearing what the people are doing through studying their singing and applauding (clapping). So, we use microphones and amplifiers to record the sounds coming out from the stadium. In this metaphor, let the singing of the people represent the *synaptic* potentials of the pyramidal neurons of the cortex. If a lot of people can join in and synchronize with the same song, the greater the volume (voltage) of the sound will be. Somewhat similarly, the more cortical neurons that fire in synchrony, the greater the voltage of the brain's electrical oscillations, i.e., the greater their amplitude and power. The claps, however, are the *action* potentials of the pyramidal neuron – very fast and hard to synchronize, and so rarely heard. An essential aspect of the EEG is not about the song (frequency and volume) that is being produced, but about where and in synchronization with which others that song is being sung (corresponding roughly to what is involved in EEG connectivity measures, such as coherence). It should be apparent from this metaphor that, just as the song and the applause of persons in a stadium may be difficult to measure and, in any event, not tell the whole story of events in the stadium, so it is with EEG activity coming from a human cranium. The physiological and technical basis of EEG should be well understood by readers who plan to use EEG measures, and such information can be found elsewhere.[50,51]

The analysis of complex information, such as the EEG, changed greatly in 1965, when the work of Cooley and Tukey[51a] made possible a faster analysis of the Fast Fourier Transform (FFT). From that time on, the old time-consuming classic techniques used to quantify the EEG spectrum were replaced.[52] By the mid-1980s the recording of brain electric activity using a digital amplifier was beginning to be customary, and a decade later it was the most-used way to acquire and store an EEG in developed countries. Today, all EEGs are digital in nature. The digital EEG (dEEG) uses a different kind of amplifier, converting analog electrical activity to a binomial language. Thus, dEEG today is really a mathematical transformation from its acquisition to a computerized storage that can be called into forms of visual and quantitative analysis.

Quantitative EEG (qEEG) refers to the process by which we can extract mathematical values from the digitized EEG and use those numbers in multiple ways. This usually involves determining the amount of energy in single frequencies (or in frequency bands) across the full spectrum of a sample of EEG (spectral analysis). There are several mathematical methods to perform a spectral analysis, but the most used is the FFT. These procedures also can be used to produce statistical values for a group of people on different EEG measures, thereby enabling the development of databases with normalized EEG measures against which one can compare the EEGs of others. This is referred to as norm-referenced EEG (nEEG). Unfortunately, the terms digital, quantitative and normative are used in the literature as if they were synonymous, but not all digitized EEG is qEEG and not all qEEG is nEEG.

The medical guild has always undervalued the qEEG, claiming it lacks the ability to localize sources of abnormality. Fortunately, the science of source localization has advanced greatly, and we can now say that EEG is another functional neuroimaging tool.[47,53] For more on qEEG and nEEG the reader is encouraged to see these references.[54–60]

DIAGNOSIS OF MTBI WITH EEG

The first paper reporting on this matter was by Jasper and colleagues in 1940,[61] allowing us to say that EEG was the first neurodiagnostic tool to demonstrate brain damage after a TBI. For such a common pathology, research regarding the value of qEEG as a diagnostic tool is surprisingly scarce. This chapter will focus on the argument that qEEG (especially nEEG) should be the gold standard in the diagnosis of MTBI and PCS, in both the acute and the long-term phases. This reasoning is based on its low cost, easy application and portability, high reliability and stability and, very importantly, its high sensitivity and specificity. For reviews the reader is referred to these references.[62–65]

Since the first reports of an EEG discriminant index for TBI by Thatcher and his group[66–68] and by Thornton,[69] similar findings have been reported for a Spanish population using a qEEG discriminant function called the Seville Independence Index (SINDI).[70] In this study, 81 patients suffering from acquired brain injury (TBIs or stroke) were almost 100% accurately classified with the SINDI, even though the mean time between injury and EEG recording was 22 months. The best discriminant values were connectivity measures of coherence and phase, demonstrating once more the original findings of Thatcher and collaborators. It is clear that qEEG measurements of connectivity can be found that enable high sensitivity and specificity far beyond 6 months post injury. This phenomenon of long-lasting effects has been called the Big Bump Theory, referring to how a single action, such as the Big Bang, can generate huge and perpetual changes – in this case in the brain (see "Big Bump Theory"),[68] especially in those patients with clinical symptoms.

In the last few years, interesting research has been done, where pre- and postinjury evaluations of the same subjects found similar EEG abnormalities to those of Thatcher et al. The first study of this kind[71] assessed 61 college student athletes at high risk of TBI using 19-channel EEG, 30 of whom actually suffered from an MTBI during the year following initial testing. A novel classification algorithm, "the support vector machine" (SVM), was applied to identify residual functional abnormalities in athletes suffering from concussion. The total accuracy was 77.1%. The discriminant function had a sensitivity of 96.7% (using linear analysis of SVM), and 80.0% (for nonlinear SVM). Another study from this research group[72] involved evaluating 160 college athletes with a 19-channel EEG prior to injury. Twenty-nine of the subjects suffered an MTBI in the next 6 months and were evaluated again 7 days after injury. EEG source localization software was used and several connectivity methods were applied. Although most of the patients were asymptomatic by day 7, and back to baseline with regard to neuropsychological measurements, qEEG analysis continued to show significant pre–post injury differences. The main abnormal findings were in connectivity and asymmetry measures. A year later this group[73] recruited and evaluated 265 athletes from the Pennsylvania State University who had no history of MTBI. During the next 12 months, everyone who suffered one concussive episode was retested around 30 days after the injury. All 30 of these MTBI subjects were asymptomatic and normal on neuropsychological testing by day 7, but on one EEG measure used (Shannon entropy of the peak frequency shifting) there was no return to normal. In a more recent study the same group tested 380 athletes before injury, 49 of whom later had an MTBI (mild concussion). Postinjury evaluation revealed a correlation between the rate of alpha suppression and both balance and clinical recovery.[74] A good overview of this research can be found in Slobounov et al.[75] Another series of reports of research in which athletes were tested before injury has been published. These studies have in common that they all used an EEG device (Brain Scope) with limited leads (four frontal, referenced to the ears). Compared to traditional EEG equipment, this is easier to carry and faster to apply on the patient, especially in the ED or any other emergency situation. The first research[76] involved 105 MTBI patients and 50 controls (also patients from the ED, but with no brain-related emergencies). The EEG data were acquired during 10 minutes with eyes closed and at rest. One to two minutes of artifact-free data were analyzed using a TBI discriminant index (automatic analysis). The discriminant function had a high sensitivity (92%) for those patients with positive computed tomography (CT) findings (complicated concussion), and only 34.6% on those with negative CT findings. The low sensitivity in the milder cases might be explained by the limited number of EEG channels used. In another interesting study,[77] 396 college athletes were assessed before injury. Of those, 28 suffered an MTBI and were tested again after injury: (on the day of injury, and 7 days and 45 days after injury). They found that by day 7 the neuropsychological testing results were back to baseline, but qEEG findings were still abnormal, especially measures of coherence (low), asymmetries (high) and power (increased in the beta band). It was not until day 45 that qEEG measures were not significantly different and approaching baseline values.

Another elegant paper,[78] using the same index and methodology on 65 MTBI athletes, reported a severity discriminant between mild and moderate concussion, with an accuracy prediction of 94% on who would return to sport before 14 days. With a larger group of 119 MTBI patients from multiple EDs, the authors[79] attempted to predict positive CT findings using the New Orleans Criteria (NOC). They reported that the qEEG TBI index had 94.7% sensitivity and the NOC had 92.1%, but a main difference was on the specificity value, where the qEEG index was 49.4% against just 23.5% using NOC. Finally, Prichep and colleagues,[80] considering the argument that there has been no objective measurement tool for diagnosing MTBI, provide an overview of this new methodology (Brain Scope), and its high sensitivity (96%) and specificity (78%) with patients assessed in the ED who had positive findings on a CT scan. They concluded that such an automatic, portable and easy to use tool is of high utility in the acute clinical setting.

It is not feasible to review here the research findings on MTBI using other neuroimaging tools, or their correlations with qEEG. For recent reviews on these issues please see these references.[46,48,75,81–86] Findings with these other tools do correlate with neuropathological findings, and with the physiopathology of MTBI. This is especially true for diffuse axonal injury, which strongly correlates with qEEG coherence and phase-lag measurements and with diffusion tension imaging, a magnetic resonance technique in which white matter (axons) is captured, also known as tractography.[87] Although a lot remains to be done regarding the diagnosis of MTBI in its acute phase, and especially in its chronic phase (or PCS), I have no doubt that the best paraclinical tool today for aiding in the diagnosis of MTBI and PCS is qEEG.

TREATING THE "SILENT EPIDEMIC"

Because we need integrative diagnosis, we also need integrative treatment.[88] There is no single therapeutic answer for most human disorders, and brain disorders are no exception. The therapies that are most used to handle PCS are cognitive training, behavioral and educational therapy, and other rehabilitation programs such as speech and motor therapy. The diagnosis of PCS is "foggy," unspecific, and based on weak pathophysiological grounds. This makes certain therapies very attractive to try to implement, especially those that directly modify brain function, either by actively stimulating the cortex or passively guiding (conditioning) brain activity based on neurophysiological data.

EEG BIOFEEDBACK

Any physiological function that can be measured can, in principle, be conditioned to a stimulus, and hence be manipulated. This is the principle of any operant conditioning therapy using biosignals. EEG biofeedback, a form of brain–computer interface and commonly called neurofeedback, has been used to treat multiple disorders.[89] Neurofeedback involves an operant conditioning learning process that uses qEEG data as the behavior to which a stimulus is to be correlated, with the goal of modifying specific brain function and its cognitive and behavioral effects. It is important to mention that neurofeedback training also can be accomplished with other tools, such as near infrared spectometry, magnetoencephalography or functional MRI. To provide neurofeedback in a proper manner, an accurate and complete diagnosis has to be made, for which nEEG[90] and a previous expert visual analysis of the EEG tracings are considered essential.

Research on the efficacy of neurofeedback with MTBI–PCS is very limited, and most published data have important shortfalls such as small numbers of subjects, heterogeneous groups, no control group and/or no objective measurements. This makes it impossible to determine the efficacy of neurofeedback in the treatment of PCS. Since the first review[91] 12 years ago, where specific suggestions for future research were given, there has not been a single Class I (prospective, randomized controlled clinical trial in a representative population) paper published on the issue. Even more surprising is the fact that in indexed publications, more reviews have been published than research articles. Only around 10 publications (two of them indexed), and four reviews[10,65,92,93] have been published since 2000.

The first reports seem to be those of Ayers,[94,95] with patients ranging across the full spectrum of severity. Positive results were reported in most of the cases, using different neurofeedback protocols. In most cases treatment involved reducing slow frequencies (<7 Hz) and reinforcing 15–18 Hz. For a review of these series of cases please see Ayers.[96] It is important to say that this research was never published in a peer-reviewed publication, and any conclusions have to be taken with caution. The reports of Thornton and collaborators[93,97,98] involved a total of eight TBI patients in the three publications. There were consistently positive findings, but the small numbers and many research design weaknesses in each of one of these reports only permit one to conclude, along with the authors, that neurofeedback seems a promising tool in the area and may be effective, but much more research needs to be done.

To the author's knowledge, since the last review in 2009[65] only two papers have been published, and one of them used an unusual "innovative electroencephalography (EEG)-based therapy,"[99] the Flexyx Neurotherapy System (FNS). The first report was by a group in Macedonia,[100] in which six patients with more than 2 days of coma (all severe TBI) were treated 2–5 years after injury. The authors measured cognitive function with the Wisconsin Card Sorting Test and the Stroop Color Word Test. They also acquired EEG data and used the Human Brain Institute Database (HBID) for nEEG. Of these six patients, one had no cognitive sequelae, and the authors failed to explain why this subject was taken into account. Most of the subjects were young (15–19 years old) and well functioning before injury. Neurofeedback therapy was applied twice a week for 20 sessions of 40 minutes each, where 4–7 Hz power was inhibited and 10–14 Hz power increases were rewarded. Before the neurofeedback session, a 15-minute session of peripheral biofeedback, based on skin conductance or heart rate variability, was applied. A complex EEG measurement considered indicative of arousal (referred to by the authors as "Brain Rate"), was acquired, and all TBI patients had a Brain Rate index lower than the norms (HBID). The results reported by the authors are vague and general. One of their conclusions was: "Along with the changes in EEG spectra, improvements of general mood, quality of sleep, and cognitive abilities were obtained. Four of our patients were considerably improved and continued with studies…". Only one patient did not show any improvements, and one must suppose that changes in the other were not significant. Although the patients were reported as improved, nowhere in the paper was it explained how they measured mood and quality of sleep. Also, as mentioned before, one of the patients had no cognitive problems, and this was not the one who did not show any improvement. So, the reader is left to believe that this patient did improve in his or her cognitive function, despite having an IQ score of 140 after injury. No objective data are given on the neuropsychological testing following treatment. I fully support their final conclusion about the need to assess the efficacy of neurofeedback in TBI patients compared to other treatment modalities in larger samples.

In the spring of 2012 Nelson and Esty,[101] using FNS, which they described as "a novel variant of EEG biofeedback," recruited seven veterans with persistent PCS and posttraumatic stress disorder (PTSD) resistant to medications. The FNS is not a conventional biofeedback process, and in fact is not totally an operant conditioned learning activity, because a very weak electrical signal is returned to the patient based on EEG activity[99]; this method is known also as low-energy neurofeedback system, although the patients were administered the Neurobehavioral Functioning Inventory (NFI) and the PTSD Symptom Scale (PSS) before and after treatment. The participants received two to three sessions per week for a total of 22–25 sessions. Of the seven subjects, only five completed treatment and posttreatment testing. Of these five, two discontinued therapy before the end of the 25 sessions (13 and 17 sessions, respectively) because of improvements in their symptoms to "minimally acceptable levels," meaning they dramatically improved. There was significant improvement on almost all measurements of the NFI and PSS. All subjects, if taking medication, substantially reduced their medication doses following treatment. As the authors concluded, even when good results are found, these should be taken as preliminary results, and larger, controlled and randomized studies are warranted.

The total number of TBI subjects treated in studies that have been published in peer-reviewed publications is no more than 150; and no more than 40 of these patients were in indexed publications (that is, indexed in Medline); this makes neurofeedback a very weak treatment option with regard to evidence-based medicine. Furthermore, not all of those subjects were MTBI-PCS patients. Although the efficacy of neurofeedback has been established as a treatment in other disorders[102,103] as well as for improving performance in healthy subjects,[104] the assumption that it is as efficacious with PCS patients is just that, and scientific proof is needed. It is desirable that in the near future more research will be completed involving larger numbers of subjects, appropriate control groups, and proper diagnosis and evaluation. This could change the present situation to one of a well-established, evidence-based reality concerning the efficacy of neurofeedback in MTBI-PCS.

TRANSCRANIAL STIMULATION TOOLS

With some exceptions where approval has been given by the Food and Drug Administration and efficacy has been proven,[105] the use of noninvasive brain stimulation (NIBS) is still considered experimental. This includes its use with MTBI. In fact, it is very much like the case of neurofeedback, where clinical research has been published on many neuropsychiatric disorders, although their cellular and molecular mechanisms are not well understood. For both modalities the potential to promote neural–synaptic plasticity has been reported.[106–108] NIBS involves different tools that use either electric or magnetic forces to stimulate the cortex from outside the cranium (see Paulus[109] for an excellent review). The idea of using electrical stimulation to improve the body has been documented since the time of the ancient Egyptians.[49]

Transcranial magnetic stimulation (TMS), or repetitive TMS (rTMS), was introduced into the clinical setting almost 30 years ago, and since then thousands of papers have been published. Its application on TBI patients is in the initial phase, with a handful of publications, most of them involving severe and comatose patients. A first review[110] concluded that, based on the data presented in that paper, TMS deserved to be investigated on TBI patients. The authors mentioned that an initial study using a modified rTMS technology was being planned using severe TBI patients during recovery from coma. This was in fact done, and the results published on a single case study[111] showed promising but inconclusive results.

There was another single case report[79] involving a young male with hypoxic encephalopathy who was in a prolonged coma, and both neurofeedback and TMS were provided. Small progress on neuropsychological testing and event-related potential results after neurofeedback (beta training), and major improvements after a TMS program, were reported. It seems clear that although NIBS therapies should not be the only treatment for rehabilitation after TBI, it can enhance and potentiate other therapeutic programs. And, although a lot of work remains to be done, a new era in neurotherapeutics appears to be on its way. For excellent reviews the reader is referred to these references.[76,112,113]

INTRACRANIAL STIMULATION

Although the main focus of this chapter is MTBI and very little has been done in the clinical setting using intracranial stimulation tools, it is important to mention that deep brain stimulation (DBS) techniques have been used in patients with severe brain injury (both traumatic and non-traumatic) for more than half a century. Probably the group with the most experience in this field is the one led by Yamamoto and Katayama from Nihon University in Japan.[114] They reported 26 cases, 21 of them in persistent vegetative state (PVS) and five in a minimally conscious state (MCS), of whom only nine had had a traumatic incident. The majority of the patients (24) had the electrodes implanted in the thalamus between 3 and 6 months after injury, which some[115] have criticized as being too early. The authors have reported that eight of the 21 PVS patients and four of the five MCS patients had significant improvement. A study[116] compared these same patients with another set of patients treated with spinal cord stimulation (SCS), and the authors concluded that DBS may be useful for both MCS and PVS, whereas SCS could be effective in MCS when the candidate selection was based on electrophysiological criteria. Another important group led by Nicholas Schiff from Weill Cornell Medical College in New York, which published a widely cited paper in *Nature* in 2007,[117] have recently published a series of single-case studies in which they concluded that DBS "significantly increase functional communication, motor performance, feeding, and object naming in the DBS on state, with performance in some domains remaining above baseline even after DBS was turned off."[118] For excellent reviews the reader is referred to these references.[119,120]

CONCLUSIONS

In a country where at least 2 million persons annually suffer from an MTBI and at least 10% of them will have permanent sequelae, with possible effects on their quality of life and their aging process,[121] it is imperative that biologically based diagnostic and prognostic tools be developed and used. There is no doubt in this author's mind that qEEG is an excellent tool, and the best available today, to aid in the diagnosis of MTBI and PCS. It is important to mention here that research is needed to differentiate between MTBI-PCS and other neuropsychiatric disorders with similar symptomatology (depression, PTSD, dementias, sleep disorders) that are not secondary to injury. However, it is very possible that these disorders share similar pathophysiological mechanisms, independent of the cause (trauma, vascular insults, endocrinologic disorders, etc.). As with all diseases, especially the chronic-degenerative disorders, it is well accepted that the cause is the sum of multiple variables. Therefore, it is ideal to have an integrative diagnosis,[79,122,123] where genetic markers,[124,125] simultaneous multi-neuroimaging tools,[48,126] molecular markers,[127,128] neuropsychological testing, clinical picture, personal history and common epidemiological data are fused in a single database. This could enable correlations to be found that might give reliable information for an etiopathogenic diagnosis, personalized treatment and accurate prognosis.

In the last decade important research has been conducted applying neurofeedback in neuropsychiatric disorders, and some progress has been made regarding MTBI. This is why we conclude that neurofeedback is a promising therapy inside an integrative management program for PCS. However, Class I evidence for this still is needed. New technology permitting neurofeedback training based on data from real-time qEEG (as in Z-score neurofeedback), and/or from low-resolution brain electromagnetic tomography (LORETA), appears to be more powerful techniques of neurofeedback,[97,129,130] and is increasingly being applied. Hopefully, in the near future publications will come from rehabilitation programs such as that at Fort Campbell, in which soldiers are being extensively tested with behavioral and psychological evaluations prior to implementation of LORETA Z-score neurofeedback.[130] Further research focusing specifically on this type of neurofeedback with MTBI-PCS is needed in order to determine its efficacy and possible superiority over conventional (surface amplitude-based) neurofeedback.

The use of TMS and other extracranial stimulating therapies[101,131,132] opened a new window on the field of clinical neuroscience, and, along with neuroimaging technologies, promises to revolutionize the field of brain research. Although the efficacy of NIBS tools in brain injury in general is still unknown, and a lot of questions on technical details are debated, there is no doubt that these technologies have an important impact on brain function and microstructure. In the near future more data on their applications in TBI can be expected, and hopefully will soon be taken into the clinic to become part of the therapeutic arsenal against this "silent epidemic" that is harming millions of the young people, the future essential pillars of our society.

ACKNOWLEDGMENT

I fully appreciate Elizabeth Soto-Cabrera MD, for her important help and insight.

REFERENCES

1. Weber JT. Altered calcium signaling following traumatic brain injury. *Front Pharmacol.* 2012;3:60.
2. Rapp PE, Curley KC. Is a diagnosis of 'mild traumatic brain injury' a category mistake? *J Trauma Acute Care Surg.* 2012;73(2):S13–S23.
3. TBI CDEs. National Institute of Neurological Disorders and Stroke, with support from the Brain Injury Association of America, the Defense and Veterans Brain Injury Center, and the National Institute of Disability and Rehabilitation Research. *NINDS TBI Common Data Elements* 2012. Accessed August 12, 2012. <http://www.commondataelements.ninds.nih.gov/TBI.aspx#tab=Data_Standards>.
4. Menon DK, Schwab K, Wright DW, Maas AI. Demographics and clinical assessment working group of the international and interagency initiative toward common data elements for research on traumatic brain injury and psychological health. Position statement: definition of traumatic brain injury. *Arch Phys Med Rehabil.* 2010;91(11):1637–1640.
5. Adelson PD, Pineda J, Bell MJ, Pediatric TBI Demographics and Clinical Assessment Working Group. Common data elements for pediatric traumatic brain injury: recommendations from the working group on demographics and clinical assessment. *J Neurotrauma.* 2012;29(4):639–653.
6. Ruff RM, Iverson GL, Barth JT, Bush SS, Broshek DK, NAN Policy and Planning Committee. Recommendations for diagnosing a mild traumatic brain injury: a National Academy of Neuropsychology education paper. *Arch Clin Neuropsychol.* 2009;24(1):3–10.
7. Agoston DV, Risling M, Bellander B. Bench-To-Bedside and bedside back to the bench; coordinating clinical and experimental traumatic brain injury studies. *Front Neurol.* 2012;3:3.
8. Al Sayegh A, Sandford D, Carson AJ. Psychological approaches to treatment of postconcussion syndrome: a systematic review. *J Neurol Neurosurg Psychiatry.* 2010;81(10):1128–1134.
9. Helmick K, Members of Consensus Conference. Cognitive rehabilitation for military personnel with mild traumatic brain injury and chronic post-concussional disorder: Results of April 2009 consensus conference. *NeuroRehabilitation;* 26(3): 239–55; 2010.
10. Thornton KE, Carmody DP. Efficacy of traumatic brain injury rehabilitation: interventions of QEEG-guided biofeedback, computers, strategies, and medications. *Appl Psychophysiol Biofeedback.* 2008;33(2):101–124.
11. Cicerone KD, Dahlberg C, Malec JF, et al. Evidence-based cognitive rehabilitation: updated review of the literature from 1998 through 2002 review article. *Arch Phys Med Rehabil.* 2005;86(8):1681–1692.
12. Cicerone KD, Langenbahn DM, Dahlberg C, et al. Evidence-based cognitive rehabilitation: updated review of the literature From 2003 through 2008 review article. *Arch Phys Med Rehabil.* 2011;92(4):519–530.
13. DoV, DoD. Department of Veterans Affairs and Department of Defense. *Clinical Practice Guideline: Management of Concussion/Mild Traumatic Brain Injury.* 2009.

Available at: <http://www.healthquality.va.gov/mtbi/concussion_mtbi_full_1_0. pdf> Accessed on 28.6.2012

14. Marshall S, Bayley M, McCullagh S, Velikonja D, Berrigan L. Clinical practice guidelines for mild traumatic brain injury and persistent symptoms. *Can Fam Physician.* 2012;58(3):257–267. e128–40.

15. Neal MT, Wilson JL, Hsu W, Powers AK. Concussions: what a neurosurgeon should know about current scientific evidence and management strategies. *Surg Neurol Int.* 2012;3:16.

16. Budzynski TH, Budzynski HK, Evans JR, Abarbanel A. *Introduction to Quantitative EEG and Neurofeedback: Advanced Theory and Applications.* San Diego: Academic Press; 2009.

17. Coben R, Evans JR. *Neurofeedback and Neuromodulation Techniques and Applications.* San Diego: Academic Press; 2011.

18. Kropotov J. *Quantitative EEG, Event-Related Potentials and Neurotherapy.* San Diego: Academic Press; 2009.

19. Nuwer MR, Hovda DA, Schrader LM, Vespa PM. Routine and quantitative EEG in mild traumatic brain injury. *Clin Neurophysiol.* 2005;116(9):2001–2025.

20. World Health Organization. *Injuries and Violence: the Facts.* Geneva, Switzerland: WHO; 2010.

21. IBAS. *Brain Injury Facts.* International Brain Injury Association. Accessed August 13, 2012. <http://www.internationalbrain.org/?q=brain-injury-facts>; 2011.

22. Langlois JA, Rutland-Brown W, Thomas KE. Traumatic brain injury in the United States: Emergency department visits, hospitalizations, and deaths 2002–2006. Atlanta, GA: Centers for Disease Control and Prevention, National Center for Injury Prevention and Control. Accessed July 12, 2012. <http://www.cdc.gov/traumaticbraininjury/pdf/blue_book.pdf>.

23. Rutland-Brown W, Langlois JA, Thomas KE, Xi YL. Incidence of traumatic brain injury in the United States, 2003. *J Head Trauma Rehabil.* 2006;21:544–548.

24. Summers CR, Ivins B, Schwab KA. Traumatic brain injury in the United States: an epidemiologic overview. *Mt Sinai J Med.* 2009;76:105–110.

25. Daneshvar DH, Riley DO, Nowinski CJ, McKee AC, Stern RA, Cantu RC. Long-term consequences: effects on normal development profile after concussion. *Phys Med Rehabil Clin N Am.* 2011;22(4):683–700. Review.

26. Fleminger S, Oliver DL, Lovestone S, Rabe-Hesketh S, Giora A. Head injury as a risk factor for Alzheimer's disease: the evidence 10 years on; a partial replication. *J Neurol Neurosurg Psychiatry.* 2003;74:857–862.

27. Bryant RA, O'Donnell ML, Creamer M, McFarlane AC, Clark CR, Silove D. The psychiatric sequelae of traumatic injury. *Am J Psychiatry.* 2010;167(3):312–320.

28. Dean PJ, O'Neill D, Sterr A. Post-concussion syndrome: Prevalence after mild traumatic brain injury in comparison with a sample without head injury. *Brain Inj.* 2012;26(1):14–26.

29. Hesdorffer DC, Rauch SL, Tamminga CA. Long-term psychiatric outcomes following traumatic brain injury: a review of the literature. *J Head Trauma Rehabil.* 2009;24(6):452–459.

30. Hoge CH, McGurk D, Thomas JL, Cox AL, Engel CC, Castro CA. Mild traumatic brain injury in U.S. Soldiers returning from Iraq. *N Engl J Med.* 2008;358 453–46.

31. Iverson GL. Outcome from mild traumatic brain injury. *Curr Opin Psychiatry.* 2005;18(3):301–317.

32. McHugh T, Laforce Jr R, Gallagher P, Quinn S, Diggle P, Buchanan L. Natural history of the long-term cognitive, affective, and physical sequelae of mild traumatic brain injury. *Brain Cogn.* 2006;60(2):209–211.

33. Nampiaparampil DE. Prevalence of chronic pain after traumatic brain injury: a systematic review. *JAMA.* 2008;300(6):711–719.

34. Ponsford JL, Ziino C, Parcell DL, et al. Fatigue and sleep disturbance following traumatic brain injury: their nature, causes, and potential treatments. *J Head Trauma Rehabil.* 2012;27(3):224–233.

35. Ryan LM, Warden DL. Post concussion syndrome. *Int Rev Psychiatry.* 2003;15(4):310–316.

36. Sayer NA. Traumatic brain injury and its neuropsychiatric sequelae in war veterans. *Annu Rev Med.* 2012;63:405–419.

37. Silver JM, McAllister TW, Arciniegas DB. Depression and cognitive complaints following mild traumatic brain injury. *Am J Psychiatry.* 2009;166:653–661. Review.

38. Sigurdardottir S, Andelic N, Roe C, Jerstad T, Schanke AK. Post-concussion symptoms after traumatic brain injury at 3 and 12 months post-injury: a prospective study. *Brain Inj.* 2009;23(6):489–497.

39. Lannsjö M, Geijerstam JL, Johansson U, Bring J, Borg J. Prevalence and structure of symptoms at 3 months after mild traumatic brain injury in a national cohort. *Brain Inj.* 2009;23(3):213–219.

40. Rohling ML, Binder LM, Demakis GJ, Larrabee GJ, Ploetz DM, Langhinrichsen-Rohling J. A meta-analysis of neuropsychological outcome after mild traumatic brain injury: re-analyses and reconsiderations of Binder et al. (1997), Frencham et al. (2005), and Pertab et al. (2009). *Clin Neuropsychol.* 2011;25(4):608–623.

41. Cernak I. The importance of systemic response in the pathobiology of blast-induced neurotrauma. *Front Neurol.* 2010;1:151.

42. Greve MW, Zink BJ. Pathophysiology of traumatic brain injury. *Mt Sinai J Med.* 2009;76:97–104.

43. Rovegno M, Soto PA, Sáez JC, von Bernhardi R. Biological mechanisms involved in the spread of traumatic brain damage. *Med Intensiva.* 2012;36(1):37–44. Article in Spanish.

44. Johnson VE, Stewart W, Smith DH. Axonal pathology in traumatic brain injury. *Exp Neurol.* 2013;246:35–43.

45. McAllister TW. Neurobiological consequences of traumatic brain injury. *Dialogues Clin Neurosci.* 2011;13(3):287–300.

46. Turken AU, Herron TJ, Kang X, et al. Multimodal surface-based morphometry reveals diffuse cortical atrophy in traumatic brain injury. *BMC Med Imaging.* 2009;31(9):20.

47. Tate DF, Shenton ME, Bigler ED. Introduction to the brain imaging and behavior special issue on neuroimaging findings in mild traumatic brain injury. *Brain Imaging Behav.* 2012;6(2):103–107.

48. Bigler ED, Maxwell WL. Neuropathology of mild traumatic brain injury: relationship to neuroimaging findings. *Brain Imaging Behav.* 2012;6(2):108–136.

49. Stahnisch FW. On the use of animal experimentation in the history of neurology. In: Finger S, Boller F, Tyler KL, eds. *Handbook of Clinical Neurology, Vol. 95 (3rd series) History of Neurology.* San Diego: Elsevier; 2010.

50. Schomer DL, Lopes da Silva FH. *Niedermeyer's Electroencephalography: Basic Principles, Clinical Applications, and Related Fields.* Philadelphia: Lippincott Williams & Wilkins; 2011.

51. Tong S, Thakor NV. *Quantitative EEG Analysis Methods and Clinical Applications.* Norwood, MA: Artech House; 2009.

51a. Cooley JW, Tukey JW. An algorithm for the machine calculation of complex Fourier series. *Math. Comput.* 1965;19:297–301. http://dx.doi.org/10.2307/2003354.

52. Dumermuth G, Fluhler H. Some modern aspects in numerical spectrum analysis of multichannel electroencephalographic data. *Med Biol Eng.* 1967;5:319–331.

53. Michel CM, Koenig T, Brandeis D, Gianotti LRR, Wackermann J. *Electrical Neuroimaging.* Cambridge: Cambridge University Press; 2009.

54. Coburn KL, Lauterbach EC, Boutros NN, Black KJ, Arciniegas DB, Coffey CE. The value of quantitative electroencephalography in clinical psychiatry: a report

by the Committee on Research of the American Neuropsychiatric Association. *J Neuropsychiatry Clin Neurosci*. 2006;18(4):460–500.

55. Gordon E, Cooper N, Rennie C, Hermens D, Williams LM. Integrative neuroscience: the role of a standardized database. *Clin EEG Neurosci*. 2005;36(2):64–75.

56. Hernandez-Gonzalez G, Bringas-Vega ML, Galán-Garcia L, et al. Cuban Human Brain Mapping Project (CHBMP). Multimodal quantitative neuroimaging databases and methods: the Cuban Human Brain Mapping Project. *Clin EEG Neurosci*. 2001;42(3):149–159.

57. Hughes JR, John ER. Conventional and quantitative electroencephalography in psychiatry. *J Neuropsychiatry Clin Neurosci*. 1999;11(2):190–208.

58. John ER, Prichep LS, Fridman J, Easton P. Neurometrics: computer-assisted differential diagnosis of brain dysfunctions. *Science*. 1988;239:162–169.

59. Prichep LS. Use of normative databases and statistical methods in demonstrating clinical utility of QEEG: importance and cautions. *Clin EEG Neurosci*. 2005;36(2):82–87.

60. Thatcher RW. Neuropsychiatry and quantitative EEG in the 21st century. *Neuropsychiatry*. 2011;1(5):495–514.

61. Jasper HH, Kershman J, Elvidge AR. Electroencephalographic studies of injury to the head. *Arch Neur Psych*. 1940;44(2):328–350.

62. Arciniegas DB. Clinical electrophysiologic assessments and mild traumatic brain injury: state-of-the-science and implications for clinical practice. *Int J Psychophysiol*. 2011;82(1):41–52.

63. O'Neil B, Naunheim RS, Prichep L, Chabot R. Quantitative brain electrical activity in the initial screening of mild traumatic brain injuries. *West J Emerg Med*. 2012;13(5):394–400. Accessed August 20, 2012. <http://escholarship.ucop.edu/uc/item/4bq6t6gj#page-1>.

64. Thatcher RW. EEG evaluation of traumatic brain injury and EEG biofeedback treatment. In: Budzinsky T, Budzinski H, Evans J, Abarbanel A, eds. *Introduction to QEEG and Neurofeedback: Advanced Theory and Applications*. San Diego: Academic Press; 2009:269–294.

65. Thornton KE, Carmody DP. Traumatic brain injury rehabilitation: QEEG biofeedback treatment protocols. *Appl Psychophysiol Biofeedback*. 2009;34(1):59–68.

66. Thatcher RW, Walker RA, Gerson I, Geisler FH. EEG discriminant analyses of mild head trauma. *Electroencephalogr Clin Neurophysiol*. 1989;73(2):94–106.

67. Thatcher RW, Cantor DS, McAlaster R, Geisler F, Krause P. Comprehensive predictions of outcome in closed head-injured patients. The development of prognostic equations. *Ann NY Acad Sci*. 1991;620:82–101.

68. Thatcher RW, North DM, Curtin RT, et al. An EEG severity index of traumatic brain injury. *J Neuropsychiatry Clin Neurosci*. 2001;13(1):77–87.

69. Thornton KE. Exploratory investigation into mild brain injury and discriminant analysis with high frequency bands (32–64 Hz). *Brain Inj*. 1999;13(7):477–488.

70. Leon-Carrion J, Martin-Rodriguez JF, Damas-Lopez J, Martin JM, Dominguez-Morales Mdel RA. QEEG index of level of functional dependence for people sustaining acquired brain injury: the Seville Independence Index (SINDI). *Brain Inj*. 2008;22(1):61–74.

71. Cao C, Tutwiler RL, Slobounov S. Automatic classification of athletes with residual functional deficits following concussion by means of EEG signal using support vector machine. *IEEE Trans Neural Syst Rehabil Eng*. 2008;16(4):327–335.

72. Cao C, Slobounov S. Alteration of cortical functional connectivity as a result of traumatic brain injury revealed by graph theory, ICA, and sLORETA analyses of EEG signals. *IEEE Trans Neural Syst Rehabil Eng*. 2010;18(1):11–19.

73. Cao C, Slobounov S. Application of a novel measure of EEG non-stationarity as 'Shannon-entropy of the peak frequency shifting' for detecting residual abnormalities in concussed individuals. *Clin Neurophysiol*. 2011;122(7):1314–1321.

74. Slobounov S, Sebastianelli W, Hallett M. Residual brain dysfunction observed one year post-mild traumatic brain injury: combined EEG and balance study. *Clin Neurophysiol.* 2012;123(9):1755–1761.

75. Slobounov S, Gay M, Johnson B, Zhang K. Concussion in athletics: ongoing clinical and brain imaging research controversies. *Brain Imaging Behav.* 2012;6(2):224–243.

76. Naunheim RS, Treaster M, English J, Casner T, Chabot R. Use of brain electrical activity to quantify traumatic brain injury in the emergency department. *Brain Inj.* 2010;24(11):1324–1329.

77. McCrea M, Prichep L, Powell MR, Chabot R, Barr WB. Acute effects and recovery after sport-related concussion: a neurocognitive and quantitative brain electrical activity study. *J Head Trauma Rehabil.* 2010;25(4):283–292.

78. Prichep LS, McCrea M, Barr W, Powell M, Chabot RJ. Time course of clinical and electrophysiological recovery after sport-related concussion. *J Head Trauma Rehabil.* 2013;28(4):266–273.

79. Pachalska M, Łukowicz M, Kropotov JD, Herman-Sucharska I, Talar J. Evaluation of differentiated neurotherapy programs for a patient after severe TBI and long term coma using event-related potentials. *Med Sci Monit.* 2011;17(10):120–128.

80. Prichep L, Jacquin A, Filipenko J, et al. Classification of traumatic brain injury severity using informed data reduction in a series of binary classifier algorithms. *IEEE Trans Neural Syst Rehabil Eng.* 2012;20(6):806–822.

81. Hunter JV, Wilde EA, Tong KA, Holshouser BA. Emerging imaging tools for use with traumatic brain injury research. *J Neurotrauma.* 2012;29(4):654–671.

82. Irimia A, Chambers MC, Torgerson CM, et al. Patient tailored connectomics visualization for the assessment of white matter atrophy in traumatic brain injury. *Front Neurol.* 2012;3:10.

83. Niogi SN, Mukherjee P. Diffusion tensor imaging of mild traumatic brain injury. *J Head Trauma Rehabil.* 2010;25(4):241–255. Review.

84. Shenton ME, Hamoda HM, Schneiderman JS, et al. A review of magnetic resonance imaging and diffusion tensor imaging findings in mildtraumatic brain injury. *Brain Imaging Behav.* 2012;6(2):137–192.

85. Sponheim AR, McGuire KA, Kang SS, et al. Evidence of disrupted functional connectivity in the brain after combat-related blast injury. *Neuroimage.* 2011;54:21–29.

86. Zhang K, Johnson B, Pennell D, Ray W, Sebastianelli W, Slobounov S. Are functional deficits in concussed individuals consistent with white matter structural alterations: combined FMRI & DTI study. *Exp Brain Res.* 2010;204(1):57–70.

87. Thatcher RW, North DM, Biver CJ. Diffusion spectral imaging modules correlate with EEG LORETA neuroimaging modules. *Hum Brain Mapp.* 2012;33(5):1062–1075.

88. Saatman KE, Duhaime AC, Bullock R, Maas AIR, Valadka A, Manley GJ. Workshop scientific team and advisory panel members. Classification of traumatic brain injury for targeted therapies. *J Neurotrauma.* 2008;25(7):719–738.

89. Birbaumer N, Ramos Murguialday A, Weber C, Montoya P. Neurofeedback and brain-computer interface clinical applications. *Int Rev Neurobiol.* 2009;86:107–117.

90. Hammond DC. The need for individualization in neurofeedback: heterogeneity in QEEG patterns associated with diagnoses and symptoms. *Appl Psychophysiol Biofeedback.* 2010;35(1):31–36.

91. Thatcher RW. EEG operant conditioning (biofeedback) and traumatic brain injury. *Clin Electroencephalogr.* 2000;31(1):38–44. Review.

92. Duff J. The usefulness of quantitative EEG (QEEG) and neurotherapy in the assessment and treatment of post-concussion syndrome. *Clin EEG Neurosci.* 2004;35(4):198–209.

93. Thornton KE, Carmody DP. Electroencephalogram biofeedback for reading disability and traumatic brain injury. *Child Adolesc Psychiatr Clin N Am.* 2005;14(1):137–162. Review.

94. Ayers M. *Electroencephalographic feedback and head trauma. Head and Neck Trauma: The Latest Information and Perspectives on Patients with a Less Than Optimal Recovery.* U.C.L.A. Neuropsychiatric Institute; 1983.
95. Ayers M. A controlled study of EEG neurofeedback training and clinical psychotherapy for right hemispheric closed head injury. *Biofeedback Self Regul.* 1993;18:3.
96. Ayers ME. Assessing and treating open head trauma, coma, and stroke using real-time digital EEG neurofeedback. In: Evans JR, Abarbanel A, eds. *Introduction to Quantitative EEG and Neurofeedback.* San Diego: Academic Press; 1999:203–223.
97. Thornton K. Improvement/rehabilitation of memory functioning with neurotherapy/QEEG biofeedback. *J Head Trauma Rehabil.* 2000;15(6):1285–1296.
98. Thornton K. The improvement/rehabilitation of auditory memory functioning with EEG biofeedback. *NeuroRehabilitation.* 2002;17(1):69–80.
99. Schoenberger NE, Shif SC, Esty ML, Ochs L, Matheis RJ. Flexyx neurotherapy system in the treatment of traumatic brain injury: an initial evaluation. *J Head Trauma Rehabil.* 2001;16(3):260–274.
100. Zorcec T, Demerdzieva A, Pop-Jordanova N. QEEG, brain rate, executive functions and neurofeedback training in patients with traumatic brain injury. *Acta Inform Med.* 2011;19(1):23–28.
101. Nelson DV, Esty ML. Neurotherapy of traumatic brain injury/posttraumatic stress symptoms in OEF/OIF Veterans. *J Neuropsychiatry Clin Neurosci.* 2012;24(2):237–240.
102. Arns M, de Ridder S, Strehl U, Breteler M, Coenen A. Efficacy of neurofeedback treatment in ADHD: the effects on inattention, impulsivity and hyperactivity: a meta-analysis. *Clin EEG Neurosci.* 2009;40(3):180–189.
103. Tan G, Thornby J, Hammond DC, et al. Meta-analysis of EEG biofeedback in treating epilepsy. *Clin EEG Neurosci.* 2009;40(3):173–179.
104. Gruzelier J, Egner T, Vernon D. Validating the efficacy of neurofeedback for optimising performance. *Prog Brain Res.* 2006;159:421–431. Review.
105. Schlaepfer TE, George MS, Mayberg H. WFSBP task force on brain stimulation. WFSBP guidelines on brain stimulation treatments in psychiatry. *World J Biol Psychiatry.* 2010;11(1):2–18.
106. Bashir S, Mizrahi I, Weaver K, Fregni F, Pascual-Leone A. Assessment and modulation of neural plasticity in rehabilitation with transcranial magnetic stimulation. *PM R.* 2010;2(12):253–268.
107. Pascual-Leone A, Freitas C, Oberman L, et al. Characterizing brain cortical plasticity and network dynamics across the age-span in health and disease with TMS-EEG and TMS-fMRI. *Brain Topogr.* 2011;24(3–4):302–315.
108. Ros T, Gruzelier JH. The immediate effects of EEG neurofeedback on cortical excitability and synchronization. In: Coben R, Evans JR, eds. *Neurofeedback and Neuromodulation Techniques and Applications.* San Diego: Elsevier; 2011:381–402.
109. Paulus W. Transcranial electrical stimulation (tES – tDCS; tRNS, tACS) methods. *Neuropsychol Rehabil.* 2011;21(5):602–617.
110. Pape TL, Rosenow J, Lewis G. Transcranial magnetic stimulation: a possible treatment for TBI. *J Head Trauma Rehabil.* 2006;21(5):437–451.
111. Pape TL, Rosenow J, Lewis G, et al. Repetitive transcranial magnetic stimulation-associated neurobehavioral gains during coma recovery. *Brain Stimul.* 2009;2(1):22–35.
112. Demirtas-Tatlidede A, Vahabzadeh-Hagh AM, Bernabeu M, Tormos JM, Pascual-Leone A. Noninvasive brain stimulation in traumatic brain injury. *J Head Trauma Rehabil.* 2012;27(4):274–292.
113. Villamar MF, Santos Portilla A, Fregni F, Zafonte R. Noninvasive brain stimulation to modulate neuroplasticity in traumatic brain injury. *Neuromodulation.* 2012;15(4):326–338.

114. Yamamoto T, Katayama Y. Deep brain stimulation therapy for the vegetative state. *Neuropsycholog Rehab.* 2005;15(3/4):406–413.
115. Sankar T, Tierney TS, Hamani C. Novel applications of deep brain stimulation. *Surg Neurol Int.* 2012;3(1):26–33.
116. Yamamoto T, Katayama Y, Obuchi T, Kobayashi K, Oshima H, Fukaya C. Deep brain stimulation and spinal cord stimulation for vegetative state and minimally conscious state. *World Neurosurg.* 2012 [Epub ahead of print].
117. Schiff ND, Giacino JT, Kalmar K, et al. Behavioural improvements with thalamic stimulation after severe traumatic brain injury. *Nature.* 2007;448(7153):600–603.
118. Schiff ND, Giacino J, Fins JJ, Machado A. Central thalamic deep brain stimulation to promote recovery from chronic posttraumatic minimally conscious state: challenges and opportunities. *Neuromodulation.* 2012;15(4):339–349.
119. Schiff ND. Moving toward a generalizable application of central thalamic deep brain stimulation for support of forebrain arousal regulation in the severely injured brain. *Ann NY Acad Sci.* 2012;1265:56–68.
120. Shah SA, Schiff ND. Central thalamic deep brain stimulation for cognitive neuromodulation: a review of proposed mechanisms and investigational studies. *Eur J Neurosci.* 2010;32(7):1135–1144.
121. De Beaumont L, Théoret H, Mongeon D, et al. Brain function decline in healthy retired athletes who sustained their last sports concussion in early adulthood. *Brain.* 2009;132(Pt 3):695–708.
122. Gordon E, Liddell BJ, Brown KJ, et al. Integrating objective gene-brain-behavior markers of psychiatric disorders. *J Integr Neurosci.* 2007;6(1):1–34.
123. Novo-Olivas CA, Pérez-Solís EE. Neuroscience in psychiatry towards an integrative and personalized medicine in the DSM-V: A proposal. *Cuad. neuropsicol.* 2009;3:1. In Spanish.
124. Jordan BD. Genetic influences on outcome following traumatic brain injury. *Neurochem Res.* 2007;32:905–915.
125. Moran LM, Taylor HG, Ganesalingam K, et al. Apolipoprotein E4 as a predictor of outcomes in pediatric mild traumatic brain injury. *J Neurotrauma.* 2009;26(9):1489–1495.
126. Korn A, Golan H, Melamed I, Pascual-Marqui R, Friedman A. Focal cortical dysfunction and blood-brain barrier disruption in patients with postconcussion syndrome. *J Clin Neurophysiol.* 2005;22(1):1–9.
127. Finnoff JT, Jelsing EJ, Smith J. Biomarkers, genetics, and risk factors for concussion. *PM R.* 2011;3:S452–S459.
128. Rostami E, Davidsson J, Ng KC, et al. A model for mild traumatic brain injury that induces limited transient memory impairment and increased levels of Axon related serum biomarkers. *Front Neurol.* 2012;3:115.
129. Cannon R, Congedo M, Lubar J, Hutchens T. Differentiating a network of executive attention: LORETA neurofeedback in anterior cingulate and dorsolateral prefrontal cortices. *Int J Neurosci.* 2009;119(3) 404–441.
130. Thatcher RW. LORETA Z-Score biofeedback and traumatic brain injury. *Neuroconnections.* 2011;4:9–14.
131. Fedorov A, Chibisova Y, Szymaszek A, Alexandrov M, Gall C, Sabel BA. Noninvasive alternating current stimulation induces recovery from stroke. *Restor Neurol Neurosci.* 2010;28(6):825–833.
132. Miniussi C, Vallar G. Brain stimulation and behavioural cognitive rehabilitation: a new tool for neurorehabilitation? *Neuropsychol Rehabil.* 2011;21(5) 553–559.

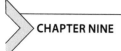

CHAPTER NINE

Treating Thought Disorders

Tanju Sürmeli

THOUGHT DISORDERS, PSYCHOSIS

A thought disorder is defined as any disturbance of thinking that affects language, communication, or thought content. Manifestations range from simple blocking and mild circumstantiality to profound loosening of associations, incoherence and delusions, characterized by a failure to follow semantic and syntactic rules that is inconsistent with the person's education, intelligence or cultural background.[1] It may involve difficulty putting cohesive thoughts together, or making sense of speech or a disturbance in one's ability to generate a logical sequence of ideas, as indicated by disordered speech and/or writing.

There are different types of thought disorders. A flight of ideas refers to language that may be difficult to understand because it switches quickly from one unrelated idea to other. Circumstantiality refers to language that may be difficult to understand, because it is long-winded and convoluted in reaching its goal. Word salad refers to words that are inappropriately strung together, resulting in gibberish.[1]

Since the early work of Bleuler,[2] Kraepelin,[3,4] and Moukas et al.,[5] thought disorder has been considered a major symptom of psychosis. Symptoms of psychosis are similar, independent of the clinical diagnosis. Patients with different diagnoses can have the same behaviors and treatment responses as with psychosis. Although psychosis is not unique to disorders such as schizophrenia, they may share a common neurophysiological substrate even though there may be various specific causes of the psychosis in different diagnostic groups. For example, thought disorders often are seen in those who have been given a diagnosis of schizophrenia or a schizophrenia-like disorder, bipolar disorder (manic episode, i.e., with psychotic symptoms), depression with psychotic features, traumatic brain injury (TBI)-induced axis I disorders (depression, bipolar disorders,

Clinical Neurotherapy.
Doi: http://dx.doi.org/10.1016/B978-0-12-396988-0.00009-X

schizophrenia and psychosis) and epilepsy,[6] and also are present to various degrees in anxiety disorders.[7–9]

Large population studies show that people with a history of epilepsy have nearly 2.5 times the risk of developing schizophrenia, and nearly three times the risk of developing a schizophrenia-like psychosis as the general population,[6] and the rate for the development of schizophrenia following a TBI is 1%.[8] Furthermore, even an initial TBI may place an individual at risk for sustaining a delayed-onset psychosis, such as schizophrenia, and for subsequent brain injuries independent of the psychosis.[10] The development of psychosis may be a delayed sequela of the pathophysiological changes resulting from either an earlier or a later TBI.[11] Persons with risk factors for developing a psychosis secondary to TBI are more likely to have had a previous congenital neurological disorder or to have sustained a head injury prior to adolescence.[12]

Lifetime incidence rates of TBI survivors who later demonstrate psychotic symptoms vary across studies, varying from 3.4% to 8.9%.[13,14] The onset of psychosis after TBI is highly variable but is generally delayed. In their study of World War II veterans, Achte et al.[15] reported that the occurrence of psychotic symptoms ranged from 2 days to 48 years after injury, with 42% experiencing their first psychotic episode 10 or more years after sustaining a missile wound to the head. Fujii and Ahmed[16] reported a range from 3 months to 19 years, with a mean onset of 5.9 years after closed head trauma. Feinstein and Ron[17] reported a mean latency of 11.7 years, with a range of 0 to 52 years.

There are several similarities between psychotic phenomena and unwanted intrusive thoughts (UITs). Garety and Hemsley[18] found that many patients with delusional beliefs scored highly (8 or more out of 10) on characteristics that are commonly associated with UITs (e.g., resistance [69%] and interference [47%]). It has also been noted that hallucinatory phenomena share many characteristics with UITs.[19] Auditory hallucinations (AHs) commonly have external precipitants,[20] as do UITs,[21] and these often increase with stress,[20] as do UITs.[22]

The co-occurrence of anxiety disorders may mediate some of the social and functional impairment well known in schizophrenia. Huppert and Smith's[23] finding that hallucinations were also related to self-reported obsessive-compulsive disorder (OCD) symptoms leads to a broader possibility: neurophysiologically, there may be an overlap between OCD symptoms and positive symptoms such as seen in schizophrenia, because the neural circuits known to relate to both types include the orbitofrontal cortex and the anterior cingulate cortex (ACC).[24,25]

Several studies show an association between thought disorders and cognitive impairment,[26–28] which suggests a common neurobiological substrate for both dysfunctions. Additionally, a meta-analysis by Kerns and Berenbaum[29] revealed a correlation between formal thought disorders (FTDs) and executive functions, and connections between thought disorders and semantic memory. Recently, thought disorders have been linked with both structural and dynamic abnormalities of the language system in the brain, which may indicate a common neurobiological basis underlying, for example, thought disorders and AHs.[30,31] Research suggesting that thought-disordered patients lack some constituent cognitive function is consonant with the notion that contextual deficits in thought-disordered patients with schizophrenia are a central issue. Defects in cognitive processing efficiency in schizophrenia seem to involve deficits in tasks that place heavy emphasis on selective attention.[32] The functions of a central executive system, elaborated on by Baddeley,[33,34] have been implicated in schizophrenia. They begin to describe coordinative functions that might be employed in selective attention, such as dividing attention, focusing on a subset, or switching attention – all of which appear demonstrably affected in patients with schizophrenia. Studies in priming also demonstrate how attention may be impaired because of disinhibited activation of semantic networks, thus impairing the ability to focus or attend to a specific subset of information. Thought-disordered subjects with high levels of impairment show inhibited semantic priming effects greater than those of less impaired thought-disorder subjects, suggesting aberrations in the activation of cognitive semantic networks.[35]

Andreasen and Grove[36] found that FTD has predictive value with regard to prognosis over several months in persons with psychiatric diagnoses. They found that negative thought disorder seems to predict the short-term outcome of schizophrenia. Patients with poverty of speech and poverty of content were more likely to have a form of schizophrenia, whereas positive forms of thought disorder were more common among the affective psychoses.[3,4,36–38]

qEEG, NEUROIMAGING STUDIES, VARETA, LORETA

Many data show that brain electrical activity reflects subtle aspects of brain function, including information processing and cognition. Many individuals suffer from disorders of these functions. An unknown but perhaps large percentage of them might benefit from intervention if precise diagnostic information were available. Although current psychological and neurological methods are not sufficiently sensitive for this purpose, electrophysiological measurements of brain functions related to information processing might be of substantial value.[39]

When looking electrophysiologically at patients with different diagnoses who share psychotic features, it has been found that those with very different clinical diagnostic labels share features that appear to be distinctive for psychosis, and it also has been demonstrated that such features do not depend upon the duration of illness or medication effects.[40] Based on a study conducted by John et al.[40] on psychotic patients that included schizophrenics, depressives and alcoholics, the authors postulated that it would be desirable to subtype psychotic patients based on their quantitative electroencephalogram; and because different subtypes may need different interventions, it would be possible to individualize treatments for the psychotic patient. One of the interventions that they specifically mentioned was neurofeedback, which would be able to target and correct the specific electrophysiological deviations (from norm) of the subtype, which, in turn, would serve to correct the specific neurotransmitter imbalances. Relevant to this, schizophrenic subtypes and their response to risperidone or to haloperidol have been identified by Czobor and Volavka.[41,42]

Abnormal EEG findings are seen in 20–60% of schizophrenic patients.[43–45] Most often, EEGs have been characterized by decreased alpha activity and/or increased beta activity.[46–49] Others have reported shifted alpha mean frequency or reduced alpha responsiveness[44,46,50] and increased slow activity.[51,52] Negative symptoms have been correlated with delta waves, especially in temporal areas,[53] coupled with decreased alpha and increased beta. Studies have shown greater coherence in patients than in healthy controls.[54,55] Increased interhemispheric coherence over frontal regions may distinguish schizophrenia patients from those suffering from bipolar depression, who are more likely to show decreased frontal coherence.[56,57] Ropohl et al.[58] found abnormally large beta oscillations localized around the left auditory cortex in a schizophrenia patient with treatment-resistant AHs. Left hemisphere source phase-locking factor (PLF) in schizophrenia was positively correlated with AH symptoms, and was modulated by delta phase. The correlation between source-evoked power and PLF found in healthy controls was reduced in schizophrenia for the left hemisphere sources.[59]

qEEG studies have shown discriminant accuracy as high as 95.67% in the detection of mild head injury,[60] and >75.8% accuracy in the prediction of outcome one year after injury.[61] These findings have been confirmed by recent studies.[62–65] Persons with major depression can be differentiated from normal controls with a specificity of 91.3% and sensitivity of 91.3%.[66] Such accuracy helps in the differential diagnosis, as between thought disorder resulting from a TBI and that caused by schizophrenia, thereby providing valuable information for the selection of treatment. Currently, the evidence for differential medical treatment is equivocal.

In region of interest analyses, structural abnormalities in the left superior temporal gyrus (STG),[67,68] the left planum temporale[69,70] and the orbitofrontal cortex[71] have been linked to a FTD in schizophrenia patients. Most findings of structural abnormalities associated with FTD were reported in the STG. Recent results point toward structural abnormalities linked to FTD beyond the STG.[31] The severity of FTD was negatively correlated with the gray matter volume of the left superior temporal sulcus, the left temporal pole, the right middle orbital gyrus and the right cuneus/lingual gyrus. Structural abnormalities specific for FTD were found to be unrelated to gray matter differences associated with schizophrenia in general. The specific gray matter abnormalities within the left temporal lobe may help to explain language disturbances included in FTD.[72] Severity of FTD was correlated with a disruption of the left semantic network in schizophrenic patients. Horn et al.'s[72] work suggests that FTD is a consequence of a frontoparietal/temporal disconnection caused by a complex interaction between structural and functional abnormalities within the left semantic network.[73]

Although the signs and symptoms of schizophrenia may be multi-faceted, neurobiological and behavioral data are beginning to show that a common element in schizophrenia is the dysregulation of emotional arousal (e.g., the hyperarousal associated with paranoid symptoms[74] and the hypoarousal associated with negative symptoms[75]), and cognitive deficits secondary to both hyper- and hypoarousal.[76]

The persistence of some level of thought disorder, even during periods of remission and drug treatment, is especially notable in schizophrenic patients. Severity of thought disorder is, in part, state- and medication-related.[77,78] Severe thought disorder, especially in schizophrenic patients, is strongly predictive of worse functional and social outcomes.[78,79] Paranoid schizophrenia tends to be related to differences in Brodmann areas (BA) 10 and 46 and the prefrontal–limbic circuit.[80,81] Although a large body of publications suggests a prefrontal deficit in schizophrenia, newer findings suggest an imbalance, or dysregulation, between the two primary components of a prefrontal–limbic negative feedback loop.[82,83] This may be related to the excitatory component of the amygdala[84,85] and the inhibitory component provided primarily by the prefrontal regions.[86,87]

Evidence from functional magnetic resonance imaging (fMRI) studies also showed that schizophrenic patients show significantly lower connectivity between left temporal cortex and left dorsolateral prefrontal cortex.[88,89] McCarthy-Jones[90] concluded that the most consistently documented areas involved in auditory verbal hallucinations are the STG, the left inferior frontal gyrus, and the arcuate fasciculus tract connecting them. It was suggested that because this neuronal geography is clear, it makes targeted neurofeedback feasible.

In a related study investigating the electrophysiology of auditory verbal hallucinations, Koutsoukos et al.[91] found theta–gamma frequency interaction differences, especially in the left temporal area, to be statistically significant for subjects experiencing such symptoms.

Based on a cluster analysis of electrophysiological measures conducted by John et al.[40] on 390 psychotic patients that included schizophrenics, depressives and alcoholics, six different clusters were identified. Using variable resolution electromagnetic tomographic analysis (VARETA – a source localization analysis of electrophysiological signals), all six clusters were found to have increased power in the excited systems, which comprised a set of subcortical regions that included limbic structures (amygdala, hippocampus, posterior cingulate), the basal ganglia and the thalamus. Cortical sources common to all clusters included the precentral gyrus, the middle and the STG. Also, they had depressed activity in the hippocampus and the occipital lobe. Low-resolution electromagnetic tomographic analysis (LORETA source analysis) studies in unmedicated patients with schizophrenia have mainly implicated slow frequencies,[92–94] probably reflecting cortical hypoactivation, and indicated a condition of abnormal functional connectivity within frontal and temporoparietal networks.[93–95] LORETA source-localization findings also support and extend the notion that the parietal lobe plays a crucial role in the pathogenesis of psychosis,[96] and that default mode network (DMN) dysfunction may be a core neurobiological feature in both schizophrenia[97] and schizophrenia-like psychosis, as sometimes seen in epilepsy.[96] In one study neuroleptic-naive patients with schizophrenia were compared to age- and sex-matched healthy controls, and data were analyzed by LORETA. Values for delta band activity were greater for patients in the left inferior temporal gyrus, right middle frontal gyrus, right superior frontal gyrus, right inferior frontal gyrus and right parahippocampal gyrus, and were negatively correlated with negative – but not positive − symptoms.[98] Phase locking in the gamma-band range has been shown to be diminished in patients with schizophrenia, and there have been reports of positive correlations between phase locking in the gamma-band range and positive symptoms, especially hallucinations. A major LORETA finding was reduced phase synchronization in schizophrenia between the left and right primary auditory cortex (Heschl's gyrus), but not between the bilateral secondary auditory cortices.[99,100] Comparisons of spectral analyses of the qEEG and LORETA of schizophrenia patients with treatment-refractory AHs, lasting for at least 2 years, with those of schizophrenia patients with nonauditory hallucinations (N-AH) in the past 2 years, showed significantly increased beta 1 and beta 2 frequency amplitude in AH compared with N-AH patients. Gamma and beta (2 and 3) frequencies were significantly correlated in AH, but not in N-AH patients. LORETA revealed significantly increased beta (1 and 2) activity in the left inferior parietal lobule and the left medial frontal gyrus in AH than in N-AH patients.[101]

The similarity between attention deficit hyperactivity disorder (ADHD) and schizophrenia was investigated in a study where matched ADHD subjects, schizophrenic patients and normal controls (100 subjects in each group) were compared using a cued GO/NOGO task. The action suppression component (generated in the supplementary motor cortex) was shown to be reduced in the ADHD group and was almost completely absent in the schizophrenia group. The conflict monitoring component was moderately reduced in ADHD and schizophrenia groups, whereas the sensory-related independent components remained practically the same in all three groups.[102]

The anatomical basis for the OCD-type thought disorder is complex and still under investigation, although ACC abnormalities are consistently being seen in the pathophysiology of OCD.[103] Anatomically, the ACC can be divided into cognitive (dorsal) and emotional (ventral) components. The dorsal part of the ACC is connected with the prefrontal and parietal cortices, as well as with the motor systems and frontal eye fields.[104] The ventral part has connections to the amygdala, the nucleus accumbens, the hypothalamus and the anterior insula. It is involved in assessing the importance and relevance of emotional and motivational information. A number of SPECT studies report hyperfrontality (increased right and left anterior prefrontal cortex activity and increased anterior cingulate gyrus activity) and increased basal ganglia activity in OCD.[105]

In a study using LORETA analysis, OCD patients who responded to antidepressants exhibited significantly lower activity in beta bands in the rostral anterior cingulate (BAs 24 and 32) and the medial frontal gyrus

(BA 10), suggesting that a distinctive pattern of activity within the medial surface of the frontal lobe predicts therapeutic response in OCD.[106] In the premedication recordings an excess current source density in the beta frequencies in the cingulate gyrus was revealed by LORETA. The beta frequencies (beta 2 [16–20 Hz], beta 3 [20–24 Hz] and beta 4 [24–28 Hz]) involved were located primarily in the middle cingulate gyrus as well as adjacent frontal and parieto-occipital regions. Other studies have found that individuals with OCD symptoms have excess beta activity in the cingulate gyrus compared to a non-OCD control group.[107] This is consistent with qEEG study findings of excess central beta.[108] The findings suggest that in addition to these regions, overactivation of the middle cingulate gyrus also plays an important role in OCD symptoms.[107] In Velikova et al.'s[109] study, the brain electrical activity of OCD patients showed increased current density for delta in the insula, and for beta in the frontal, parietal and limbic lobes. OCD subjects also had decreased interhemispheric coherence and reduced coupling between delta and beta frequencies. They concluded that in OCD increased frontal beta is consistent with previous evidence of frontal dysfunction.

PSYCHOPHARMACOLOGICAL TREATMENT

Psychopharmacological treatment can suppress psychotic symptoms in most patients with schizophrenia, but about 20% remain resistant to the antipsychotic effects of neuroleptic therapy and continue to manifest delusions and hallucinations as well as FTD.[110] The challenge of treatment-resistant schizophrenia continues despite the advent of a second-generation class of antipsychotics. The widespread off-label use of combination therapies of two, three or even four antipsychotic drugs is an indication that many clinicians still encounter a substantial number of patients who do not adequately respond to the approved doses of antipsychotic medications.[110] The comorbidity of OCD in schizophrenia may contribute to treatment resistance. Among 118 outpatients with schizophrenia, 8.8% had clinically significant OCD symptoms as measured by the Yale–Brown Obsessive Compulsive Scale (Y-BOCS).[111] The higher the Y-BOCS score, the greater the positive symptoms measured by the positive and negative syndrome scale (PANSS), especially delusions. Some studies have found a higher prevalence of OCD symptoms up to 25% in schizophrenia.[112] Treatment of this comorbidity may be complicated by the fact that, according to a series of case reports, the use of atypical antipsychotics in monotherapy may be associated with the de novo appearance of, or the aggravation of, preexisting OCD symptoms in a small proportion of patients with schizophrenia.[113] On the other hand, the addition of atypicals to selective serotonin reuptake inhibitors (SSRIs) has been shown to increase the response of OCD patients who have failed to respond adequately to SSRIs.

With OCD, a moderate amount of evidence suggests that atypical antipsychotic medications have clinically important effects when used as augmentation therapy for 8–16 weeks in patients with OCD resistant to standard treatment. Only risperidone, olanzapine and quetiapine have been studied. The evidence for benefit with risperidone and quetiapine is stronger than for olanzapine.[114]

Typical antipsychotic medications are commonly used to control TBI-induced agitation and psychosis. However, there are no controlled antipsychotic medication studies, or evidence other than case studies, concerning psychosis after TBI. Case studies (varying between one and nine patients) of atypical antipsychotic agents such as clozapine, risperidone and olanzapine given to TBI patients showed mixed results.[115–117]

It is evident that more effective treatment modalities are needed in treatment-resistant schizophrenia, or any form of thought disorder, to address the needs of patients who remain substantially symptomatic and disabled even with the use of currently available antipsychotic agents.

SCIENTIFIC EVIDENCE OF NONMEDICATION TREATMENT MODELS IN PSYCHOSIS

Electroconvulsive Therapy

The use of electroconvulsive therapy (ECT) to treat schizophrenia was introduced in 1938. A review of studies of combined ECT and antipsychotics for schizophrenia did not necessarily address whether this approach is effective in cases of treatment resistance.[118] A review of the literature on the efficacy of ECT[119] involving placebo-controlled studies showed minimal support for effectiveness with either depression or schizophrenia during the course of treatment (i.e., only for some patients, on some measures, and sometimes perceived only by psychiatrists but not by other raters), and no evidence, for either diagnostic group, of any benefits beyond the treatment period. There are no placebo-controlled studies evaluating the hypothesis that ECT prevents suicide, and no robust evidence from other kinds of studies to support that hypothesis.

Repetitive Transcranial Magnetic Stimulation (rTMS)

Investigation of the influence of rTMS on functional brain responses in healthy subjects has revealed an increased connectivity between the right temporoparietal cortex and the dorsolateral prefrontal cortex and the angular gyrus in subjects who had received rTMS. These findings have been interpreted as indicators of normalization of functional connectivity between these regions, which might support therapeutic effects of rTMS, e.g., for schizophrenic patients.[120] Neuroimaging studies have implicated left temporoparietal hyperactivity during AHs,[121] and related therapeutic studies have shown reduced severity of hallucinations with low-frequency rTMS (putatively reducing cortical excitability) with the stimulation coil applied midway between T3 and P3 (using the 10–20 EEG international system).

Two randomized, double-blind, sham-controlled trials of treat-ment-refractory AHs in patients with well-defined treatment-resistant schizophrenia produced conflicting results. In one study no significant improvement occurred in total mean PANSS score, either in its positive or its AH subscales, among active-treatment patients compared to controls.[122] In the other study[123] a significant improvement in the mean PANSS positive subscale score occurred in active-treatment patients, regardless of which hemisphere was stimulated, compared to controls. However, a meta-analysis study indicated that rTMS at 1 Hz applied to the temporo-parietal region once on several consecutive days may reduce AHs.[124]

In another study, low-frequency rTMS (0.9 Hz, 100% of motor thresh-old, 20 min) applied to the left temporoparietal cortex was used for 10 days in the treatment of medication-resistant AHs in schizophrenia. They found a significant improvement in total and positive symptoms (PANSS), and on the hallucination scales, and a decrease in current densi-ties (LORETA) for the beta 1 and beta 3 bands in the left temporal lobe, whereas an increase was found for the beta 2 band contralaterally.[125]

Slow rTMS, at a frequency of 1 Hz, has been proposed as a treatment for AHs. Some meta-analyses have supported this approach, reporting a substantial effect size (d values 0.515–0.88) of low-frequency rTMS on hal-lucinations.[126–129] However, results have been inconsistent, with two recent studies reporting no effect.[129,130]

The systems involved in speech generation and perception are broad and involve frontal as well as temporoparietal areas.[131] Only a few stud-ies have examined low-frequency rTMS targeting these broader brain regions. Although increased activation has been reported in Broca's area,[132] its right homologue,[133] Heschl's gyrus,[99,134,135]and the middle and STGs,[131,136,137] stimulation of these areas with rTMS was not found to be more effective than sham stimulation.[138–142] High-frequency rTMS stimulation (putatively increasing neuronal excitability) over the prefrontal cortex has shown some promise in improving negative symptoms in schizophrenia.[143] Based on three meta-analyses conducted on the effects of rTMS on negative symptoms,[127–144] a mild to moderate effect size was observed. The effect size increased when only AHs were targeted, and when the stimulation time was increased.[145]

The evidence generally suggests that rTMS can modulate cortical excitability to improve refractory auditory verbal hallucinations in schizophrenia.

Transcranial Direct Current Stimulation (tDCS)

Hasan et al.'s[146] study concerned schizophrenia patients who were clinically stable and who were divided into two groups. One group consisted of patients who had had a single psychotic episode (lasting at least 1 month), no relapse, and duration of psychosis <2 years (recent-onset schizophrenia). The second group included patients with more than two psychotic episodes, at least one relapse, and a duration of psychosis >2 years (multiepisode schizophrenia). These latter patients displayed a more chronic course of schizophrenia. The patient groups were matched with healthy subjects. Schizophrenia patients with multiple psychotic episodes displayed significant deficient long-term potentiation, such as plasticity, as reflected in a reduced motor-evoked potential increase after anodal tDCS, compared to healthy subjects and patients with recent-onset schizophrenia.

In healthy adults, probabilistic association learning, which involves a gradual learning of cue–outcome associations, activates a frontostriatal network. Studies of probabilistic association learning in schizophrenia have shown frontostriatal dysfunction, although considerable heterogeneity in performance has also been reported. Anodal tDCS to the dorsolateral prefrontal cortex has been shown to improve probabilistic association learning in healthy adults[147] and might be predicted to do so in schizophrenic patients. Although anodal tDCS failed to improve probabilistic association learning based on the performance of the whole healthy sample, greater variance in the active relative to the sham conditions suggested that a subset of people may respond to treatment.

In a first single-case pilot study Homan and colleagues[148] found improvements in clinical symptoms accompanied by a decrease in regional cerebral blood flow in the frontal and temporal lobes, indicating that tDCS can have a specific neurobiological effect.

It has been suggested that the application of tDCS with inhibitory stimulation over the left temporoparietal cortex and excitatory stimulation over the left dorsolateral prefrontal cortex could affect hallucinations and negative symptoms, respectively. In the study by Brunelin et al.,[149] 30 patients with schizophrenia and medication-refractory auditory verbal hallucinations were randomly allocated to receive either 20 minutes of active 2-mA tDCS or sham stimulation twice a day on five consecutive days. The authors assessed the efficacy of tDCS administered to the left temporoparietal junction ("inhibitory" cathodal tDCS) and the left dorsolateral prefrontal cortex ("excitatory" anodal tDCS) in reducing the severity of refractory auditory verbal hallucinations in patients with schizophrenia. They also assessed the impact of this technique on other refractory schizophrenia symptoms. Auditory verbal hallucinations were robustly reduced by tDCS after 10 active sessions over five days' tDCS compared to sham stimulation. There was a mean diminution of 31%, compared with an 8% reduction after 10 sham sessions. At the end of the trial, six patients (40%) could still be categorized as responders (defined as a >50% reduction in Auditory Hallucinations Rating Scale score), and this has not been the case in rTMS studies.[127–129] The beneficial effect on hallucinations lasted for up to 3 months. The authors also observed an amelioration of other symptoms with tDCS, as measured by the positive and negative syndrome scale (d = 0.98, 95% CI 0.22–1.73), especially for the negative and positive dimensions. No effect was observed on the dimensions of disorganization or grandiosity. The results show promise for tDCS in treating refractory auditory verbal hallucinations and other selected manifestations of schizophrenia.

Cranial Electrotherapy Stimulation (CES)

In one study it was found that anxiety and depression scores improved significantly in a CES treatment group but not in a placebo (sham treated) group, or in a "wait in line" control group of persons with mild TBI.[150] In another study evidence was found that CES reduces aggression in violent neuropsychiatric patients (16 schizophrenia, 10 schizoaffective disorders, one psychosis, two bipolar disorder).[151]

With regard to mechanisms through which this treatment modality may work, Feusner et al.'s[152] study provides evidence that CES stimulation may result in cortical deactivation, as well as altering brain connectivity in the DMN. In patients with anxiety and those with depression, one possibility is that alterations in the DMN may have a therapeutic effect of disengaging worry or rumination-promoting internal dialogue,[153] and/or promoting attention to external stimuli.

Deep Brain Stimulation

Deep brain stimulation (DBS) is a surgical treatment in which a device called a neurostimulator delivers tiny electrical signals to the areas of the brain that control movement. DBS has emerged as a treatment for severe cases of therapy-refractory OCD, and promising results have been reported. However, the published results are limited and the method is currently experimental.[154] Although no DBS studies have been conducted in schizophrenia, in cases where OCD is comorbid with schizophrenia, DBS may prove to be an effective treatment modality.

Computer-Based Cognitive Training

Cognitive training is an important aim of treatment for patients with schizophrenia. In a multicenter study, 64 patients with schizophrenia were investigated before and after completing a 5-week course of computer-based cognitive training using the program "Cogpack." Besides improvements in cognitive function (primary effect), patients enjoyed the training and reported increased self-esteem and progress in using computers (secondary effects). Computer-based anxiety scores at the onset of treatment did not exceed normal values. After completion of the training, these scores were significantly reduced and subjective reports of wellbeing significantly increased.[155]

Treating Thought Disorders with Neurofeedback and Biofeedback

Dr Andrew Abarbanel, in discussing how neurofeedback is useful in ADHD, stated that neural networks controlling the attention processes could be adjusted by neuromodulation, and in the long term could be transformed into a stable state, with longer-lasting results than with pharmacological treatment. He further postulated that this form of neuromodulation (neurofeedback) would be useful in depression, OCD and schizophrenia, because different behavior processes are controlled by similar neuropsychological mechanisms that can be self-modulated.[156]

In all forms of biofeedback operant and, in some cases classical, conditioning is considered to be the basic mechanism through which effects are mediated.

In 2000 Eric Kandel[157] won a Nobel Prize for showing that the synaptic mechanisms of classical conditioning and operant conditioning (including RNA/DNA mechanisms) are universal throughout the animal kingdom, including humans. There are also sensitization and habituation, which are scientifically understood but not generally effective, or do not have long-lasting effects and do not involve the same plasticity mechanism as operant and classical conditioning. Evidence of this plasticity was demonstrated in an fMRI study conducted by Ghaziri et al.,[158] who conducted fMRI feedback training in healthy subjects using an attention paradigm with a sham control. In the active treatment, group scores on the Integrated Visual & Auditory (IVA) full scale attention quotient (which is based on measures of both visual and auditory attention) significantly increased in comparison to baseline, and IVA subtest scores on auditory attention were also significantly higher following neurofeedback. For participants in the sham group, scores on visual attention were greater after training, but no difference in overall attention performance was noted. More importantly, a significantly greater than baseline increase in gray matter volume was found for the active neurofeedback group in a number of cortical areas. These were located in the right hemisphere (RH; inferior, middle and superior frontal gyri; inferior parietal lobule; inferior temporal gyrus), and in the left hemisphere (LH; inferior and superior frontal gyri; inferior and STGs; superior parietal lobule). With regard to white matter, significant increases in fractional anisotropy were measured in the superior longitudinal fasciculus (LH), inferior longitudinal fasiculus (LH) anterior limb of the internal capsule (LH), anterior corona radiata (RH), cingulum (RH) and (LH), and corpus callosum (genu, body, splenum). No change in gray and white matter was noted for members of the sham and control groups. These findings suggest that neurofeedback therapy can induce changes in brain regions implicated in attention. Their findings also indicate that neurofeedback therapy can produce modifications in white matter tracts involved in attentional processes. Ros et al.[159] were able to show that at around 30 minutes after training, neurofeedback induced a statistically significant upregulation of functional connectivity within the dorsal anterior cingulate/mid-cingulate cortex of the salience network in the experimental group, but not in the sham group. Therefore, by using fMRI neurofeedback and a placebo-control group, they were able to extend the findings of Ros et al.[160] demonstrating that the adult cortex is sufficiently plastic that a mere half-hour of targeted volitional activity (i.e., neurofeedback) is capable of intrinsically reconfiguring the brain's functional activity to last above and beyond – or at least as long as – the period of training itself.

There has been some reported research using fMRI neurofeedback and other forms of neurofeedback with clinical populations. For example, in a pilot study with real-time functional magnetic resonance imagining conducted by Ruiz et al.,[161] schizophrenic patients were able to train the self-activation of the right insula, resulting in improved performance on a face recognition task.

There is empirical evidence that neurofeedback can help with brain regulation in ADHD, impaired social skills of children with ADHD,[162–164] seizure disorder,[165] substance abuse,[166–169] depression,[170–173] personality and mood instability,[174,175] and can significantly improve or redress many of the symptoms of patients with postconcussion syndrome (PCS),[176–179] as well as improving similar symptoms in non-PCS patients.[179]

Various theories have been proposed as to why neurofeedback can be helpful in so many disorders. One reason is that several disorders may stem from dysregulation in the same neural regions or networks. For example, DMN dysfunction is seen in the pathophysiology of schizophrenia, epilepsy, anxiety/depression and ADHD.[180]

The FPO2 site has been found to be relevant in the treatment of both fear and anxiety problems. It is a site that has been found to access the amygdala, which is a structure often disturbed or dysregulated in both schizophrenia and anxiety. FPO stands for frontal pole orbital (prefrontal) and "2" signifies the right side of the brain. This site is off the standard 10–20 system and sits at the juncture of the right brow bone and the top of the nose, in the inner corner of the eye socket.[176–179,181]

Another theory is that by engaging principally with the DMN, the salience network, and the central executive network, thought disorders can be treated. This is based on a model that postulates that much of psychopathology is traceable to dysregulation of the interaction among these three resting state networks. There is some speculation that infra-low-frequency neurofeedback training may provide the most direct access to the dynamics of these interactions.[182]

Recently there have been some applications of an EEG inverse solution to neurofeedback. Using LORETA modeling, it is possible train a functional area of the brain, for example the anterior cingulate (cognitive division) to improve sustained attention. Possible applications of the technique include the discovery and treatment of epileptic foci, the rehabilitation of specific brain regions damaged as a consequence of TBI, and, in general, the training of any spatially specific cortical electrical activity.[183] LORETA neurofeedback in the ACC appears to induce long-term cortical changes and produces significant positive increases in working memory and processing speed scores.[184]

As stated previously, because OCD symptoms and positive symptoms overlap, and because the neural circuits related to these symptoms are common, the training of these circuits may be especially important in the treatment of both OCD and thought disorders. An uncontrolled study by Sürmeli and Ertem[185] gave a detailed description of the neurofeedback protocols used that have been found to be helpful in OCD.

We have found that with neurofeedback, a general rule is to link the patient's symptoms to deviant Z-scores noted at scalp electrode sites above cortical regions with known functional specializations related to the patient's symptoms.[186,187] The importance of proper location and frequency band selection was also shown by Moore in a review of two OCD studies he conducted, where he found that pure alpha training did not produce any results. He concluded that this was because there were two OCD subgroups, neither of which would have been expected to benefit from alpha training.[188]

In an OCD study conducted by Sürmeli and Ertem[185] the case study group assessed showed improvement in scores on the Y-BOCS. The magnitude of the improvement was 21.53 points, which was almost double the 10.64-point average improvement seen with drug treatment by Ackerman and Greenland.[189] Furthermore, after 2 years of follow-up, of the 36 original patients 19 remained symptom free or improved; nine had developed mild symptoms that did not interfere with their daily functioning and who did not feel the need to seek treatment; and five had relapsed. Of the two patients who received medication during treatment, one was in the group that did not respond to treatment. That patient also did not respond to medication and was in the follow-up relapse group. The other patient who received medication responded well to neurofeedback treatment and remained improved and medication free.

In a study on PCS, 20 out of 40 drug-free patients had some sort of psychotic symptom (20 with paranoia, one with visual hallucinations and four with AHs). All of these patients' symptoms resolved after neurofeedback treatment without antipsychotics being given.[176]

If Leff and Vaughn's[190] finding that the likelihood of relapse in schizophrenic persons is significantly greater in those living in high-stress homes than in those living in low-stress homes is accurate, we may conclude that psychosocial stress can induce psychosis,[191] and that a schizophrenic person's ability to cope with stress is one of the important factors in preventing relapse.[192]

Initial studies show that some schizophrenic patients can learn to cope with stress by using relaxation therapy combined with forms of biofeedback. In one study, a biofeedback group reduced its postsession electromyographic (EMG) levels by 40%. There are several controlled[193,194] and uncontrolled[195–198] studies of successful stress reduction with biofeedback in schizophrenia. Hawkins et al.,[199] using relaxation therapy and thermal biofeedback in a controlled study of 40 long-term inpatients with schizophrenia, found no significant differences in anxiety reduction between the experimental group and the control group. One-year follow-up and post hoc analyses, however, indicated a subgroup of "anxious" schizophrenics who showed a substantial reduction in anxiety following treatment with biofeedback and relaxation.

In the 1960s Von Hilsheimer and Quirk[200] reportedly restored schizophrenics to normal life at the Clark Psychiatric Institute at Queen Street Hospital, in Toronto, Canada. Of 150 patients, 143 were discharged after self-regulation galvanic skin resistance training. This group had an average hospitalization time of 9 years (maximum 45 years). After the biofeedback treatment, they remained out of hospital for a follow-up period of three years.[200]

Although these were biofeedback paradigms and not neurofeedback, they demonstrate the feasibility of operant conditioning with schizophrenia; and the path is clear to examine the efficacy of neurofeedback therapeutic interventions in schizophrenia and the schizotypal spectrum.[201]

Nine schizophrenic patients participated in a study by Schneider and Pope[202] that explored whether EEG feedback techniques could effect changes in the EEG similar to those associated with neuroleptic-induced improvement. During five sessions, each patient was presented with feedback signals that continuously reflected the discrepancy between characteristics of the patient's EEG power spectral profile and spectral profile characteristics associated by past research with neuroleptic-induced clinical improvement. Significant within-session changes were observed for two of three EEG power spectrum bands of interest. However, no significant session-to-session EEG changes were observed. The results suggest that the EEG of schizophrenics can be temporarily altered using feedback techniques, in a way that mimics the EEG changes that have been shown to occur with neuroleptic-induced clinical improvement.

Slow cortical potentials (SCPs) are considered to reflect the regulation of attention resources and cortical excitability in cortical neuronal networks. Impaired attentional functioning, as found in patients with schizophrenic disorders, may co-vary with impaired SCP regulation. In controlled studies on SCPs, neurofeedback treatment has shown improvement in cognitive functions in schizophrenia patients.[203–205]

In review articles[206,207] it has been concluded that in view of the affirmative evidence and advances in understanding the functional significance of EEG rhythms, the undertaking of therapeutic regimens with electrocortical operant conditioning is warranted in the schizophrenia spectrum. The positive findings using rTMS in schizophrenia,[208–210] where statistically significant decreases in AHs have been reported when the left temporoparietal cortex and left dorsolateral prefrontal cortex were stimulated, have raised the possibility that neurofeedback, which is a safer way to modulate brain activity, could be an alternative treatment option for schizophrenia.[211]

The effect of neurofeedback treatment for sleep problems in chronic schizophrenia patients has been shown in a controlled multiple case study only.[212] However, although neurofeedback has been extensively studied in the treatment of many disorders, there have been few published uncontrolled case reports on its clinical effects in the treatment of schizophrenia.[211,213]

In the paper by Sürmeli et al.[211] a group of 51 schizophrenic patients were treated with neurofeedback. In this study subjects with a PANSS total score of 70 or above were included (range: 76–156; between 70 and 79: two subjects; 80–89: nine subjects; 90–99: eight subjects; 100–109: five subjects; 110–119: nine subjects; 120–129: five subjects; 130–139: five subjects; and >140: five subjects). The results showed that 47 out of 48 participants showed clinical improvement after neurofeedback treatment, as indicated by changes in their PANSS scores, where the group's mean score of 110.24 (SD 21.62) decreased to 19.56 (SD 26.78). This change was found to be statistically significant. The participants who were able to take the Minnesota Multiphasic Personality Inventory (MMPI) and the Test of Variables of Attention (TOVA) showed significant improvements in these measures as well. Forty of the subjects were followed up for more than 22 months, two for 1 year, one for 9 months, and three for between 1 and 3 months after completion of neurofeedback. The average reduction in PANSS scores was 83% (SD 23), which was above the 20% change seen when only antipsychotic medications were used. In the study, 94% of the subjects complied with the neurofeedback regimen, and of those who needed medication, 68% complied with their drug treatment when followed for up to 2 years. In the Clinical Antipsychotic Trials of Intervention Effectiveness (CATIE) study, the efficacy of the pharmacological treatment on the primary measure, which was the subject staying in the study until completion, was only 26%.[214–216] In a study conducted by Schummer and von Stietz, after a patient was treated with neurofeedback to reduce his coherence abnormalities, his treatment dose of apiprazole was reduced from 20 mg to 7.5 mg, with an improvement of functioning giving him the ability to graduate from college.

When reading much of the literature on efficacy of various treatments with schizophrenic patients, it is useful to have information concerning the rating scales used.

The PANSS is the most commonly used clinical rating scale in registration trials of new antipsychotic medications.[217] Clinical trials testing the acute efficacy of antipsychotics ordinarily have certain thresholds for eligibility, such as a PANSS total score of at least 70 or 80 (although sometimes lower thresholds have been used). It is commonly observed that the baseline PANSS total score for participants in acute schizophrenia trials averages around 90, give or take 10 points. A PANSS total score of more than 120 would be considered very high and likely incompatible with being able to participate in a placebo-controlled clinical trial of monotherapy. Although mean change in PANSS total scores is often the primary outcome measure in a registration trial, it is more clinically relevant to know how many patients achieved a certain degree of improvement. A "responder analysis" can help address this, and inform the clinician about the proportion of patients who achieved a certain reduction in psychopathology, for example a 20% (barely perceptible), 30% (modest improvement) or 40% (relatively robust improvement) decrease in their PANSS total score from baseline. Clinically, it may be quite relevant to know that in a clinical trial 45% of the patients receiving the antipsychotic "responded," compared to 15% for placebo. This 30% difference in response rates would be considered attributable to the medication.[214,218,219]

The efficacy of the biofeedback treatment methods that have been used in schizophrenia likely falls into the range "possibly efficacious" to "probably efficacious" according to the guidelines jointly established by the Association for Applied Psychophysiology and Biofeedback and the International Society for Neurofeedback and Research (Table 9.1).[214]

Table 9.1 Published Studies on Biofeedback in Schizophrenia

Authors	Treatment Type	N	In/ outpatient	Controls/groups	Sessions	Outcome
Schnieder SJ, Pope AT. [202]	NF to mimic neuroleptic–induced EEG changes	9	Out	None	5	Significant within session changes. Not significant between session changes
Cortoos A, Verstraeten E, Joly J, et al. [212]	NF Effect of NF on sleep	13	In	NF Group Control group	40	Sleep quality improved
Bolea AS. [213]	NF Clinical study	1	In	None	130	Improvement in symptomatology and neuropsychological tests. Subject discharged to community living and improvements lasted for 2 years. NF was administered to more than 70 inpatients with chronic schizophrenia who had been hospitalized for as long as 20 years
Sürmeli T, Ertem, A, Eralp E, Kos, IH. [211]	NF Clinical study	51	Out	None	58,8 (average)	Statistically significant improvement in PANSS MMPI, TOVA, with improvements seen up to 2 year follow–up in majority of cases

Author	Protocol	Sessions	In/Out	Controls	N	Outcome
Schneider F, Rockstroh B, Heimann H et al.[203]	SCP	12	In	12 Healthy controls	20	Difference with controls (poorer learning), however in the last 3 sessions no difference with controls
Hardman E, Gruzelier J, Cheesman K, et al.[204]	SCP Reducing left right asymmetry in slow potential negativity in F3, F4	16	Out	8 Coached to use emotional strategies, 8 no strategy	3	Significant learning in both groups
Gruzelier J, Hardman E, Wild J, Zaman R.[205]	SCP Reducing left right asymmetry in slow potential negativity in C3, C4	16	Out	None	10	Patients were able to learn and control interhemispheric asymmetry. Ratings of anxiety and tension on the positive and negative symptom scale were closely related to reduced performance. A follow-up examination of case studies revealed that one participant evidenced a 50% reduction on a global psychopathology score. Another participant evidenced EEG readings that suggested the prior conditioning had persisted over 3 months
Acosta FX, Yamamoto J.[195]	EMG Biofeedback	6	Out	None	10+	Reduced EMG

(Continued)

Table 9.1 (Continued)

Authors	Treatment Type	N	In/ outpatient	Controls/groups	Sessions	Outcome
Nigl AJ, Jackson B. [220]	EMG Biofeedback	10	In	2 Groups Normal controls	6	All groups significantly reduced level of muscle tension. Length of hospitalization decreased in group that received biofeedback
Weiner [196]	EMG Biofeedback	6	Out	None	Operant paradigm 22	Easier to increase than reduce EMG
Keating [197]	EMG Biofeedback	4	In	None		EMG reduced, anxiety reduced in 3 subjects
Pharr OM, Coursey RD. [194]	EMG Biofeedback (frontalis and forearm extensor muscles)	30	In	Randomly assigned to: progressive relaxation group control group	1 orientation 6 active	Tension–Anxiety Scale of the Profile Mood states – not significant Nurses' Observation Scale for Inpatient Evaluation – Social Competence and Social Interest Factors Significant Improvement
Hawkins RC 2nd, Doell SR, Lindseth P, et al. [199]	Thermal biofeedback and relaxation therapy	40	In	Randomly assigned to: biofeedback, relaxation, biofeedback and relaxation, and minimal treatment control	10	No between-group differences. One-year follow-up and post hoc analyses indicated a subgroup of "anxious" schizophrenics who showed substantial reduction in anxiety following treatment with biofeedback and relaxation
Stien F, Nicolic S. [192]	Stress management, including biofeedback	1	Out	None	7	Improvement of 7 out of 20 items of the State–Trait Anxiety Inventory

Finally, all of the studies of EEG biofeedback in schizophrenia to date have used EEG biofeedback as an add-on to antipsychotic treatment regimens, so any statements of efficacy would have to acknowledge that EEG biofeedback has not been used as a stand-alone treatment for schizophrenia.

The criteria for Levels of Evidence of Efficacy of levels 1–5 are as follows:

- **Level 1: Not empirically supported**. This classification is assigned to those treatments that have only been described and supported by anecdotal reports and/or case studies in non-peer-reviewed journals.
- **Level 2: Possibly efficacious**. This classification is considered appropriate for those treatments that have been investigated in at least one study that had sufficient statistical power and well-identified outcome measures, but lacked randomized assignment to a control condition internal to the study.
- **Level 3: Probably efficacious**. Treatment approaches that have been evaluated and shown to produce beneficial effects in multiple observational studies, clinical studies, wait-list control studies, and within-subject and between-subject replication studies merit this classification.
- **Level 4: Efficacious**. In order to be considered "efficacious", a treatment must meet the following criteria:
  - In a comparison with a no-treatment control group, alternative treatment group or sham (placebo) control group using randomized assignment, the investigational treatment is shown to be statistically significantly superior to the control condition, or the investigational treatment is equivalent to a treatment of established efficacy in a study with sufficient power to detect moderate differences.
  - The studies have been conducted with a population treated for a specific problem, for which inclusion criteria are delineated in a reliable, operationally defined manner.
  - The study used valid and clearly specified outcome measures related to the problem being treated.
  - The data are subjected to appropriate data analysis.
  - The diagnostic and treatment variables and procedures are clearly defined in a manner that permits replication of the study by independent researchers; and
  - The superiority or equivalence of the investigational treatment has been shown in at least two independent studies'.
- **Level 5: Efficacious and specific**. To meet the criteria for this classification, the treatment needs to be demonstrated to be statistically

superior to a credible sham therapy, pill or bona fide treatment in at least two independent studies (LaVaque et al. 2002, p. 280).[221]

Example Case Study: This Case Study as an "Illustration" of neurofeedback Treatment

To end this chapter with an illustration of successful neurofeedback treatment, a case study is presented below.

A 27-year-old woman previously diagnosed with bipolar disorder and psychosis was treated for 4 years. Her symptoms started with some obsessive thoughts. Her problems included obsessions, hearing voices, communicating with people on the television, talking to herself out loud, laughing inappropriately, not getting pleasure from life, not being able to do housework, and not being able to attend her college classes. One of the psychiatrists from the local government hospital put her on depakote and olanzepine. She had four psychotic episodes while on medication, and her condition did not improve.

When she came to our center she was "washed out" of all medication in preparation for her qEEG recording. During the washout she became fully psychotic. However, her baseline qEEG was able to be recorded, medication-free. Based on her qEEG, the NxLink database suggested a diagnosis of schizophrenia (and not bipolar disorder), which was in agreement with the clinical judgment of the examining physician.

Here it is important to note that, although her illness could not be differentiated clinically between bipolar disorder and schizophrenia, her qEEG findings were able to suggest a similarity to the brain electrical activity seen in schizophrenia, and not that seen in bipolar disorder.[222]

After her psychotic episode, risperidone 3 mg/day was administered and her qEEG was re-recorded (Figure 9.1). Her psychotic episode, coupled with the medication, may have increased theta and theta hypercoherence.

Based on these findings, we decided to reduce theta and theta hypercoherence with neurofeedback. With this treatment regimen the obsessive thoughts and AHs disappeared, as did her talking to people via the TV. Her talking to herself and laughing inappropriately also disappeared. She functioned much better and was able to continue her college courses. These changes were observed clinically also. Her PANSS positive score decreased from 18 to 2, her negative score from 42 to 2, and her global scores from 90 to 2, reducing her total score from 150 to 60. Her MMPI results showed similar improvement. The schizophrenia scale T-score

Baseline (unmedicated)   Psychosis Developed Risperidone
                                                          Re-introduced

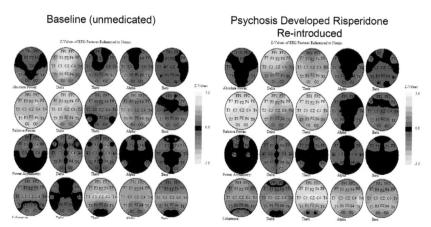

Figure 9.1 As can be seen, the psychotic episode increased theta activity. The coherence increase may be related to a drug effect or to the exacerbation of the illness. However, her baseline qEEG was able to be recorded, medication free.

decreased from 80 to 49. Other MMPI scores that showed improvement were psychasthenia T-score (81 to 44), psychopathic deviation T-score (79 to 40), paranoia T-score (74 to 45) and depression T-score (73 to 43). Following the treatment she functioned much better with only 2 mg risperidone per day and was stable for 2 years. After 2 years the patient was lost to follow-up.

CONCLUSIONS

The current treatment of choice for thought disorders is medication. However, a major drawback of pharmacological treatment is that this group is not very compliant with treatment. According to the CATIE study, about 74% of the schizophrenia patients who have discontinued the first medication prescribed will have a relapse within a year.[215]

There is a lack of studies investigating the efficacy of long-term drug treatment. Most studies are rarely longer than 12 weeks, and those that have looked into long-term use fail to show efficacy.[223] However, treatment periods with these drugs most often are longer than the durations that have been investigated by clinical studies. The currently available evidence does not provide enough information to predict which antipsychotic will provide the best treatment with the fewest side effects. Therefore, current drug selection involves a trial and error approach by the clinician.[206] Another issue is that a "one size fits all" treatment approach (usually with antipsychotic medications) may not be beneficial for a particular patient population, and more personalized treatments may be needed.[211]

The idea of "personalized" treatment is consistent with subclusters of dysregulation indicated by qEEG analyses, but qEEG is not yet widely used.[1] Neurofeedback protocols derived from qEEG analyses enable a tailoring of treatment protocols to specific brain regions and their functional status in a more individualized manner than can currently be provided by medications.

The clinical studies with schizophrenia performed by Bolea[213] and Sürmeli et al.,[211] and studies done with OCD,[224] are limited in that they are not controlled or blinded. However, recent comparisons between randomized controlled studies and randomized observational studies have shown that there is no great difference in treatment effects between the two, and that observational studies do provide relevant treatment information.[225–228]

The evidence of the effectiveness of neurofeedback as a treatment modality for thought disorders is increasing. Although efficacy is being shown clinically and reported in clinical case series, there is a lack of placebo-controlled studies of treatment of thought disorders using neurofeedback. This may be a result of the difficulty of applying the "gold-standard" placebo control to neurofeedback. A first reason for this is that if the sham control is not designed properly, subjects usually are able to identify the sham treatment, thereby breaking the blinding.[229] A second factor is an ethical one. According to the Helsinki accords, sham or placebo-controlled studies are ethically acceptable only for those disorders for which no effective treatment is available. Therefore, an active treatment control group (treatment equivalence) design is most appropriate for those clinical studies examining disorders for which there is a known, effective treatment.[230] Relevant to this, the use of sham feedback (placebo) in evaluating the efficacy of neurofeedback in the ADHD population was declared unethical by the University of California, San Diego.[231] This being the case, successful controlled neurofeedback studies are being conducted where efficacy is being demonstrated by comparing neurofeedback results to those found in a control group treated by some other treatment known to be effective.[170] In the treatment of thought disorders, it follows that according to Helsinki criteria the appropriate studies would be comparing neurofeedback to drugs approved by the Food and Drug Administration for thought disorder (e.g., antipsychotics).

With the growing importance of personalized medicine, these types of treatments (such as neurofeedback) may become more common in the future. This issue has recently been addressed by the Report of the National Advisory Mental Health Council's Workgroup in its August 2010 report. According to the report, its definition of "personalized" is as follows:

> *Personalized means that there is something known about the individual that differentially predicts how he or she will respond to a given treatment. Evidence-based treatment algorithms are helpful, but too general, with little tailoring based on individual differences (e.g., genomic variations), and supported by very little actual evidence beyond acute treatment.[232]*

According to Elkins et al.,[233] among the most frequently used complementary and alternative therapies, biofeedback is substantial, with 30% use among psychiatric inpatients (9% of them schizophrenics). So, we may conclude that biofeedback has been gaining importance among psychiatric illnesses. This chapter ends with a quote from Lamb,[234] who noted that many schizophrenic patients are neglected because clinicians conclude that they have lost the ability to cope independently in a normal environment. Lamb continued: "If mental health professionals pursue goals and use techniques that are not consistent with clinical reality, the recently revived interest in the chronically mentally ill will be lost out of frustration, staff burnout, and the disappointed hope of the administrators and the general public" (p 1007).

REFERENCES

1. Sadock BJ, Sadock VA, Ruiz P, Kaplan HI. *Kaplan & Sadock's comprehensive textbook of psychiatry*. 9th ed. Philadelphia, PA: Wolters Kluwer Health/Lippincott Williams & Wilkins; 2009.
2. Bleuler E. In: Zinkin J, ed. *Dementia Praecox or the Group of Schizophrenias*. New York, NY: International Universities Press; 1911.
3. Kraepelin E. In: Ross Diefendorf A, ed. *Clinical Psychiatry: A Textbook for Students and Physicians*. 7th ed. New York, NY: Macmillan; 1915.
4. Kraepelin E. In: Barclay RM, ed. *Dementia Praecox and Paraphrenia*. Edinburgh, Scotland: E. S. Livingstone; 1919.
5. Moukas G, Stathopoulou A, Gourzis P, Beratis IN, Beratis S. Relationship of 'prodromal' symptoms with severity and type of psychopathology in the active phase of schizophrenia. *Compr Psychiatry*. 2010;51(1):1–7.
6. Qin P, Xu H, Laursen TM, Vestergaard M, Mortensen PB. Risk for schizophrenia and schizophrenia-like psychosis among patients with epilepsy: population based cohort study. *BMJ*. 2005;331(7507):23. Epub 2005 Jun 17.
7. McAllister TW, Ferrell RB. Evaluation and treatment of psychosis after traumatic brain injury. *NeuroRehabilitation*. 2002;17(4):357–368.
8. Schwarzbold M, Diaz A, Martins ET, et al. Psychiatric disorders and traumatic brain injury. *Neuropsychiatr Dis Treat*. 2008;4(4):797–816.

9. Jolley S, Garety P, Bebbington P, et al. Attributional style in psychosis-the role of affect and belief type. *Behav Res Ther.* 2006;44(11):1597–1607.

10. Carlsson GS, Svardsudd K, Welin L. Long-term effects of head injuries sustained during life in three male populations. *J Neurosurg.* 1987;67:197–205.

11. Gualteri CT, Cox DR. The delayed neurobehavioral sequelae of traumatic brain injury. *Brain Inj.* 1991;5:219–232.

12. Fujii DE, Ahmed I. Risk factors in psychosis secondary to traumatic brain injury. *J Neuropsychiatry Clin Neurosci.* 2001;13:61–69.

13. Violin A, De Mol J. Psychological sequelae after head traumas in adults. *Acta Neurochir (Wien).* 1987;85:96–102.

14. Achte K, Jarho L, Kyykka T, Vesterinen E. Paranoid disorders following war brain damage. *Psychopathology.* 1991;24:309–315.

15. Achte KA, Hillbom E, Aalberg V. Psychoses following war injuries. *Acta Psychiatr Scand.* 1969;45:1–18.

16. Fujii DE, Ahmed I. Psychosis secondary to traumatic brain injury. *Neuropsychiatry Neuropsychol Behav Neurol.* 1996;9:133–138.

17. Feinstein A, Ron M. A longitudinal study of psychosis due to a general medical condition: establishing predictive and construct validity. *J Neuropsychiatry Clin Neurosci.* 1998;10:448–452.

18. Garety PA, Hemsley DR. *Delusions: Investigations into the Psychology of Delusional Reasoning.* Hove, UK: Psychology Press; 1994.

19. Morrison AP, Haddock G, Tarrier N. Intrusive thoughts and auditory hallucinations: a cognitive approach. *Behav Cogn Psychother.* 1995;23:265–280.

20. Nayani TH, David AS. The auditory hallucination: a phenomenological survey. *Psychol Med.* 1996;26:177–189.

21. Parkinson L, Rachman SJ. The nature of intrusive thoughts. *Adv Behav Res Ther.* 1981;3:101–110.

22. Horowitz M. Intrusive and repetitive thoughts after experimental stress. *Arch Gen Psychiatry.* 1975;78:86–92.

23. Huppert JD, Smith TE. Anxiety and schizophrenia: the interaction of subtypes of anxiety and psychotic symptoms. *CNS Spectrum.* 2005;10(9):721–731.

24. Cottraux J, Gerard D. Neuroimaging and neuroanatomical issues in obsessive-compulsive disorder. In: Swinson RP, Antony MM, Rachman S, Richeter MA, eds. *Obsessive-Compulsive Disorder: Theory, Research, and Treatment.* New York, NY: Guilford Press; 1998:154–180.

25. Silbersweig DA, Stern E, Frith C, et al. A functional neuroanatomy of hallucinations in schizophrenia. *Nature.* 1995;378:176–179.

26. Czernikiewicz A. Evaluation of language disorders in the group of patients with paranoid schizophrenia. *Psychiatr Pol.* 1990;24(2):141–145.

27. Sponheim SR, Surerus-Johnson C, Dieperink ME, Spoont M. Generalized cognitive dysfunction, symptomatology, and specific cognitive processes in relation to functioning of schizophrenia patients. *Schizophr Res.* 2003;64(2–3):191–193.

28. Subotnik KL, Nuechterlein KH, Green MF, et al. Neurocognitive and social cognitive correlates of formal thought disorder in schizophrenia patients. *Schizophr Res.* 2006;85(1–3):84–95. Epub 2006 Apr 19.

29. Kerns JG, Berenbaum H. Cognitive impairments associated with formal thought disorder in people with schizophrenia. *J Abnorm Psychol.* 2002;111(2):211–224.

30. Strik W, Dierks T. Neurophysiological mechanisms of psychotic symptoms. *Eur Arch Psychiatry Clin Neurosci.* 2008;258(suppl 5):66–70.

31. Horn H, Federspiel A, Wirth M, et al. Structural and metabolic changes in language areas linked to formal thought disorder. *Br J Psychiatry.* 2009;194(2):130–138.

32. Schatz J. Cognitive processing efficiency in schizophrenia: generalized vs. domain specific deficits. *Schizophr Res.* 1998;30(1):41–49.

33. Baddeley AD. Exploring the central executive. *Q J Exp Psychol A*. 1996;49(A):5–28.

34. Baddeley AD. Is working memory still working? *Am Psychol*. 2001;56:851–864.

35. Aloia MS, Gourovitch ML, Missar D, Pickar D, Weinberger DR, Goldberg TE. Cognitives substrates of thought disorder II: specifying a candidate cognitive mechanism. *Am J Psychiatry*. 1998;155(12):1677–1684.

36. Andreasen N, Grove W. Thought, language, and communication in schizophrenia: diagnosis and prognosis. *Schizophr Bull*. 1986;12(3):348–359.

37. Winokur G, Morrison J, Clancy J, Crowe R. The Iowa 500: familial and clinical findings favor two kinds of depressive illness. *Compr Psychiatry*. 1973;14(2):99–106.

38. Morrison J, Clancy J, Crowe R, Winokur G. The Iowa 500; I. diagnostic validity in mania, depression, and schizophrenia. *Arch Gen Psychiatry*. 1972;27(4):457–461.

39. John ER, Karmel BZ, Corning WC, et al. Neurometrics. *Science*. 1977;196(4297):1393–1410.

40. John ER, Prichep LS, Winterer G, et al. Electrophysiological subtypes of psychotic states. *Acta Psychiatr Scand*. 2007;116:17–35.

41. Czobor P, Volavka J. Pretreatment EEG predicts shortterm response to haloperidol treatment. *Biol Psychiatry*. 1991;30:927–942.

42. Czobor P, Volavka J. Quantitative EEG effect of risperidone in schizophrenic patients. *J Clin Psychopharm*. 1993;13:332–342.

43. Small JG. Psychiatric disorders and EEG. In: Niedermeyer E, Lopes da Silva F, eds. *Electroencephalography: Basic Principles, Clinical Applications, and Related Fields*. Baltimore, MD: Williams & Wilkins; 1993:581–596.

44. Small JG, Milstein V, Sharpley PH, Klapper M, Small IF. Electroencephalographic findings in relation to diagnostic constructs in psychiatry. *Biol Psychiatry*. 1984;19(4):471–487.

45. Ellingson RJ. The incidence of EEG abnormality among patients with mental disorders of apparently nonorganic origin: a critical review. *Am J Psychiatry*. 1954;111:263–275.

46. Itil TM. Qualitative and quantitative EEG findings in schizophrenia. *Schizophr Bull*. 1977;3(1):61–79. Review.

47. John ER, Prichep LS, Fridman J, Easton P. Neurometrics: computer-assisted differential diagnosis of brain dysfunctions. *Science*. 1988;239(4836):162–169.

48. Dierks T, Maurer K, Ihl R, et al. Evaluation and interpretation of topographic EEG data in schizophrenic patients. In: Mauer K, ed. *Topographic Brain Mapping of EEG and Evoked Potentials*. Berlin, Heidelberg: Springer-Verlag; 1989:507–517.

49. Merrin EL, Floyd TC. Negative symptoms and EEG alpha activity in schizophrenic patients. *Schizophr Res*. 1992;8(1):11–20.

50. Colombo C, Gambini O, Macciardi F, et al. Alpha reactivity in schizophrenia and in schizophrenic spectrum disorders: demographic, clinical and hemispheric assessment. *Int J Psychophysiol*. 1989;7:47–54.

51. Morihisa JM, Duffy FH, Wyatt RJ. Brain electrical activity mapping (BEAM) in schizophrenic patients. *Arch Gen Psychiatry*. 1983;40:719–728.

52. Galderisi S, Maj M, Mucci A, et al. QEEG alpha1 changes after a single dose of high-potency neuroleptics as a predictor ofshort-term response to treatment in schizophrenia patients. *Biol Psychiatry*. 1994;35:367–374.

53. Gattaz WF, Mayer S, Ziegler P, et al. Hypofrontality on topographic EEG in schizophrenia: correlations with neuropsychological and psychopathological parameters. *Eur Arch Psychiatry Clin Neurosci*. 1992;241:328–332.

54. Nagase Y, Okubo Y, Matsuura M, Kojima T, Toru M. EEG coherence in unmedicated schizophrenic patients: topographical study of predominantly never medicated cases. *Biol Psychiatry*. 1992;32:1028–1034.

55. Weller M, Montagu JD. EEG coherence in schizophrenia: a preliminary study. *Electroencephalogr Clin Neurophysiol*. 1980;49:100–101.

56. John ER, Prichep LS. Principles of neurometric analysis of EEG and evoked potentials. In: Niedermeyer E, Lopes da Silva F, eds. *EEG: Basic Principles, Clinical Applications, and Related Fields*. Baltimore, MD: Williams & Wilkins; 1993:989–1003.

57. Hughes JR, John ER. Conventional and quantitative electroencephalography in psychiatry. *J Neuropsychiatry Clin Neurosci*. 1999;11:190–208.

58. Ropohl A, Sperling W, Elstner S, et al. Cortical activity associated with auditory hallucinations. *Neuroreport*. 2004;15(3):523–526.

59. Spencer KM. The functional consequences of cortical circuit abnormalities on gamma oscillations in schizophrenia: insights from computational modeling. *Front Hum Neurosci*. 2009;3:33–60. http://dx.doi.org/10.3389/neuro.09.033.2009 Epub 2009 Oct 20.

60. Thatcher RW, Walker RA, Gerson I, Geisler F. EEG discriminant analyses of mild head trauma. *EEG Clin Neurophysiol*. 1989;73:93–106.

61. Thatcher RW, Cantor DS, McAlaster R, Geisler F, Krause P. Comprehensive predictions of outcome in closed head injury: the development of prognostic equations. *Ann NY Acad Sci*. 1991;620:82–104.

62. Prichep L, Jacquin A, Filipenko J, et al. Classification of traumatic brain injury severity using informed data reduction in a series of binary classifier algorithms. *IEEE Trans Neural Syst Rehabil Eng*. 2012:26. [Epub ahead of print].

63. Prichep LS, McCrea M, Barr W, Powell M, Chabot RJ. Time course of clinical and electrophysiological recovery after sport-related concussion. *J Head Trauma Rehabil*. 2012:14. [Epub ahead of print].

64. Arciniegas DB. Clinical electrophysiologic assessments and mild traumatic brain injury: state-of-the-science and implications for clinical practice. *Int J Psychophysiol*. 2011;82(1):41–52. Epub 2011 Mar 16.

65. Cao C, Tutwiler RL, Slobounov S. Automatic classification of athletes with residual functional deficits following concussion by means of EEG signal using support vector machine. *IEEE Trans Neural Syst Rehabil Eng*. 2008;16(4):327–335.

66. Knott V, Mahoney C, Kennedy S, Evans K. EEG power, frequency, asymmetry and coherence in male depression. *Psychiatry Res*. 2001;106(2):123–140.

67. Shenton ME, Kikinis R, Jolesz FA, et al. Abnormalities of the left temporal lobe and thought disorder in schizophrenia. A quantitative magnetic resonance imaging study. *N Engl J Med*. 1992;327(9):604–612.

68. Subotnik KL, Bartzokis G, Green MF, Nuechterlein KH. Neuroanatomical correlates of formal thought disorder in schizophrenia. *Cogn Neuropsychiatry*. 2003;8(2):81–88.

69. Rossi A, Serio A, Stratta P, et al. Planum temporale asymmetry and thought disorder in schizophrenia. *Schizophr Res*. 1994;12(1):1–7.

70. Barta PE, Pearlson GD, Brill II LB, et al. Planum temporale asymmetry reversal in schizophrenia: replication and relationship to gray matter abnormalities. *Am J Psychiatry*. 1997;154(5):661–667.

71. Nakamura M, Nestor PG, Levitt JJ, et al. Orbitofrontal volume deficit in schizophrenia and thought disorder. *Brain*. 2008;131(Pt 1):180–195. Epub 2007 Dec 3.

72. Horn H, Federspiel A, Wirth M, et al. Gray matter volume differences specific to formal thought disorder in schizophrenia. *Psychiatry Res*. 2010;182:183–186.

73. Horn H, Jann K, Federspiel A, et al. Semantic network disconnection in formal thought disorder. *Neuropsychobiology*. 2012;66:14–23.

74. Williams LM, Das P, Harris AW, et al. Dysregulation of arousal and amygdala-prefrontal systems in paranoid schizophrenia. *Am J Psychiatry*. 2004;161:480–489.

75. Merrin EL, Floyd TC. Negative symptoms and EEG alpha in schizophrenia: a replication. *Schizophr Res*. 1996;19:151–161.

76. Mujica-Parodi LR, Corcoran C, Greenberg T, Sackeim HA, Malaspina D. Are cognitive symptoms of schizophrenia mediated by abnormalities in emotional arousal? *CNS Spectr*. 2002;7:58–60, 65–69.

77. Docherty N, Schnur M, Harvey PD. Reference performance and positive and negative thought disorder: a follow-up study of manics and schizophrenics. *J Abnorm Psychol.* 1988;97(4):437–442.

78. Harrow M, Marengo JT. Schizophrenic thought disorder at follow-up: its persistence and prognostic significance. *Schizophr Bull.* 1986;12(3):373–393.

79. Bowie CR, Harvey PD. Communication abnormalities predict functional outcomes in chronic schizophrenia: differential associations with social and adaptive functions. *Schizophr Res.* 2008;103(1–3):240–247.

80. Radulescu AR, Rubin D, Strey HH, Mujica-Parodi LR. Power spectrum scale invariance identifies prefrontal dysregulation in paranoid schizophrenia. *Hum Brain Mapp.* 2012;33(7):1582–1593.

81. Dean B, Keriakous D, Scarr E, Thomas EA. Gene expression profiling in Brodmann's area 46 from subjects with schizophrenia. *Australian New Zealand J Psychiatry.* 2007;41(4):308–320.

82. Ragland JD, Laird AR, Ranganath C, Blumenfeld RS, Gonzales SM, Glahn DC. Prefrontal activation deficits during episodic memory in schizophrenia. *Am J Psychiatry.* 2009;166:863–874.

83. Yoon JH, Minzenberg MJ, Ursu S, et al. Prefrontal cortex dysfunction is associated with disrupted coordinated brain activity in schizophrenia: relationship to impaired cognition, behavioral disorganization and global function. *Am J Psychiatry.* 2008;165:1006–1014.

84. Floresco SB, Tse MT. Dopaminergic regulation of inhibitory and excitatory transmission in the basolateral amygdala-prefrontal cortical pathway. *J Neurosci.* 2007;27:2045–2057.

85. LeDoux J. The emotional brain, fear, and the amygdala. *Cell Mol Neurobiol.* 2003;23:727–738.

86. Phelps EA, Delgado MR, Nearing KI, LeDoux JE. Extinction learning in humans: role of the amygdala and vmPFC. *Neuron.* 2004;43:897–905.

87. Rosenkranz JA, Moore H, Grace AA. The prefrontal cortex regulates lateral amygdala neuronal plasticity and responses to previously conditioned stimuli. *J Neurosci.* 2003;23:11054–11064.

88. Lawrie SM, Buechel S, Whalley HC, et al. Reduced frontotemporal functional connectivity in schizophrenia associated with auditory hallucinations. *Biol Psychiatry.* 2002;51:1008–1011.

89. Burns J, Jop D, Bastin ME, et al. Structural disconnectivity in schizophrenia: a diffusion tensor magnetic resonance imaging study. *Br J Psychiatry.* 2003;182:439–443.

90. McCarthy-Jones S. Taking back the brain: could neurofeedback training be effective for relieving distressing auditory verbal hallucinations in patients with schizophrenia? *Schizophr Bull.* 2012;38(4):678–682.

91. Koutsoukos E, Angelopoulos E, Maillis A, Papadimitriou GN, Stefanis C. Indication of increased phase coupling between theta and gamma EEG rhythms associated with the experience of auditory verbal hallucinations. *Neurosci Lett.* 2013;534:242–245. http://dx.doi.org/10.1016/j.neulet.2012.12.005 Epub 2012 Dec 20.

92. Mientus S, Gallinat J, Wuebben Y, et al. Cortical hypoactivation during resting EEG in schizophrenics but not in depressives and schizotypal subjects as revealed by low resolution electromagnetic tomography (LORETA). *Psychiatry Res.* 2002;116:95–111.

93. Pascual-Marqui RD, Lehmann D, Koenig T, et al. Low resolution brain electromagnetic tomography (LORETA) functional imaging in acute, neuroleptic-naive, first-episode, productive schizophrenia. *Psychiatry Res.* 1999;90:169–179.

94. Saletu B, Anderer P, Saletu-Zyhlarz GM. EEG topography and tomography (LORETA) in the classification and evaluation of the pharmacodynamics of psychotropic drugs. *Clin EEG Neurosci.* 2006;37:66–80.

95. Winterer G, Egan MF, Rädler T, Coppola R, Weinberger DR. Event-related potentials and genetic risk for schizophrenia. *Biol Psychiatry.* 2001;50(6):407–417.

96. Canuet L, Ishii R, Pascual-Marqui RD, et al. Resting-state EEG source localization and functional connectivity in schizophrenia-like psychosis of epilepsy. *PLoS One.* 2011;6(11):e27863. http://dx.doi.org/10.1371/journal.pone.0027863 Epub 2011 Nov 18.

97. Woodward ND, Rogers B, Heckers S. Functional resting-state networks are differentially affected in schizophrenia. *Schizophr Res.* 2011;130(1–3):86–93. http://dx.doi.org/10.1016/j.schres.2011.03.010

98. Itoh T, Sumiyoshi T, Higuchi Y, Suzuki M, Kawasaki Y. LORETA analysis of three-dimensional distribution of δ band activity in schizophrenia: relation to negative symptoms. *Neurosci Res.* 2011;70(4):442–448. http://dx.doi.org/10.1016/j.neures.2011.05.003

99. Mulert C, Kirsch V, Pascual-Marqui R, McCarley RW, Spencer KM. Long-range synchrony of γ oscillations and auditory hallucination symptoms in schizophrenia. *Int J Psychophysiol.* 2011;79(1):55–63. http://dx.doi.org/10.1016/j.ijpsycho.2010.08.004

100. Pascual-Marqui RD, Lehmann D, Koukkou M, et al. Assessing interactions in the brain with exact low-resolution electromagnetic tomography. *Philos Transact A Math Phys Eng Sci.* 2011;369(1952):3768–3784. http://dx.doi.org/10.1098/rsta.2011.0081

101. Lee SH, Wynn JK, Green MF, et al. Quantitative EEG and low resolution electromagnetic tomography (LORETA) imaging of patients with persistent auditory hallucinations. *Schizophr Res.* 2006;83(2–3):111–119. Epub 2006 Mar 9.

102. Kropotov J. What is unique and common in physiology of schizophrenia and ADHD: The ERP study. Abstracts of SAN Meeting/Neuroscience Letters 500S 2011.

103. Bush C, Luu P, Posner MI. Cognitive and emotional influences in anterior cingulate cortex. *Trends Cogn So.* 2000;4:215–222.

104. Gevensleben H, Holl B, Albrecht B, et al. Neurofeedback training in children with ADHD: 6-month follow-up of a randomized controlled trial. *Eur Child Adolesc Psychiatry.* 2010;19:715–724.

105. Can C, Birbaumer N, Strehl U. Long term effects after feedback of slow cortical potentials and of theta-beta-amplitudes in children with attention-deficit/hyperactivity disorder. *Int J Bioelectromagn.* 2008;10:209–232.

106. Fontenelle LF, Mendlowicz MV, Ribeiro P, Piedade RA, Versiani M. Low-resolution electromagnetic tomography and treatment response in obsessive-compulsive disorder. *Int J Neuropsychopharmacol.* 2006;9(1):89–94. Epub 2005 Jun 7.

107. Sherlin L, Congedo M. Obsessive-compulsive dimension localized using low-resolution brain electromagnetic tomography (LORETA). *Neurosci Lett.* 2005;387(2):72–74.

108. Prichep LS, Mas F, Hollander E, et al. Quantitative electroencephalographic subtyping of obsessive-compulsive disorder. *Psychiatry Res.* 1993;50(1):25–32.

109. Velikova S, Locatelli M, Insacco C, Smeraldi E, Comi G, Leocani L. Dysfunctional brain circuitry in obsessive-compulsive disorder: source and coherence analysis of EEG rhythms. *Neuroimage.* 2010;49(1):977–983. http://dx.doi.org/10.1016/j.neuroimage.2009.08.015

110. Nasrallah H, White R. Treatment-Resistant vs Pseudo-Resistant Schizophrenia. Retrieved from < www.medscape.com/editorial/cmetogo/5743 > Release Date: July 20, 2006.

111. Ongur D, Goff DC. Obsessive-compulsive symptoms in schizophrenia: associated clinical features, cognitive function and medication status. *Schizophr Res.* 2005;75(2–3):349–362.

112. Green AI, Canuso CM, Brenner MJ, Wojcik JD. Detection and management of comorbidity in patients with schizophrenia. *Psychiatr Clin N Am.* 2003;26:115–139.
113. Faucher S, Dardennes R, Ghaem O, Guelfi JD. Obsessive-compulsive symptoms treatment in schizophrenia [in French, English abstract]. *Can J Psychiatry.* 2005;50:423–428.
114. Southern California/RAND Evidence-based Practice Center. Efficacy and Comparative Effectiveness of Off-Label Use of Atypical Antipsychotics. AHRQ Publication No. 07-EHC003-EF January. Retrieved from < www.ahrq.gov > ; 2007.
115. Michals ML, Crismon ML, Roberts S, Childs A. Clozapine response and adverse effects in nine brain-injured patients. *J Clin Psychopharmacol.* 1993;13(3):198–203.
116. Arciniegas DB, Harris SN, Brousseau KM. Psychosis following traumatic brain injury. *Int Rev Psychiatry.* 2003;15(4):328–340.
117. Guerreiro DF, Navarro R, Silva M, Carvalho M, Gois C. Psychosis secondary to traumatic brain injury. *Brain Inj.* 2009;23(4):358–361.
118. Braga RJ, Petrides G. The combined use of electroconvulsive therapy and antipsychotics in patients with schizophrenia. *J ECT.* 2005;21:75–83.
119. Read J, Bentali R. The effectiveness of electroconvulsive therapy: a literature review. *Epidemiologia Psychiatria Sociale.* 2010:333–347.
120. Gromann PM, Tracy DK, Giampietro V, Brammer MJ, Krabbendam L, Shergill SS. Examining frontotemporal connectivity and rTMS in healthy controls: implications for auditory hallucinations in schizophrenia. *Neuropsychology.* 2012;26(1):127–132. http://dx.doi.org/10.1037/a0026603
121. Silbersweig DA, Stern E, Frith C, et al. A functional neuroanatomy of hallucinations in schizophrenia. *Nature.* 1995;378(6553):176–179.
122. Fitzgerald PB, Benitez J, Daskalakis JZ, et al. A double-blind sham-controlled trial of repetitive transcranial magnetic stimulation in the treatment of refractory auditory hallucinations. *J Clin Psychopharmacol.* 2005;25:358–362.
123. Lee SH, Kim W, Chung YC, et al. A double blind study showing that two weeks of daily repetitive TMS over the left or right temporoparietal cortex reduces symptoms in patients with schizophrenia who are having treatment-refractory auditory hallucinations. *Neurosci Lett.* 2005;376:177–181.
124. Hoffman RE, Gueorguieva R, Hawkins KA, et al. Temporoparietal transcranial magnetic stimulation for auditory hallucinations: safety, efficacy and moderators in a fifty patient sample. *Biol Psychiatry.* 2005;58:97–104.
125. Horacek J, Brunovsky M, Novak T, et al. Effect of low-frequency rTMS on electromagnetic tomography (LORETA) and regional brain metabolism (PET) in schizophrenia patients with auditory hallucinations. *Neuropsychobiology.* 2007;55(3–4):132–142. Epub 2007 Jul 19.
126. Aleman A, Sommer IE, Kahn RS. Efficacy of slow repetitive transcranial magnetic stimulation in the treatment of resistant auditory hallucinations in schizophrenia: a meta-analysis. *J Clin Psychiatry.* 2007;68(3):416–421.
127. Freitas C, Fregni F, Pascual-Leon A. Meta-analysis of the effects of repetitive transcranial magnetic stimulation (rTMS) on negative and positive symptoms in schizophrenia. *Schizophr Res.* 2009;108:11–24.
128. Matheson SL, Green MJ, Loo C, Carr VJ. Quality assessment and comparison of evidence for electroconvulsive therapy and repetitive transcranial magnetic stimulation for schizophrenia: a systematic meta-review. *Schizophr Res.* 2010;118(1–3):201–210. http://dx.doi.org/10.1016/j.schres.2010.01.002
129. Slotema CW, Blom JD, Hoek HW, Sommer IE. Should we expand the toolbox of psychiatric treatment methods to include repetitive transcranial magnetic stimulation (rTMS)? A meta-analysis of the efficacy of rTMS in psychiatric disorders. *J Clin Psychiatry.* 2010;71(7):873–884. http://dx.doi.org/10.4088/JCP.08m04872gre

130. de Jesus DR, Gil A, Barbosa L, et al. A pilot double-blind sham-controlled trial of repetitive transcranial magnetic stimulation for patients with refractory schizophrenia treated with clozapine. *Psychiatry Res.* 2011;188(2):203–207. http://dx.doi.org/10.1016/j.psychres.2010.11.022

131. Jardri R, Pouchet A, Pins D, Thomas P. Cortical activations during auditory verbal hallucinations in schizophrenia: a coordinate-based meta-analysis. *Am J Psychiatry.* 2011;168(1):73–81. http://dx.doi.org/10.1176/appi.ajp.2010.09101522

132. McGuire PK, Shah GM, Murray RM. Increased blood flow in Broca's area during auditory hallucinations in schizophrenia. *Lancet.* 1993;342:703–706.

133. Sommer IE, Diederen KM, Blom JD, et al. Auditory verbal hallucinations predominantly activate the right inferior frontal area. *Brain.* 2008;131:3169–3177.

134. Dierks T, Linden DE, Jandl M, et al. Activation of Heschl's gyrus during auditory hallucinations. *Neuron.* 1999;22:615–621.

135. van de Ven VG, Formisano E, Röder CH, et al. The spatiotemporal pattern of auditory cortical responses during verbal hallucinations. *Neuroimage.* 2005;27:644–655.

136. Hoffman RE, Pittman B, Constable RT, Bhagwagar Z, Hampson M. Time course of regional brain activity accompanying auditory verbal hallucinations in schizophrenia. *Br J Psychiatry.* 2011;198:277–283.

137. Shergill SS, Brammer MJ, Williams SCR, Murray RM, McGuire PK. Mapping auditory hallucinations in schizophrenia using functional magnetic resonance imaging. *Arch Gen Psychiatry.* 2000;57:1033–1038.

138. Schonfeldt-Lecuona C, Gron G, Walter H, et al. Stereotaxic rTMS for the treatment of auditory hallucinations in schizophrenia. *Neuroreport.* 2004;15:1669–1673.

139. Hoffman RE, Hampson M, Wu K, et al. Probing the pathophysiology of auditory/verbal hallucinations by combining functional magnetic resonance imaging and transcranial magnetic stimulation. *Cereb Cortex.* 2007;17:2733–2743.

140. Schreiber S, Dannon PN, Goshen E, Amiaz R, Zwas TS, Grunhaus L. Right prefrontal rTMS treatment for refractory auditory command hallucinations: a neuroSPECT assisted case study. *Psychiatry Res.* 2002;116:113–117.

141. Loo CK, Sainsbury K, Mitchell P, Hadzi-Pavlovic D, Sachdev PS. A sham-controlled trial of left and right temporal rTMS for the treatment of auditory hallucinations. *Psychol Med.* 2009;40:541–546.

142. Vercammen A, Knegtering H, Bruggeman R, et al. Effects of bilateral repetitive transcranial magnetic stimulation on treatment resistant auditory-verbal hallucinations in schizophrenia: a randomized controlled trial. *Schizophr Res.* 2009;114:172–179.

143. Brunelin J, Szekely D, Costes N, et al. Theta burst stimulation in the negative symptoms of schizophrenia and striatal dopamine release: an iTBS-[11C]raclopride PET case study. *Schizophr Res.* 2011;131:264–265.

144. Dlabac-de Lange JJ, Knegtering R, Aleman A. Repetitive transcranial magnetic stimulation for negative symptoms of schizophrenia: review and meta-analysis. *J Clin Psychiatry.* 2010;71:411–418.

145. Prikryl R, Ustohal L, Prikrylova-Kucerova H, Ceskova E. Occurrence of robust psychotic symptoms after initial rTMS treatment session. *J ECT.* 2011;27(3):265–266. http://dx.doi.org/10.1097/YCT.0b013e3181f665bc

146. Hasan A, Nitsche MA, Herrmann M, et al. Impaired long-term depression in schizophrenia: a cathodal tDCS pilot study. *Brain Stimul.* 2012;5(4):475–483. http://dx.doi.org/10.1016/j.brs.2011.08.004 Epub 2011 Sep 5.

147. Vercammen A, Rushby JA, Loo C, Short B, Weickert CS, Weickert TW. Transcranial direct current stimulation influences probabilistic association learning in schizophrenia. *Schizophr Res.* 2011;131(1–3):198–205. http://dx.doi.org/10.1016/j.schres.2011.06.021 Epub 2011 Jul 13.

148. Homan P, Kindler J, Federspiel A, et al. Muting the voice: a case of arterial spin labeling-monitored transcranial direct current stimulation treatment of auditory verbal hallucinations. *Am J Psychiatry*. 2011;168(8):853–854.

149. Brunelin J, Mondino M, Gassab L, et al. Examining Transcranial Direct-Current Stimulation (tDCS) as a Treatment for Hallucinations in Schizophrenia. *Am J Psychiatry*. 2012;169:719–724.

150. Kirsch D. CES for mild traumatic brain injury. *Pract Pain Manag*. 2008:70–77.

151. Childs A, Price L. Cranial electrotherapy stimulation reduces aggression in violent neuropsychiatric patients. *Prim Psychiatry*. 2007;14(3):50–56.

152. Feusner JD, Madsen S, Moody TD, et al. Effects of cranial electrotherapy stimulation on resting state brain activity. *Brain Behav*. 2012;2(3):211–220.

153. Hamilton JP, Furman DJ, Chang C, Thomason ME, Dennis E, Gotlib IH. Default-mode and task-positive network activity in major depressive disorder: implications for adaptive and maladaptive rumination. *Biol Psychiat*. 2011;70:327–333.

154. Blomstedt P, Sjöberg RL, Hansson M, Bodlund O, Hariz MI. Deep brain stimulation in the treatment of obsessive-compulsive disorder. *World Neurosurg*. 2012 Oct 5. pii: S1878–8750(12)01105–9. doi: 10.1016/j.wneu.2012.10.006. [Epub ahead of print].

155. Bender S, Resch F, Weisbrod M, Oelkers-Ax R. Specific task anticipation versus unspecific orienting reaction during early contingent negative variation. *Clin Neurophysiol*. 2004;115(8):1836–1845.

156. Abarbanel A. Gates, states, rhythms and resonances: the scientific basis of neurofeedback training. *J Neurotherapy*. 1995;1:15–38.

157. Kandel ER. The molecular biology of memory storage: a dialogue between genes and synapses. *Science*. 2001;294:1030–1038.

158. Ghaziri J, Tucholka A, Larue V, et al. Neurofeedback training induces changes in white and gray Matter. *Clin EEG Neurosci*. 2013:26. [Epub ahead of print].

159. Ros T, Théberge J, Frewen PA, et al. Mind over chatter: plastic up-regulation of the fMRI salience network directly after EEG neurofeedback. *Neuroimage*. 2013;65:324–335. doi: 0.1016/j.neuroimage.2012.09.046. Epub 2012 Sep 26.

160. Ros T, Munneke MA, Ruge D, Gruzelier JH, Rothwell JC. Endogenous control of waking brain rhythms induces neuroplasticity in humans. *Eur J Neurosci*. 2010;31(4):770–778. http://dx.doi.org/10.1111/j.1460–9568.2010.07100.x

161. Ruiz S, Lee S, Soekadar S, et al. Acquired self-control of insula cortex modulates emotion recognition and brain network connectivity in schizophrenia. *Hum Brain Mapp*. 2013;34(1):200–212. http://dx.doi.org/10.1002/hbm.21427 Epub 2011 Oct 22.

162. Arns M, de Ridder S, Strehl U, Breteler M, Coenen A. Efficacy of neurofeedback treatment in ADHD: the effects on inattention, impulsivity and hyperactivity: a meta-analysis. *Clin EEG Neurosci*. 2009;40(3):180–189.

163. Mayer K, Wyckoff SN, Strehl U. One size fits all? slow cortical potentials neurofeedback: a review. *J Atten Disord*. 2013;17(5):393–409. [Epub ahead of print].

164. Hodgson K, Hutchinson AD, Denson L. Nonpharmacological treatments for ADHD: a meta-analytic review. *J Atten Disord*. 2012 [Epub ahead of print].

165. Tan G, Thornby J, Hammond DC, et al. Meta-analysis of EEG biofeedback in treating epilepsy. *Clin EEG Neurosci*. 2009;40(3):173–179.

166. Horrell T, El-Baz A, Baruth J, et al. Neurofeedback effects on evoked and induced EEG gamma band reactivity to drug-related cues in cocaine addiction. *J Neurother*. 2010;14(3):195–216.

167. Sokhadze TM, Cannon R, Trudeau DL. EEG biofeedback as a treatment for substance use disorders: review, rating of efficacy and recommendations for future research. *Appl Psychophysiol Biofeedback*. 2008;33:1–28. [PubMed: 18214670].

168. Trudeau DL. A review of the treatment of addictive disorders byEEG biofeedback. *Clin Electroencephalogr.* 2000;31(1):13–26.

169. Scott WC, Brod TM, Sideroff S, Kaiser D, Saga M. Type-specific EEG biofeedback improves residential substance abuse treatment. Presented at the American Psychiatric Association Annual Meeting. <http://eegbiofeedback.com/research.html> ; 2002 Accessed 19.06.10.

170. Choi SW, Chi SE, Chung SY, Kim JW, Ahn CY, Kim HT. Is alpha wave neurofeedback effective with randomized clinical trials in depression? A pilot study. *Neuropsychobiology.* 2011;63:43–51.

171. Baehr E, Rosenfeld JP, Baehr R. The clinical use of an alpha symmetry protocol in the neurofeedback treatment of depression: two case studies. *J Neurotherapy.* 1997;2(3):10–23.

172. Baehr E, Rosenfeld JP, Baehr R. The clinical use of an alpha symmetry protocol in the eurofeedback treatment of depression: follow-up study one to five years post therapy. *J Neurotherapy.* 2001;4(4):11–18.

173. Rosenfeld JP. An EEG biofeedback protocol for affective disorders. *Clin Electroencephalogr.* 2000;31(1):7–12.

174. Sürmeli T, Ertem A. QEEG guided neurofeedback therapy in personality disorders: 13 case studies. *Clin EEG Neurosci.* 2009;40(1):5–10.

175. Sterman MB. Physiological origins and functional correlates of EEG rhythmic activities: implications for self-regulation. *Biofeedback Self Regul.* 1996;21(1):3–33.

176. Sürmeli T, Ertem A. Efficacy of QEEG and neurofeedback in the assessment and treatment of post concussive syndrome: a clinical case series. *Biol Psychol.* 2012 in Review.

177. Thatcher RW. Normative EEG databases and biofeedback. *J Neurotherapy.* 1998;2(4):8–39.

178. Thatcher RW. EEG operant conditioning (biofeedback) and traumatic brain injury. *Clin Electroencephalogr.* 2000;31(1):38–44.

179. Duff J. The usefulness of QEEG and neurotherapy in the assessment and treatment of post-concussion syndrome. *Clin EEG Neurosci.* 2004;35:4.

180. Broyd SJ, Demanuele C, Debener S, Helps SK, James CJ, Sonuga-Barke EJ. Default-mode brain dysfunction in mental disorders: a systematic review. *Neurosci Biobehav Rev.* 2009;33(3):279–296.

181. Fisher S. FPO2 and the regulation of fear. *ISNR J Newsletter.* 2006;15:117.

182. Othmer SF, Othmer S. Interhemispheric EEG training: clinical experience and conceptual models. In: Evans JR, ed. *Handbook of Neurofeedback.* New York: Haworth Press; 2007:109–136.

183. Congedo M, Lubar JF, Joffe D. Low-resolution electromagnetic tomography neurofeedback. *IEEE Trans Neural Syst Rehabil Eng.* 2004;12(4):387–397.

184. Cannon R, Lubar J. Long-term effects of neurofeedback training in anterior cingulate cortex: a short follow-up report. *J Neurotherapy.* 2011;15(2):130–150.

185. Sürmeli T, Ertem A. Obsessive compulsive disorder and the efficacy of qEEG-guided neurofeedback treatment: a case series. *Clin EEG Neurosci.* 2011;42(3):195–201.

186. Thatcher RW, North O, Corea R, et al. An EEG severity index of traumatic brain injury. *J Neuropsychia: Clin Neurosci.* 2001;13:77–87.

187. Thatcher RW, Biver CL, Gomez-Molina IF, et al. Estimation of the EEG power spectrum by MRI T2 relaxation time in traumatic brain injury. *Clin Neurophysiology.* 2001;112:729–745.

188. Moore NC. A review of EEG biofeedback treatment of anxiety disorders. *Clin Electroencephalogr.* 2000;31:1–6.

189. Ackerman DL, Greenland S. Multivariate meta-analysis of controlled drug studies for obsessive-compulsive disorder. *J Clin Psychopharmacol.* 2002;22:309–317.

190. Leff J, Vaughn C. The role of maintenance therapy and relatives' expressed emotion in relapse of schizophrenia: a two-year follow up. *Br J Psychiatry*. 1981;139:102–104.

191. Van Winkel R, Stefanis NC, Myin-Germeys I. Psychosocial stress and psychosis. a review of the neurobiological mechanisms and the evidence for gene-stress interaction. *Schizophr Bull*. 2008;34:1095–1105.

192. Stein F, Nikolic S. Teaching stress management techniques to a schizophrenic patient. *Am J Occup Ther*. 1989;43(3):162–169.

193. Van Hassel J, Bloom L, Gonzalez A. Anxiety management with schizophrenic outpatients. *J Clin Psychol*. 1982;38:280–285.

194. Pharr OM, Coursey RD. The use and utility of EMG biofeedback with chronic schizophrenic patients. *Biofeedback Self Regul*. 1989;14(3):229–245.

195. Acosta FX, Yamamoto J. Application of electromyographic biofeedback to the relaxation training of schizophrenic, neurotic, and tension headache patients. *J Consult Clin Psychol*. 1978;46(2):383–384.

196. Weiner H. On altering muscle tension with chronic schizophrenics. *Psychol Rep*. 1979;44:527–534.

197. Keating C. *Exploration of a Combined Program of Electromyographic Biofeedback and Progressive Relaxation as a Treatment Approach with Schizophrenics. Unpublished doctoral dissertation*. East Lansing: Michigan State University; 1981.

198. Wentworth-Rohr I. Biofeedback for schizophrenia and neurosis. *Frontiers of Psychiatry, Roche Report*. 1981;11:6–11.

199. Hawkins II RC, Doell SR, Lindseth P, Jeffers V, Skaggs S. Anxiety reduction in hospitalized schizophrenics through thermal biofeedback and relaxation training. *Percept Mot Skills*. 1980;51(2):475–482.

200. Von Hilsheimer G, Quirk DA. Using biofeedback to treat the untreatable. <http://www.drbiofeedback.com/sections/library/articles/untreatable.html> 1988 Accessed 15.06.10.

201. Gruzelier JH. Theory, methods and new directions in the psychophysiology of the schizophrenic process and schizotypy. *Int J Psychophysiol*. 2003;48(2):221–245. Review.

202. Schneider SJ, Pope AT. Neuroleptic-like electroencephalographic changes in schizophrenics through biofeedback. *Biofeedback Self Regul*. 1982;7(4):479–490.

203. Schneider F, Rockstroh B, Heimann H, et al. Self-regulation of slow cortical potentials in psychiatric patients: schizophrenia. *Biofeedback Self Regul*. 1992;17(4):277–292.

204. Hardman E, Gruzelier J, Cheesman K, et al. Frontal interhemispheric asymmetry: self regulation and individual differences in humans. *Neurosci Lett*. 1997;221(2–3):117–120.

205. Gruzelier J, Hardman E, Wild J, Zaman R. Learned control of slow potential interhemispheric asymmetry in schizophrenia. *Int J Psychophysiol*. 1999;34(3):341–348.

206. Gruzelier J. Self regulation of electrocortical activity in schizophrenia and schizotypy: a review. *Clin Electroencephalogr*. 2000;31(1):23–29. Review.

207. Gruzelier JH. Theory, methods and new directions in the psychophysiology of the schizophrenic process and schizotypy. *Int J Psychophysiol*. 2003;48(2):221–245. Review.

208. Rollnik JD, Huber TJ, Mogk H, et al. High frequency repetitive transcranial magnetic stimulation (rTMS) of the dorsolateral prefrontal cortex in schizophrenic patients. *Neuroreport*. 2000;11(18):4013–4015.

209. d'Alfonso AA, Aleman A, Kessels RP, et al. Transcranial magnetic stimulation of left auditory cortex in patients with schizophrenia: effects on hallucinations and neurocognition. *J Neuropsychiat Clin Neurosci*. 2002;14(1):77–79.

210. Hoffman RE, Hawkins KA, Gueorguieva R, et al. Transcranial magnetic stimulation of left temporoparietal cortex and medication-resistant auditory hallucinations. *Arch Gen Psychiatry*. 2003;60(1):49–56.

211. Sürmeli T, Ertem A, Eralp E, Kos IH. Schizophrenia and the efficacy of qEEG-guided neurofeedback treatment: a clinical case series. *Clin EEG Neurosci.* 2012;43(2):133–144.

212. Cortoos A, Verstraeten E, Joly J, Cluydts R, De Hert, M, Peuskens, J. The impact of neurofeedback training on sleep quality in chronic schizophrenia patients: a controlled multiple case study. Unpublished manuscript. Society of Applied Neuroscience Annual meeting, 2006. Retrieved from <http://applied-neuroscience.org/index.php?option=com_content&view=article&id=64: 2006-san-programme&catid=64 > : previous-conferences.

213. Bolea AS. Neurofeedback treatment of chronic inpatient schizophrenia. *J Neurotherapy: Investig Neuromodulation, Neurofeedback Appl Neurosci.* 2010;14(1).

214. Lieberman JA, Stroup TS, McEvoy JP, et al. Effectiveness of antipsychotic drugs in patients with chronic schizophrenia. *N Engl J Med.* 2005;353:1209–1223.

215. Kane JM. Pharmacologic advances in the treatment of schizophrenia post-CATIE: an expert interview. *Med Psychiatry Ment Health.* 2006;11:1.

216. Janicak PG. The CATIE study and its implications for antipsychotic drug use. *Essent Psychopharmacol.* 2006;7(1):53–63.

217. Kay SR, Fiszbein A, Opler LA. The positive and negative syndrome scale (PANSS) for schizophrenia. *Schizophr Bull.* 1987;13(2):261–276.

218. Citrome L. Comparison of intramuscular ziprasidone, olanzapine, or aripiprazole for agitation: a quantitative review of efficacy and safety. *J Clin Psychiatry.* 2007;68:1876–1885.

219. Citrome L. Compelling or irrelevant? Using number needed to treat can help decide. *Acta Psychiatr Scand.* 2008;117:412–419.

220. Nigl AJ, Jackson B. Electromyograph biofeedback as an adjunct to standard psychiatric treatment. *J Clin Psychiatry.* 1979;40(10):433–436.

221. La Vaque TJ, Hammond DC, Trudeau D, et al. Template for developing guidelines for the evaluation of the clinical efficacy of psychophysiological interventions. *Appl Psychophysiol Biofeedback.* 2002;27(4):273–281. http://dx.doi.org/10.102 3/A:1021061318355

222. Prischep LS, John ER. Neurometrics: clinical applications Vol. 2 of Handbook of Electroencephalography and Clinical Neurophysiology. In: Lopes Da Silva FH, Storm van Leeuwen W, Remond A, eds. *Clinical Applications of Computer Analysis of EEG and other Neurophysiological Variables.* Amsterdam, The Netherlands: Elsevier; 1986:153–170.

223. Duncan B, Antonuccio DO. A patient bill of rights for psychotropic prescription: a call for a higher standard of care. *Int J Clin Med.* 2011;2:353–359.

224. Sürmeli T, Ertem A, Eralp E, Kos IH. Obsessive compulsive disorder and the efficacy of qEEG-guided neurofeedback treatment: a case series. *Clinical EEG and Neuroscience.* 2011;42(3):195–201.

225. Kaplan BJ, Giesbrecht G, Shannon S, Mcleod K. Evaluating treatments in health care: the instability of a one-legged stool. *BMC Med Res Methodol.* 2011;11:65.

226. Benson K, Hartz AJ. A comparison of observational studies and randomized, controlled trials. *N Engl J Med.* 2000;342(25):1878–1886.

227. Concato J, Shah N, Horwitz RI. Randomized, controlled trials, observational studies, and the hierarchy of research designs. *N Engl J Med.* 2000;342(25):1887–1892.

228. Britton A, McPherson K, KcKee M, Sanderson C, Black N, Bain C. Choosing between randomized and nonrandomized studies: a systematic review. *Health Technol Assess (Rockv).* 1998;2(13):1–124.

229. Hammond DC. Placebos and neurofeedback: a case for facilitating and maximizing placebo response in neurofeedback treatments. *J Neurotherapy.* 2011;15:94–114.

230. La Vaque TJ, Rossiter T. The ethical use of placebo controls in clinical research: the Declaration of Helsinki. *Applied Psychophysiology and Biofeedback*. 2001;26(1):23–37.
231. Duric NS, Assmus J, Gundersen DI, Elgen IB. Neurofeedback for the treatment of children and adolescents with ADHD: a randomized and controlled clinical trial using parental reports. *BMC Psychiatry*. 2012;12:107.
232. Report of the National Advisory Mental Health Council's Workgroup. From Discovery To Cure (NAMHC report). Accelerating the Development of New and Personalized Interventions for Mental Illness. August 2010.
233. Elkins G, Rajab MH, Marcus J. Complementary and alternative medicine use by psychiatric inpatients. *Psychol Rep*. 2005;96:163–166.
234. Lamb R. Some reflections on treating schizophrenics. *Arch Gen Psychiatry*. 1986;43:1007–1011.

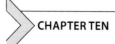

CHAPTER TEN

Treating Chronic Pain Disorders

Erbil Dursun and Nigar Dursun

Chronic pain is a common problem and expensive to treat. The success rate of all the available treatments for this condition is limited, because it rarely responds to the therapeutic measures that are successful in treating acute pain.[1] For the majority of patients, the currently used treatments can not eliminate pain adequately.[2] Besides, most of the pharmacological treatments used for chronic pain often have adverse effects, especially dependence on pain medications. For these reasons, as the mechanisms of pain become better understood, new interventions that may affect pain at the cortical level are being developed.[3–5]

For many years, biofeedback and relaxation therapies have been used in addition to medical approaches to treat acute and chronic pain syndromes. The term biofeedback covers a group of therapeutic procedures that use electronic or electromechanical instruments to properly measure, process and feed back to patients in the form of auditory and/or visual signals using information about their normal and/or abnormal neuromuscular and autonomic activity.[6] Biofeedback is used to help patients develop a greater awareness of and an increase in voluntary control over their physiological processes, which are otherwise involuntary and unfelt. In psychiatry, biofeedback has been used in a wide range of clinical conditions, such as motor weakness,[7,8] balance and gait disturbances,[9,10] spasticity,[11] neurogenic bladder[12] and bowel dysfunction,[13,14] and speech[15] and swallowing problems.[16] It has also been used in the management of various acute and chronic painful conditions, such as temporomandibular joint dysfunction,[17] headaches,[18] lower back pain[19] and patellofemoral pain syndrome.[20,21] In addition, biofeedback treatment is also suggested to be helpful in the management of fibromyalgia syndrome (FMS).[22]

Electroencephalographic (EEG) biofeedback is an operant conditioning procedure that can alter the amplitude, frequency or coherence of the neurophysiological dynamics of the brain. Therapeutic application of EEG

Clinical Neurotherapy.
Doi: http://dx.doi.org/10.1016/B978-0-12-396988-0.00010-6

biofeedback is often referred to as neurofeedback, and it has various clinical applications, such as migraine,[23,24] epilepsy,[25] attention deficit hyperactivity disorder (ADHD),[26–28] alcohol abuse,[29] sleep disorders[30] and chronic fatigue.[31] Sensorimotor rhythm (SMR) training is a commonly applied neurofeedback protocol that is normally associated with a quiet body and an active mind, and appears to facilitate thalamic inhibitory mechanisms.[32] On the other hand, studies in epileptic patients with SMR training showed significantly increased EEG spindle densities during sleep and prolonged sleep episodes, and a related decrease in state conversions.[33,34] In this way, SMR treatment suppresses some of the pathological consequences of epilepsy and potentially reduces vulnerability to a convulsion.

As described by the International Association for the Study of Pain (IASP), pain is an unpleasant sensory and emotional experience associated with actual or potential tissue damage, or is described in terms of such damage. According to IASP, pain is unquestionably a sensation in a part or parts of the body, but it is also always unpleasant, and therefore also an emotional experience. The IASP website continues: "Many people report pain in the absence of tissue damage or any likely pathophysiological cause; usually this happens for psychological reasons. There is usually no way to distinguish their experience from that due to tissue damage if we take the subjective report. If they regard their experience as pain, and if they report it in the same ways as pain caused by tissue damage, it should be accepted as pain."

If pain is considered only as a symptom associated with physical damage, and is understood as a simple response to physical damage, then nociception must be transmitted via a simple channel directly to a "pain perception area" in the brain. If we consider it like this, pain must be thought of as being related only to physical damage that occurs in the periphery. In this regard the brain is seen as a passive perceiver of sensory information. Melzak and Wall[35] integrated the physiological and psychological aspects of pain according to the gate control theory of pain. This theory declares that the dorsal horn of the spinal cord acts like a gate, regulating the flow of impulses from the peripheral nerve fibers to the brain. The gate is influenced by peripheral fiber activity and by descending influences from the central nervous system. Thus, this system explains how pain stimuli are adjusted in the spinal cord before moving to the brain. At present, as we better understand the mechanisms of pain in relation to the brain itself, our perceptions regarding pain are changing from the periphery and spinal cord to the brain itself. Supraspinal mechanisms are increasingly accepted as playing a major role in the representation and modulation of pain.[36]

Nociceptive stimuli are influenced on many levels in the brain, such as the cortex, insula, anterior cingulate and thalamus. Hyperalgesia is related to changes at the site of injury as well as to hyperexcitability in the central nervous system, which results in long-term changes to the nervous system, known as plasticity.[37] This hyperexcitability is also known as central sensitization and leads to increased activity at higher brain centers. It is likely perceived as more intense and prolonged pain.[38] A number of pathophysiological processes are suggested as responsible for the diffuse pain of FMS, including central pain processing systems, the hypothalamo-pituitary–adrenal axis and the autonomic nervous system, in which central pain syndromes are the most productive area of research.[39] There is increased tenderness to pressure in FMS, and augmentation of pain caused by central mechanisms. Augmentation of pain, such as windup,[40] or weakened effects of descending antinociceptive pathways, are examples of central mechanisms.[41] FMS patients have not only sensitivity to pressure stimuli but also decreased nociceptive thresholds with regard to heat, cold, electrical stimuli and even sound. The review by Williams and Clauw[39] focuses on their current understanding of FMS as a prototypical central pain syndrome. They stress that the terms central augmentation or central pain threshold are different from central sensitization, and because the tenderness or hyperalgesia occurs far away from the area of pain, central augmentation or central pain are likely to be more suitable terms for what is seen in FMS.

Deactivation of inhibitory processes in the central nervous system arouses interest.[38,42–44] Because the caudate nucleus and thalamus are both involved in signaling the occurrence of noxious events, low regional cerebral blood flow, which indicates decreased functional activity, is a marker for impaired inhibition of nociceptive transmission by these brain structures.[38] In chronic pain states, thalamic blood flow is reduced, whereas acute pain increases thalamic blood flow.[45,46] In a controlled study[47] the total Fibromyalgia Impact Questionnaire (FIQ) score in patients was positively correlated with blood flow in the parietal lobe, including the postcentral cortex. This correlation was seen in the areas of significant hyperfusion. Also the total FIQ score was negatively correlated with blood flow in a left anterior temporal cluster, one of the areas of significant hypoperfusion. The authors concluded that brain perfusion abnormalities in patients with FMS are correlated with the clinical severity of the disease. Mountz et al.[46] measured resting-state regional cerebral blood flow in the hemithalami and left and right heads of the caudate nucleus in

10 untreated women with FMS and seven normal control women using single-photon emission CT (SPECT). They also evaluated pain thresholds at tender and control points. Regional cerebral blood flow in the left and right hemithalami and the left and right heads of the caudate nucleus was found to be significantly lower in women with FMS, as were lower pain threshold levels. The authors concluded that abnormal pain perception in women with FMS might result from a functional abnormality within the central nervous system. Kwiatek et al.[45] measured regional cerebral blood flow using improved SPECT and advanced complementary analytic techniques in resting female FMS patients and in age-, gender-, and education-matched healthy controls. They confirmed that thalamic regional cerebral blood flow is reduced in FMS, but to a statistically significant extent only on the right. Low thalamic regional cerebral blood flow has been observed not only in patients with FMS, but also in patients with other chronic pain disorders, such as chronic neuropathic pain, metastatic cancer and mononeuropathy.[38] It may be that low thalamic regional cerebral blood flow, which indicates decreased functional activity, is a marker for impaired inhibition of nociceptive transmission by brain structures such as the caudate nucleus and thalamus.

Several studies suggest that P300 indicates the activation of inhibitory processes in the central nervous system, and a reduced P300 amplitude may demonstrate a deficit in these inhibitory mechanisms.[48] It was reported that P300 amplitudes were reduced in clinical conditions such as alcoholism, ADHD and Alzheimer's disease.[49–51] Hada et al.[52] declared that the lower P3a amplitude and weaker sources in alcoholics suggests disorganized inefficient brain functioning, and this global electrophysiological pattern suggests cortical disinhibition perhaps reflecting underlying central nervous system hyperexcitability in alcoholics.[52] Reduced P300 amplitudes are seen in patients with FMS, and sertraline was shown to increase the amplitude of P300 within 8 weeks.[53,54] SMR training increases P300 amplitudes, which supports the observation that SMR training facilitates thalamocortical inhibitory mechanisms.[55]

These findings have important implications regarding treatment, because the pain of tissue or nerve damage can be attacked at the site of the injury where it is initiated, as well as at central nervous system sites where it is maintained.[38] Interventions that reprogram or interrupt central sensitization could provide significant relief for some individuals with chronic pain, and the understanding that pain experience is modulated at many levels of the central nervous system opens the door to interventions that might affect pain at the cortical level, including treatments such as neurofeedback.[56] On the other hand, with regard to P300, we can assume that neurofeedback treatment may play an inhibitory role on the central nervous system, and this may alter central augmentation in FMS. In this way, we can hypothesize that neurofeedback treatment will be effective in alleviating the symptoms and signs of FMS.

Ibric and Dragomirescu[57] discusses 147 chronic pain patients, 10 of whom were presented as case studies. All of the 147 patients had little resolution of pain with other treatment modalities. The 10 case study patients had diagnoses including reflex sympathetic dystrophy, headache, neuropathy, myofascial pain, left inguinal pain, chronic lower back and leg pain, and FMS. In all cases the neurofeedback treatment involved SMR enhancement as well as theta and high beta discouragement. The patients had positive improvements after the neurofeedback treatment. The authors noted that the results of neurofeedback were highly dependent on the number of sessions: when sessions numbered 19 or fewer, the rate of success was very reduced, but when the patients had completed more than 19 sessions of neurofeedback training, the success rate was evident.

In our rater-blinded controlled study[5] involving 40 patients with FMS randomized into either a neurofeedback (enhanced SMR activity and decreased theta activity) or a control (escitalopram treatment) group, each neurofeedback session was 30 minutes long and the patients had five sessions per week. Each patient was trained at the same time of day for 4 weeks. The symptoms of FMS and the clinical grading scales were noted at baseline, and at the second, fourth, eighth, 16th and 24th weeks for both groups. The Visual Analogue Scale (VAS) for pain, VAS for fatigue, FIQ and Short Form-36 (SF-36), Hamilton Depression Scale (HDS), Beck Depression Scale (BDS), Hamilton Anxiety Scale (HAS) and Beck Anxiety Scale (BAS) were applied. Also, the mean amplitudes of alpha, beta 1, beta 2, theta, delta, SMR and theta/SMR ratios were recorded at baseline and at the second, fourth, eighth, 16th and 24th weeks in the neurofeedback group. VAS pain and VAS fatigue scores were significantly decreased by the end of the study period in the two groups. However, the values of the neurofeedback group were significantly lower than in the control group at all posttreatment assessments, even at the end of the 24th week. These findings emphasize the positive effects of neurofeedback on pain and fatigue, with the reorganization of the brain structures perhaps owing to facilitation of the thalamocortical inhibitory mechanisms.

Besides pain, patients with FMS have many other diagnostic symptoms, such as fatigue, sleep difficulties, a swollen feeling in tissues, paresthesias, cognitive dysfunction, dizziness, increased tenderness in multiple points, morning stiffness, psychological disorders, abdominal pain, dysmenorrhea, irritable bowel syndrome, headaches and restless legs syndrome. There is evidence for central sensitization in these conditions.[58] A neurogenic form has also developed, suggesting that functional dysregulation of central pain pathways could account for many of the clinical manifestations of FMS.[45] The frequent joining of chronic pain with several other chronic disabilities may not be coincidental. A meta-analysis shows that the brain network for acute pain perception in normal subjects is at least partially distinct from that seen in chronic clinical pain conditions, and that chronic pain engages brain regions critical for cognitive/emotional assessments, implying that this component of pain may be a distinguishing feature between chronic and acute pain.[36] There are brain regions that reduce their activity during task performance, and these regions are the component members of the default-mode network. Raichle et al.[59] used quantitative metabolic and circulatory measurements from positron-emission tomography to obtain the oxygen extraction fraction regionally throughout the brain. Areas of activation were prominent by their absence, and increases indicated deactivations. Baliki et al.[60] proposed that long-term pain alters the functional connectivity of cortical regions known to be active at rest. They demonstrated that chronic pain has a widespread impact on overall brain function, where the default-mode network shown by functional magnetic resonance imaging is imbalanced and disrupted, and disorders of the default-mode network may account for the development of accompanying cognitive and behavioral impairments. Therefore, neurofeedback's effect in positively altering the brain functions may be founded on its supporting effect in the correction of this cortical disruption.

As neurofeedback improves attention deficits, Caro and Winter[61] reasoned that FMS patients with cognitive and attention complaints might benefit from an EEG-based modality. In their experience many FMS symptoms correlate with one another. Because of this, they speculated that if neurofeedback positively improved cognitive symptoms in FMS, it might also improve somatic complaints. They included 15 FMS patients with attention problems who completed 40 or more neurofeedback sessions where the SMR protocol was used, which augmented 12–15 Hz brain waves while simultaneously inhibiting 4–7 Hz brain waves (theta) and 22–30 Hz brain waves (high beta). Sixty-three FMS patients who received standard medical treatment but who did not receive EEG biofeedback were included as controls. The neurofeedback group showed significant improvements in visual attention, tenderness, pain and fatigue.

Albeit not statistically significant, there was also a trend toward improvement in psychological distress and morning stiffness.

In an uncontrolled clinical trial, Mueller et al.[62] prospectively followed 30 FMS patients through a brainwave-based intervention known as EEG-driven stimulation. Besides this, patients had also other treatments, including massage therapy, physical therapy and surface electromyographic neuromuscular retraining. Before and after treatment and during an extended follow-up, comparison of the number of positive tender points and pain thresholds, psychological and physical functioning indices, and specific FMS symptom ratings revealed statistically significant improvements. In our study,[5] post-treatment assessments revealed that neurofeedback and control treatments caused significant improvements in depressive symptoms and anxiety; i.e., all the depression and anxiety scores (HDS, BDS, HAS and BAS) showed significant improvements in both the neurofeedback and the SF control groups, but the neurofeedback group displayed greater benefits than controls. In addition, FIQ and SF-36 revealed significant improvements in both of the groups, but the values of the neurofeedback group were significantly better than those of the escitalopram treatment group during the whole study period. These findings underline the positive effects of the neurofeedback treatment on psychosocial aspects, quality of life and physical functioning, in addition to other symptomatology of FMS. On the other hand, the therapeutic efficacy of neurofeedback was found to begin in the second week and reached its maximum effect in the fourth week, whereas the improvements in escitalopram treatment were also detected to begin in the second week but reached its maximum effect at the eighth week. This early effect of neurofeedback may be related to a faster brain plasticity process and certainly can be considered one of the advantages of this treatment.

Pain may be associated with relatively lower amplitudes of slower wave (delta, theta and alpha) activity and relatively higher amplitudes of faster wave (beta) activity.[56] Morphine treatment alters brain waves in the low-frequency range (2–4 Hz) during the first 300 ms after stimulus, whereas active brain waves remain unchanged after placebo treatment.[63] The results show significant slowing of the EEG in spinal cord-injured patients with neuropathic pain, consistent with the presence of thalamocortical dysrhythmia.[64] Intense painful stimulation causes an increase in beta wave activity and tends to reduce mostly alpha (slower) wave activity.[56] Mueller et al.[62] obtained statistically significant reductions in delta, theta and alpha waves after treatment. The relative predominance of low-frequency (delta, theta and low alpha) activity detected at the beginning of treatment had normalized by the end of treatment. In our study,[5] no statistically significant changes were noted regarding mean amplitudes of EEG rhythms. However, the theta/SMR ratio showed a significant decrease by the fourth week compared to baseline in the neurofeedback group. The detected decrease in theta/SMR ratio is important and may show a concrete finding concerning neurofeedback treatment. Thus, SMR neurofeedback treatment may have a facilitator effect on thalamic inhibitory mechanisms by arranging brain activity via increasing the slower waves and decreasing the faster waves of the brain. Further well-organized controlled studies with higher patient numbers are needed to verify this finding.

Pain is regulated by interactions between ascending and descending pathways, and brain mechanisms are increasingly being accepted as having a major role in the modulation of pain. Understanding these mechanisms is crucial if fully effective treatments for clinical pain conditions are to be developed.[36]

The etiologic factors of chronic pain syndromes and the relationship between chronic pain and central nervous system mechanisms need to be clarified in future investigations. Because the EEG is an important physiological tool, studies that use more quantitative EEG evaluations with respect to pain would be very helpful. On the other hand, it is obvious that scientific data are insufficient for neurofeedback interventions regarding pain modulation. Many well-designed controlled prospective studies with larger patient populations must be carried out in order to be certain about the role of neurofeedback interventions on pain management and its therapeutic mechanisms.

REFERENCES

1. Bennett RM. Emerging concepts in the neurobiology of chronic pain: evidence of abnormal sensory processing in fibromyalgia. *Mayo Clin Proc.* 1999;74(4):385–398.
2. Turk DC. Clinical effectiveness and cost-effectiveness of treatments for patients with chronic pain. *Clin J Pain.* 2002;18(6):355–365.
3. Fregni F, Freedman S, Pascual-Leone A. Recent advances in the treatment of chronic pain with non-invasive brain stimulation techniques. *Lancet Neurol.* 2007;6:188–191.
4. Green AL, Wang S, Bittar RG, et al. Deep brain stimulation for pain relief: a meta-analysis. *J Clin Neurosci.* 2005;12:515–519.
5. Kayiran S, Dursun E, Dursun N, Ermutlu N, Karamürsel S. Neurofeedback intervention in fibromyalgia syndrome; a randomized, controlled, rater blind clinical trial. *Appl Psychophysiol Biofeedback.* 2010;35(4):293–302.
6. Dursun E. Biofeedback. In: Stone JH, Blouin M, eds. *International Encyclopedia of Rehabilitation.* Available online: <http://cirrie.buffalo.edu/encyclopedia/article.php?id=23&language=en>.
7. Intiso D, Santilli V, Grasso MG, Rossi R, Caruso I. Rehabilitation of walking with electromyographic biofeedback in foot-drop after stroke. *Stroke.* 1994;25(6):1189–1192.

8. Wissel J, Ebersbach G, Gutjahr L, Dahlke F. Treating chronic hemiparesis with modified biofeedback. *Arch Phys Med Rehabil.* 1989;70(8):612–617.

9. Dursun E, Dursun N, Alican D. Effects of biofeedback treatment on gait in children with cerebral palsy. *Disabil Rehabil.* 2004;26(2):116–120.

10. Petrofsky JS. The use of electromyogram biofeedback to reduce Trendelenburg gait. *Eur J Appl Physiol.* 2001;85(5):491–495.

11. Nash J, Neilson PD, O'Dwyer NJ. Reducing spasticity to control muscle contracture of children with cerebral palsy. *Dev Med Child Neurol.* 1989;31(4):471–480.

12. Middaugh SJ, Whitehead WE, Burgio KL, Engel BT. Biofeedback in treatment of urinary incontinence in stroke patients. *Biofeedback Self Regul.* 1989;14(1):3–19.

13. Chiarioni G, Salandini L, Whitehead WE. Biofeedback benefits only patients with outlet dysfunction, not patients with isolated slow transit constipation. *Gastroenterology.* 2005;129(1):86–97.

14. Ho YH, Tan M. Biofeedback therapy for bowel dysfunction following low anterior resection. *Ann Acad Med Singapore.* 1997;26(3):299–302.

15. Draizar A. Clinical EMG feedback in motor speech disorders. *Arch Phys Med Rehabil.* 1984;65(8):481–484.

16. Denk DM, Kaider A. Videoendoscopic biofeedback: a simple method to improve the efficacy of swallowing rehabilitation of patients after head and neck surgery. *ORL J Otorhinolaryngol Relat Spec.* 1997;59(2):100–105.

17. Crider A, Glaros AG, Gevirtz RN. Efficacy of biofeedback-based treatments for temporomandibular disorders. *Appl Psychophysiol Biofeedback.* 2005;30(4):333–345.

18. Stokes DA, Lappin MS. Neurofeedback and biofeedback with 37 migraineurs: a clinical outcome study. *Behav Brain Funct.* 2010;6:9.

19. Neblett R, Mayer TG, Brede E, Gatchel RJ. Correcting abnormal flexion-relaxation in chronic lumbar pain: responsiveness to a new biofeedback training protocol. *Clin J Pain.* 2010;26(5):403–409.

20. Dursun N, Dursun E, Kili Z. Electromyographic biofeedback-controlled exercise versus conservative care for patellofemoral pain syndrome. *Arch Phys Med Rehabil.* 2001;82(12):1692–1695.

21. Yip SL, Ng GY. Biofeedback supplementation to physiotherapy exercise programme for rehabilitation of patellofemoral pain syndrome: a randomized controlled pilot study. *Clin Rehabil.* 2006;20(12):1050–1057.

22. Babu AS, Mathew E, Danda D, Prakash H. Management of patients with fibromyalgia using biofeedback: a randomized control trial. *Indian J Med Sci.* 2007;61(8):455–461.

23. Kropp P, Siniatchkin M, Gerber WD. On the pathophysiology of migraine–links for 'empirically based treatment' with neurofeedback. *Appl Psychophysiol Biofeedback.* 2002;27(3):203–213.

24. Siniatchkin M, Hierundar A, Kropp P, Kuhnert R, Gerber WD, Stephani U. Selfregulation of slow cortical potentials in children with migraine: an exploratory study. *Appl Psychophysiol Biofeedback.* 2000;25(1):13–32.

25. Saxena VS, Nadkarni VV. Nonpharmacological treatment of epilepsy. *Ann Indian Acad Neurol.* 2011;14(3):148–152.

26. Lofthouse N, Arnold LE, Hurt E. Current status of neurofeedback for attention-deficit/hyperactivity disorder. *Curr Psychiatry Rep.* 2012;14(5):536–542.

27. Monastra VJ. Quantitative electroencephalography and attention-deficit/hyperactivity disorder: Implications for clinical practice. *Curr Psychiatr Rep.* 2008;10:432–438.

28. Monastra VJ, Monastra DM, George S. The effects of stimulant therapy, EEG biofeedback, and parenting style on the primary symptoms of attention-deficit/hyperactivity disorder. *Appl Psychophysiol Biofeedback.* 2002;27(4):231–249.

29. Sokhadze TM, Cannon RL, Trudeau DL. EEG biofeedback as a treatment for substance use disorders: review, rating of efficacy, and recommendations for further research. *Appl Psychophysiol Biofeedback.* 2008;33(1):1–28.

30. Hammer BU, Colbert AP, Brown KA, Ilioi EC. Neurofeedback for insomnia: a pilot study of Z-score SMR and individualized protocols. *Appl Psychophysiol Biofeedback.* 2011;36(4):251–264.

31. Hammond DC. Treatment of chronic fatigue with neurofeedback and self-hypnosis. *NeuroRehabilitation.* 2001;16(4):295–300.

32. Sterman MB. Physiological origins and functional correlates of EEG rhythmic activities: implications for self-regulation. *Biofeedback Self Regul.* 1996;21:3–33.

33. Sterman MB, Howe RD, MacDonald LR. Facilitation of spindle-burst sleep by conditioning of electroencephalographic activity while awake. *Science.* 1970;167:1146–1148.

34. Sterman MB, Shouse MN. Quantitative analysis of training, sleep EEG, and clinical response to EEG operant conditioning in epileptics. *Electroencephalogr Clin Neurophysiol.* 1980;49:558–576.

35. Melzack R, Wall PD. Pain mechanisms: a new theory. *Science.* 2005;50:971–979.

36. Apkarian AV, Bushnell MC, Treede RD, Zubieta JK. Human brain mechanisms of pain perception and regulation in health and disease. *Eur J Pain.* 2005;9(4):463–484.

37. Dubner R, Ruda MA. Activity-dependent neuronal plasticity following tissue injury and inflammation. *Trends Neurosci.* 1992;15(3):96–103.

38. Pillemer SR, Bradley LA, Crofford LJ, Moldofsky H, Chrousos GP. The neuroscience and endocrinology of fibromyalgia. *Arthritis Rheum.* 1997;40(11):1928–1939.

39. Williams DA, Clauw DJ. Understanding fibromyalgia: lessons from the broader pain research community. *J Pain.* 2009;10(8):777–791.

40. Staud R, Price DD, Robinson ME, Mauderli AP, Vierck CJ. Maintenance of windup of second pain requires less frequent stimulation in fibromyalgia patients compared to normal controls. *Pain.* 2004;110:689–696.

41. Leffler AS, Hansson P, Kosek E. Somatosensory perception in a remote pain-free area and function of diffuse noxious inhibitory controls (DNIC) in patients suffering from long-term trapezius myalgia. *Eur J Pain.* 2002;6:149–159.

42. Howe RC, Sterman MB. Cortical-subcortical EEG correlates of suppressed motor behavior during sleep and waking in the cat. *Electroencephalogr Clin Neurophysiol.* 1972;32(6):681–695.

43. Lautenbacher S, Rollman GB. Possible deficiencies of pain modulation in fibromyalgia. *Clin J Pain.* 1997;13(3):189–196.

44. Staud R, Vierck CJ, Cannon RL, Mauderli AP, Price DD. Abnormal sensitization and temporal summation of second pain (wind-up) in patients with fibromyalgia syndrome. *Pain.* 2001;91(1–2):165–175.

45. Kwiatek R, Barnden L, Tedman R, et al. Regional cerebral blood flow in fibromyalgia: single-photon-emission computed tomography evidence of reduction in the pontine tegmentum and thalami. *Arthritis Rheum.* 2000;43(12):2823–2833.

46. Mountz JM, Bradley LA, Modell JG, et al. Fibromyalgia in women. Abnormalities of regional cerebral blood flow in the thalamus and the caudate nucleus are associated with low pain threshold levels. *Arthritis Rheum.* 1995;38(7):926–938.

47. Guedj E, Cammilleri S, Niboyet J, et al. Clinical correlate of brain SPECT perfusion abnormalities in fibromyalgia. *J Nucl Med.* 2008;49(11):1798–1803.

48. Zhang XL, Cohen HL, Porjesz B, Begleiter H. Mismatch negativity in subjects at high risk for alcoholism. *Alcohol Clin Exp Res.* 2001;25(3):330–337.

49. Ozdag MF, Yorbik O, Ulas UH, Hamamcioglu K, Vural O. Effect of methylphenidate on auditory event related potential in boys with attention deficit hyperactivity disorder. *Int J Pediatr Otorhinolaryngol.* 2004;68(10):1267–1272.

50. Pokryszko-Dragan A, Słotwiński K, Podemski R. Modality-specific changes in P300 parameters in patients with dementia of the Alzheimer type. *Med Sci Monit.* 2003;9(4):130–134.

51. Van der Stelt O, Geesken R, Gunning WB, Snel J, Kok A. P3 scalp topography to target and novel visual stimuli in children of alcoholics. *Alcohol*. 1998;15(2):119–136.
52. Hada M, Porjesz B, Begleiter H, Polich J. Auditory P3a assessment of male alcoholics. *Biol Psychiatry*. 2000;48(4):276–286.
53. Alanoğlu E, Ulaş UH, Ozdağ F, Odabaşi Z, Cakçi A, Vural O. Auditory event-related brain potentials in fibromyalgia syndrome. *Rheumatol Int*. 2005;25(5):345–349.
54. Ozgocmen S, Yoldas T, Kamanli A, Yildizhan H, Yigiter R, Ardicoglu O. Auditory P300 event related potentials and serotonin reuptake inhibitor treatment in patients with fibromyalgia. *Ann Rheum Dis*. 2003;62(6):551–555.
55. Egner T, Gruzelier JH. Learned self-regulation of EEG frequency components affects attention and event-related brain potentials in humans. *Neuroreport*. 2001;12(18):4155–4159.
56. Jensen MP, Hakimian S, Sherlin LH, Fregni F. New insights into neuromodulatory approaches for the treatment of pain. *J Pain*. 2008;9(3):193–199.
57. Ibric VL, Dragomirescu LG. Neurofeedback in pain management. In: Budzynski T, Budzynski H, Evans J, Abarbanel A, eds. *Introduction to Quantitative EEG and Neurofeedback–Advanced Theory and Applications*. New York, NY: Elsevier; 2008:417–451.
58. Yunus MB. Role of central sensitization in symptoms beyond muscle pain, and the evaluation of a patient with widespread pain. *Best Pract Res Clin Rheumatol*. 2007;21(3):481–497.
59. Raichle ME, MacLeod AM, Snyder AZ, Powers WJ, Gusnard DA, Shulman GL. A default mode of brain function. *Proc Natl Acad Sci USA*. 2001;98(2):676–682.
60. Baliki MN, Geha PY, Apkarian AV, Chialvo DR. Beyond feeling: chronic pain hurts the brain, disrupting the default-mode network dynamics. *J Neurosci*. 2008;28(6):1398–1403.
61. Caro XJ, Winter EF. EEG biofeedback treatment improves certain attention and somatic symptoms in fibromyalgia: a pilot study. *Appl Psychophysiol Biofeedback*. 2011;36:193–200.
62. Mueller HH, Donaldson CC, Nelson DV, Layman M. Treatment of fibromyalgia incorporating EEG-driven stimulation: a clinical outcomes study. *J Clin Psychol*. 2001;57(7):933–952.
63. Lelic D, Olesen AE, Brock C, Staahl C, Drewes AM. Advanced pharmaco-EEG reveals morphine induced changes in the brain's pain network. *J Clin Neurophysiol*. 2012;29(3):219–225.
64. Boord P, Siddall PJ, Tran Y, Herbert D, Middleton J, Craig A. Electroencephalographic slowing and reduced reactivity in neuropathic pain following spinal cord injury. *Spinal Cord*. 2008;46(2):118–123.

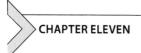

CHAPTER ELEVEN

Treating Addiction Disorders

Estate M. Sokhadze, David L. Trudeau and Rex L. Cannon

INTRODUCTION

This chapter focuses on the history and future potential of neurofeedback applications in substance use disorder (SUD). Neurofeedback has been used for more than 40 years in the treatment of alcoholism and other addictions but is still a less than mainstream intervention. The treatment of addictive disorders employs various individual- and group-based psychotherapeutic interventions, case management, residential structure, values-based programs, incentive-based (contingency management) therapy, cognitive–behavioral therapies (CBTs), pharmacological interventions, motivational techniques and other methods. Addictive disorders are complex and associated with other comorbid mental conditions, and it seems unlikely that a single approach will satisfy the needs of patients with SUD.

It is important to emphasize that neurofeedback is currently used mostly as an add-on treatment to other established addiction treatment therapies, namely 12-step programs and/or CBTs, or other types of psychotherapies or residential programs. Neurotherapy is not validated as a stand-alone therapy for addictive disorders. As noted, many addicted individuals have comorbid mental conditions, and these need to be considered when designing a treatment plan that incorporates neurotherapy. These include conditions such as mild traumatic brain injury (mTBI), anxiety disorders, including posttraumatic stress disorder (PTSD), affective disorders, depression or attention deficit hyperactivity disorder (ADHD), which may require separate neurofeedback treatment for those specific conditions either preceding neurofeedback treatment for addiction, or incorporated into it. Such conditions may require separate assessments during the course of therapy to determine response and the need to change protocols or seek other treatments, i.e., medication or psychotherapy, to integrate into the treatment plan.

SUDs include disorders related to the taking of a drug of abuse (including alcohol) and represent the most common psychiatric conditions that can

Clinical Neurotherapy.
Doi: http://dx.doi.org/10.1016/B978-0-12-396988-0.00011-8

result in serious impairments of cognition and behavior. Acute and chronic drug abuse results in significant alterations in brain activity[1] detectable with quantitative electroencephalography (qEEG) methods. The treatment of addictive disorders by EEG biofeedback (neurofeedback) was first popularized by the work of Eugene Peniston (often referred to as the Peniston Protocol).[2–4] This approach used independent auditory feedback to enhance two slow brainwave frequencies, alpha (8–13 Hz) and theta (4–8 Hz) during an eyes closed condition to produce a hypnagogic state. Prior to neurofeedback, the patient was taught to use what amounts to success imagery (of sobriety, refusing offers of alcohol, living confident and happy) as he or she drifted down into the "alpha/theta" state. Repeated sessions resulted in long-term abstinence and changes in personality test results. Because the method worked well for alcoholics, it was tried in subjects with cannabis dependence and stimulant dependence – but with limited success until the work of Scott and Kaiser.[5,6] The latter described treating stimulant-abusing subjects first with EEG biofeedback protocols commonly used with attention deficit disorders (ADDs), followed by the Peniston Protocol. They reported substantial improvements in program retention and long-term abstinence rates. This approach has become known widely as the Scott–Kaiser modification of the Peniston Protocol. A third approach to neurofeedback in SUD has been qEEG-guided neurofeedback, although the efficacy of this method has not been as extensively studied.

STUDIES OF EEG BIOFEEDBACK IN SUBSTANCE ABUSE TREATMENT

The Peniston Protocol (alpha/theta feedback)

The early studies on self-regulation of the alpha rhythm elicited substantial interest in potential clinical applications of alpha biofeedback for SUD treatment.[7] Several uncontrolled case studies and reviews on alpha EEG training for alcohol and drug abuse treatment were reported, but the impact of alpha biofeedback training as a SUD therapy was not significant.[8–17] The bulk of the literature to date regarding EEG biofeedback in addictive disorders is focused on simultaneous alpha and theta biofeedback. The technique involves the simultaneous measurement of occipital alpha (8–13 Hz) and theta (4–8 Hz), with feedback by separate auditory tones for each of those frequencies representing amplitudes greater than preset thresholds. The subject is encouraged to relax and to increase the amount of time the signal is heard, that is, to increase the amount of time that the amplitude of each defined bandwidth exceeds the threshold.

Alpha/theta feedback training was first employed and described by Elmer Green and colleagues[18] at the Menninger Clinic. The method was based on Green's observations of single-lead EEG during meditative states in practiced meditators. He had noted that increased theta amplitude occurred following initially increased alpha amplitude, and then a drop-off of alpha amplitude (theta/alpha crossover). When feedback of the alpha and theta signals was provided to subjects, states of profound relaxation and reverie were reported to occur. The method was seen as useful in augmenting psychotherapy and individual insight.[19] It could be seen as using a brainwave signal feedback to enable a subject to maintain a particular state of consciousness similar to a meditative or hypnotic, relaxed state over a 30- or 40-minute feedback session.

The first reported use of alpha/theta feedback in SUD treatment was in an integrated program at Topeka Veterans Affairs (VA) hospital, which included group and individual therapies. Daily 20-minute EEG biofeedback sessions (integrated with electromyographic biofeedback and temperature control biofeedback) were conducted over 6 weeks, resulting in free, loose associations, heightened sensitivity and increased suggestibility. Patients discussed their insights and experiences associated with biofeedback in therapy groups several times a week, augmenting expressive psychotherapy.[20,21] These initial studies advanced the utility of biofeedback-induced theta states in promoting insight and attitude change in alcoholics, with the assumption that biofeedback-induced theta states are associated with heightened awareness and suggestibility, and that such heightened awareness and suggestibility would enhance recovery. Outcome data regarding abstinence were not reported.

In the first reported randomized controlled study of alcoholics treated with alpha/theta EEG biofeedback, Peniston and Kulkosky[2] described positive outcome results. Their subjects were inpatients in a VA hospital treatment program, and all were men with established chronic alcoholism and multiple past failed treatments. Following a skin temperature biofeedback pretraining phase, Peniston's experimental subjects (n = 10) completed 15 30-minute sessions of eyes closed occipital alpha/theta biofeedback. Compared to a traditionally treated alcoholic control group (n = 10) and nonalcoholic controls (n = 10), alcoholics receiving brainwave biofeedback showed significantly greater percentage increases in the time that their EEG records contained alpha and theta rhythms, and greater increases in alpha rhythm amplitudes (single-lead measurements at international 10–20 system site O1). The experimentally treated subjects showed reductions in Beck Depression Inventory scores compared to the control groups. Control subjects who received standard treatment alone showed increased levels of circulating beta-endorphin, an index of stress, whereas the EEG biofeedback group did not. Follow-up data at 13 months indicated significantly more sustained prevention of relapse in alcoholics who completed alpha/theta brainwave training than in the control alcoholics. Successful relapse prevention was defined as "not using alcohol for more than 6 contiguous days" during the follow-up period. In a further report on the same control and experimental subjects, Peniston and Kulkosky[3] described substantial changes in personality test results in the experimental group compared to the controls. That is, the experimental group showed improvements in psychological adjustment on 13 scales of the Millon Clinical Multiaxial Inventory, compared to the traditionally treated alcoholics who improved on only two scales and became worse on one scale. On the 16-PF personality inventory, the neurofeedback training group demonstrated improvement on seven scales, compared to only one scale among the traditional treatment group. This small study used controls and blind outcome evaluation. Actual outcome figures of 80% positive outcome for the treatment group versus 20% for the traditional treatment control condition were reported at 4 years' follow-up.

With two exceptions, the protocol described by Peniston at the Fort Lyons VA facility cited above is similar to that initially employed by Twemlow and colleagues at the Topeka VA facility and by Elmer Green at the Menninger Clinic. The exceptions were (1) temperature training and (2) script. Peniston introduced temperature biofeedback training as a pre-conditioning relaxation exercise, and an induction script to be read at the start of each session. This latter protocol is the one that has become known as the Peniston Protocol (sometimes referred to also as Peniston Brain Wave Training Protocol), and has become the focus of research in subsequent studies. More specifically, subjects are first taught deep relaxation by skin temperature biofeedback using autogenic phrases and have at least five sessions of temperature feedback. Peniston used the criteria of attaining 94° before moving on to EEG biofeedback. They then are instructed in EEG biofeedback and, in an eyes closed and relaxed condition, receive auditory signals from EEG apparatus using the international 10–20 electrode site system's O1 site and a single electrode. A standard induction script using suggestions to relax and "sink down" into reverie is read.

When alpha (8–12 Hz) brain waves exceed a preset amplitude threshold, a pleasant tone is heard, and, by learning to produce this tone voluntarily, the subject becomes progressively relaxed. Then, when theta brain waves (4–8 Hz) are produced at sufficiently high amplitude, a second tone is heard, the subject becomes even more relaxed, and, according to Peniston, enters a hypnagogic state of free reverie and high suggestibility. Following the session, with the subject in a relaxed and suggestible state, a therapy session is conducted between subject and therapist where the contents of the imagery experienced are explored.[2–4,22,23]

A number of case series have replicated the initial findings of Peniston in terms of personality, mood and long-term abstinence with alcoholics.[24–29] However, attempts to employ alpha/theta with mixed substance abuse, especially stimulants, has not met with the same success. For a complete review of studies and a critical discussion, please see the review paper listed in the references.[30] It should also be noted that slow cortical potential feedback has been employed in alcoholics. Similar positive results have been claimed,[24–29] although no controlled studies have been reported. These studies indicate that applied psychophysiological approaches, mostly based on alpha/theta biofeedback protocols, are a valuable alternative or supplement to conventional substance abuse treatment.

The Scott–Kaiser Modification of the Peniston Protocol

It should be noted that psychostimulant (cocaine, methamphetamine) addictions may require various approaches, and neurofeedback protocols other than alpha/theta training. Cocaine-dependent persons become cortically underaroused during protracted abstinence. qEEG changes, such as a decrease in high beta (18–26 Hz) power, are typical of withdrawal from cocaine. Cocaine abusers who are still taking the drug often show low amounts of delta and excess alpha and beta activity, whereas chronic methamphetamine abusers usually exhibit excessive delta and theta activity.[30] Thus, cocaine and methamphetamine users may need different EEG biofeedback protocols, at least at the beginning stages of neurofeedback therapy.

Scott and Kaiser[5,6] describe combining a protocol commonly used for attentional training (beta and/or sensorimotor rhythm (SMR) augmentation with theta suppression) with the Peniston Protocol (alpha/theta training) in a population of subjects with mixed substance abuse but containing many stimulant abusers. Their beta protocol is similar to that used in ADHD.[31] It was used until measures of attention normalized, and then the standard Peniston Protocol (without temperature training) was applied.[6] Their study group was substantially different from that reported in either the Peniston or the replication studies. The rationale for their study was based in part on reports of substantial alterations in qEEG seen in stimulant abusers and associated with early treatment failure. This, in turn, had seemed likely to be associated with marked frontal neurotoxicity and alterations in dopamine receptor mechanisms. Additionally, pre-existing ADHD has been associated with stimulants as the "drugs of choice" in adult substance abusers, independent of stimulant-associated qEEG changes. These findings of chronic EEG abnormality and a high incidence of pre-existing ADHD in stimulant abusers suggested that they might be less able to engage in the hypnagogic and auto-suggestive Peniston Protocol. Furthermore, it was considered that eyes-closed alpha feedback as a starting protocol may be deleterious in stimulant abusers because the most common EEG abnormality in crack cocaine addicts is excess frontal alpha.[32]

Using their approach, Scott et al. in 2005[6] reported a substantial improvement in measures of attention and personality similar to those reported by Peniston and Kulkosky. A total of 121 inpatient drug program subjects were randomized to condition and were followed up at one year. Prior to treatment, members of the experimental and control groups were evaluated and matched for the presence of attentional and cognitive deficits, personality states and traits. The experimental group underwent an average of 13 SMR-beta (12–18 Hz) neurofeedback training sessions, followed by 30 alpha/theta sessions during the first 45 days of treatment. The control group received treatment as usual at the same center. Treatment retention was significantly better in the neurotherapy group and was positively associated with the initial SMR-beta training outcomes. The experimental group showed normalization of attentional variables following the SMR-beta portion of the neurofeedback, but the control group showed no improvement. Experimental subjects demonstrated significant changes (p < .005) beyond the control subjects on five of the 10 scales of the Minnesota Multiphasic Personality Inventory-2. Subjects in the experimental group were also more likely to stay in treatment longer, and more likely to complete treatment than the control group. Finally, the 1-year sustained abstinence levels were significantly higher for the experimental group than for the control group.[6]

The approach of beta training in conjunction with alpha/theta training has been applied with impressive results in a treatment program aimed at homeless crack cocaine abusers at a mission in Houston, Texas.[33] A total of 270 male addicts received 30 sessions of a protocol similar to the Scott–Kaiser modification. One-year follow-ups of 94 treatment completers indicate that 95.7% of subjects were maintaining a regular residence, 93.6% were employed/in school or training, and 88.3 % had had no arrests subsequent to the training. Self-report depression scores dropped by 50% and self-report anxiety scores by 66%. Furthermore, 53.2% reported no alcohol or drug use 12 months after neurofeedback, and 23.4% used drugs or alcohol only one to three times after their stay. This was a substantial improvement over the 30% or less expected recovery in this group. The remaining 23.4% reported using drugs or alcohol more than 20 times over the year. Urinalysis results corroborated self-reports of drug use. The treatment program saw substantial changes in length of stay and completion. After the introduction of SMR-beta neurofeedback treatment to the mission regimen, the length of stay tripled, beginning at 30 days on average and culminating at 100 days after the addition of alpha/theta neurotherapy. In a later study the authors reported follow-up results on 87 subjects after completion of all neurofeedback training.[33] The follow-up measures of drug screening results, length of residence and self-reported depression scores showed significant improvement. It should be noted that this study had several limitations, i.e., neurofeedback was positioned only as an adjunct therapy to all the other faith-based treatments for crack cocaine-abusing homeless persons enrolled in this residential shelter mission; in addition, it was an uncontrolled study. Yet the improvement in program retention is impressive and may well be causally related to the improved outcomes.

qEEG-guided Neurotherapy

A number of qEEG abnormalities have been described as specific to suspected neurotoxicities associated with chronic stimulant abuse (reviewed in[30,34]). These studies, based on reasonably uniform abstinence times and employing different EEG technology and analytical approaches, have remarkably similar and striking findings of alpha relative amplitude excess and delta relative amplitude deficit. Excess alpha amplitude with slowing of alpha frequency has been reported to be associated with chronic cannabis abuse. Clinically it may make good sense to consider specific neurotherapy treatment of these qEEG aberrations, either in place of or preceding alpha/theta therapy.

Neurotherapy approaches can be attractive alternatives for coexisting or underlying conditions in SUD clients who have high-risk behaviors for medication treatment, such as overdosing, abuse or poor compliance. Although there are no systematic published studies of the effects of neurotherapy treatment for co-occurring depression, mTBI, ADHD, PTSD or drug neurotoxicity on the course and outcome of addictive disorders, there have been several recent reports of neurotherapy for addictions based on qEEG findings. These, in turn, may be related to treatment of comorbidities. Basically, this technique involves the use of qEEG to identify patterns of EEG that deviate from standardized norms, thereby allowing individualized neurofeedback training protocols to be developed. Whereas historically alpha/theta training has been the accepted approach to treating alcohol and drug dependency, there are some theoretical bases to suggest that qEEG-guided training is a viable alternative that may lead to similar outcomes regarding personality change and abstinence rates. Future directions for qEEG-guided neurotherapy could include determination of those most likely to benefit from a particular treatment or combination of treatments, as well as assisting in the prediction of long-term abstinence. Preliminary results of qEEG-guided neurofeedback therapy as an outpatient treatment approach in drug- and alcohol-dependent patients are promising.[26,35] Gurnee[35] presented data on a series of 100 sequential participants with SUD treated by qEEG-based neurotherapy. There was marked heterogeneity of qEEG subtypes and corresponding symptom complexes in the group. In this clinically derived scheme, qEEGs that deviated from normative databases, mainly with excess alpha amplitude, were associated more often with depression and ADD. Those with deficient alpha amplitude were associated with anxiety, insomnia and alcohol/drug abuse. Excess beta amplitude was associated with anxiety, insomnia and alcohol/drug abuse. Central abnormalities were interpreted as mesial frontal dysfunction and associated with anxiety, rumination and obsessive–compulsive symptoms. The therapeutic approach was to base neurotherapy on correcting qEEG abnormalities, i.e., to train beta excess amplitude down when present, while monitoring symptoms.

INTEGRATING NEUROTHERAPY WITH OTHER THERAPIES

Pharmacotherapies

Pharmacological interventions for SUD have wide acceptance in certain situations. Aversive therapies for alcohol dependence, such as disulfuram, or neuropeptide-blocking therapy such as naltrexone, have been employed in alcoholics. New drugs designed to reduce alcohol consumption or binge drinking, or produce aversive reactions, regularly become available. There has been no study on the combined effects of neurofeedback with these therapies, but there is little reason to believe that there would be any negative interactions. There is a possibility, however, that alpha/theta neurofeedback could potentiate aversive drug therapies for alcoholics.

Opioid substitution, i.e., methadone maintenance or agonist/antagonist therapies for opioid addiction, are well accepted and widely acknowledged as efficacious. There is no study of neurofeedback per se in conjunction with these pharmacotherapies, but there is no obvious reason why it could not be used in cases where there is a comorbidity such as anxiety or ADHD, where sedative-type medications or stimulants may be less than desirable because of the risk of abuse.

Although effective agonist and antagonist pharmacotherapies as well as symptomatic treatments exist for opioid dependence, neither agonists nor antagonists have been approved as uniquely effective for the treatment of stimulant abuse or dependence.[36] There is no current evidence supporting the clinical use of pharmacological agents in the treatment of cocaine dependence.[37,38] However, there is continued interest in developing pharmacotherapies that may be effective in treatments for stimulant abuse. Below we discuss how opiate substitute pharmacotherapy could be combined with neurofeedback in opioid-dependent patients.

Rationale for Application of Neurofeedback in Opiate Addicts Enrolled in Maintenance Treatment

Opiate Drug Addiction

Opioid dependence is a neurobehavioral disorder characterized by a repeated compulsive seeking or use of an opioid medication. It is accompanied by well-described physical dependence with a withdrawal syndrome and tolerance. Opiate addiction includes not only abuse of illicit heroin and other opium derivates, but also the less commonly recognized problem of misuse and chronic abuse of prescription opioid pain relief medications, such as hydrocodone, oxycodone, codeine, etc. Dependence on and abuse of the prescription opioid drugs is now a major health problem, with prescription opioid abuse exceeding cocaine abuse in young people.[39,40] Opiate dependence is less prevalent in the general population than nicotine or alcohol dependence but represents a severe public health problem because it often runs a malignant course, with severe medical and

psychosocial morbidity and high mortality rates.[41–43] Methadone maintenance programs, despite positive results, have not kept pace with the
rising prevalence of opioid addiction. Buprenorphine was identified as
a viable option for the maintenance treatment of individuals addicted
to opioids, and the enactment of the Drug Addiction Treatment Act of
2000 has now enabled physicians in the United States to offer specifically approved formulations of buprenorphine for the treatment of opioid
addiction.[42] Maintenance treatment with buprenorphine tablets (Subutex)
has been associated with reductions in heroin and other opiate use; however, concerns exist with regard to intravenous misuse and other diversions.[44] A buprenorphine/naloxone formulation (Suboxone) for sublingual
use was designed to reduce this misuse risk while retaining buprenorphine's efficacy and safety. A fixed-combination formulation containing a
buprenorphine:naloxone ratio of 4:1 (hereafter referred to as Suboxone)
was approved for use in the European Union in 2006 and is available in
many countries for the management of opioid dependence.[45–52] However,
despite low physical symptoms of withdrawal, Suboxone-treated opioid-
dependent patients still demonstrate vulnerability to stress responses and
distorted emotional regulation.[53–57] Additionally, craving and physiological
arousal in response to drug-cues may contribute to the high rates of non-
compliance and relapse among opioid-dependent individuals undergoing
Suboxone maintenance treatment.

Craving, Attentional Bias and Cue Reactivity Connection in Opiate Addiction

Current concepts of addiction recognize craving as a central driving force
for continuing drug use. Craving, considered as a multidimensional construct,[58–60] is the result of an associative learning process, when environmental stimuli are repeatedly paired with drug consumption. In this
process, drug-related stimuli acquire excessive incentive–motivational value,
and evoke expectations of drug consumption and memories of past drug
euphoria.[61,62] Craving has been known to play an important role in ongoing drug use, relapse, and prognosis of treatment.[63–66] The cue-reactivity
paradigm has been among the most prominent methods for investigating
drug craving. It also is possible that treatment status may affect neurobiological responses to drug cues that are eliciting craving. If treatment status does affect reactivity to drug cues, such effects might be most readily
apparent in electrophysiological responses reflecting activity of the brain
structures implicated in integrating motivational or affective responses.

Conceptually, psychophysiological findings indicate that craving is a complex phenomenon involving both cognitive and affective processes. Craving has been described as an important clinical precipitant of relapse in opioid abusers and may be a useful additional outcome for developing new drug abuse therapies. Furthermore, high levels of craving during treatment or during cue-induced challenges predict poor treatment response and later relapse to drug abuse.

The results of an event-related potential (ERP) study[67] revealed robust significant positive correlations between heroin cue-evoked ERP amplitudes and self-reported craving for heroin. Recent studies conclude that automatic and perhaps unconscious processes may be related to the experience of craving.[68] These findings are in agreement with the theory of craving, which suggests that stimuli and mental representations associated with drug use produce the quality of "incentive salience," and therefore automatically capture the attention of the drug-dependent individual.[63] These processes should be reflected in the evoked EEG responses at the frontal and frontocentral sites known to be sensitive indicators of orienting to significant cues. According to modern theoretical models, cue reactivity might be resulting from a process of associative learning when previously neutral stimuli acquire incentive–motivational properties following repeated pairing with drug taking. These drug-associated stimuli can elicit both subjective reports of craving and increased negative affect.[69,70] Conditioned stimuli thus play a critical role in both ongoing drug-seeking behavior and during abstinence, when craving may perpetuate further drug use and relapse. Drug addicts exposed to pharmacotherapy exhibit less craving for drugs, suggesting that a greater understanding of the role of explicit orienting of attention to drug-related stimuli in drug-seeking behavior will ultimately help the development of more effective behavioral and neurotherapeutic approaches.

Emotional Abnormalities in Addiction

It has been shown that emotional abnormalities such as dysphoria and dysthymia are typical for addicts.[71–74] Addicted individuals could be affected by a dysregulation associated with changes in emotional reactivity to natural positive reinforcers.[75] Sensitization to drugs and counter-adaptation are hypothesized to contribute to dysregulation of hedonic homeostasis and observed abnormalities in brain reward systems.[76–79] Heightened physiological reactivity (including EEG responses) on exposure to drug-related cues, and attenuated physiological reactivity to naturally rewarding emotional cues, are common for addictions. Several studies also report increased physiological responsiveness to stress in addicts.[69,76] Furthermore, functional magnetic resonance imaging data have shown that addicted patients are less sensitive to pleasant stimuli, a condition usually referred to as anhedonia.[80] There is emerging evidence suggesting that emotional processes may have an important role in the predisposition to drug abuse and in the development of addiction, and that emotional alterations (both premorbid and those resulting from chronic drug use) may compromise the effectiveness of treatment approaches in addiction. Nonetheless, studies that have examined the experience of emotions in opiate-dependent patients, especially with regard to natural positive affective stimuli, are limited in number.[47–49,81,82] Because emotional deficits may have detrimental effects on the personal and social relationships of drug-dependent individuals, efforts aimed at preventing or treating compulsive drug-taking behavior should be more focused on regulating addicts' emotions and provide ways of learning to adapt during emotional states.

Neurobiology of Craving, Cue Reactivity and Anhedonia

Correlations between self-reported "urge to use" during viewing of heroin-related cues and increased regional blood flow in the orbitofrontal cortex (OFC), inferior frontal cortex (IFC), right precuneus and left insula were noted in a positron emission tomography (PET) scan study of heroin addicts.[83] A number of other neuroimaging studies have stressed the importance of mesolimbic and mesocortical systems in the control and regulation of addictive behaviors.[54,75,81,84–89] Involvement of these systems implies that dopaminergic projections of the ventral tegmental area to the nucleus accumbens, amygdala, hippocampus, anterior cingulate cortex (ACC) and prefrontal cortex (PFC) play a major role in the motivational and rewarding effects of addictive drugs.[64–66] The mesolimbic system is involved in the reinforcing effects of drugs and conditioned responses during craving, and this system is also responsible for emotional and motivational changes during withdrawal.[85] The mesocortical system is involved in the attribution of incentive salience to environmental stimuli associated with drug use.[59,63,90–94] Exposure to such drug-related cues results in cravings, leading to compulsive drug use and relapse. Neuroimaging investigations of the neurobiological correlates of drug cue-elicited craving have shown that the neural structures involved in cue-reactivity and craving appear to be similar for all drugs of abuse. The most prominent brain regions found to be activated by visual cue exposure are the ACC, the OFC and the dorsolateral PFC.[95–97]

Among related studies only a few have investigated the neuroanatomic substrate of acute heroin and opiate craving. PET studies[98,99] in 12 abstinent opioid-dependent subjects used auditory personal craving memory scripts and reported activation of the left medial PFC and left ACC. In some ERP studies, cue-evoked P300 and slow positive waves (SPW) were thought to reflect allocation of attention and effort during a variety of cognitive processing tasks, and these have also been shown to be indicative of motivational significance of affect-related processes.[100,101] However, research on P300 and other ERPs in opiate-addicted individuals is limited.[102] Franken[67] examined ERPs in heroin-dependent patients and controls while exposed to neutral and heroin-related pictures, and found larger SPW on heroin cues than on neutral cues in heroin addicts, indicating the motivational relevance of heroin cues. Recent studies on how individual drugs of abuse initiate their habit-forming actions have revealed that disparate drugs activate a common reward circuitry in the brain. Although different drugs (heroin, cocaine, nicotine, alcohol and cannabis) have distinct chemical actions, their habit-forming actions and the elements of their withdrawal symptoms appear to have a common denominator, namely, similar effects in "hijacking"[55,103] the brain mechanisms of reward.

Conceptual Approach to Treatment of Opiate Addiction Using Neurofeedback

Monitoring cue-reactivity, craving and emotional states in controlled environments before, during and after neurotherapy with opiate-dependent patients should be considered an important objective. To improve replacement therapy outcomes and prevent the risk of relapse, it should be feasible to modify the cognitive, attentional, affective and behavioral mechanisms that mediate the motivational and emotional processes involved in drug-cue reactivity. Thus, the goal would be to modify the overlearned and consolidated response to drugs and drug-associated conditioned stimuli[104] that are often accompanied by craving and negative affect. According to Volkow et al.,[89] effective monitoring and modification of cue-reactivity is considered an efficient treatment strategy to prevent the progression of drug abuse into drug dependence, and lower the chance of relapse in drug-dependent addicts in treatment. An effective treatment approach for opioid dependence might consist of emphasizing the risk associated with exposure to drug-related stimuli and environments, along with cognitive, behavioral and neurofeedback-based regulation of responses to these stimuli in a controlled and monitored environment, where both subjective reports of craving and physiological responses are recorded and analyzed in real time. Some of our earlier studies looked at the relationship between a drug-cue-induced attentional bias and treatment status in a group of cocaine abusers enrolled in neurofeedback treatment.[30,34,105–109] We found decreased cue-reactivity to drug- and stress-related cues after neurofeedback treatment.[110] So far, only one study has been reported where neurofeedback was used in a group of methadone-maintained opioid-dependent addicts.[111]

Modification of Cue-Reactivity and Affect Using Pharmacotherapy and Neurofeedback Training

We propose that attentional bias and reactivity toward opiate drug-related cues in patients with opioid dependence are very common, and that the extent of the attentional bias, cue-reactivity and craving would change depending on the current clinical conditions of patients on Suboxone replacement therapy enrolled in neurofeedback treatment. We propose that treated patients, specifically those on opioid substitution therapy combined with neurofeedback therapy and positive emotion training, would show a smaller attentional bias than before treatment. This would result from the reduction in the motivational salience of drug-related cues, albeit through different moderating mechanisms, i.e., either by reducing craving (opioid substitution therapy) or by modifying behavior using neurofeedback aimed at training positive emotions. In line with findings from other studies,[89,112] opioid substitution therapy, with either methadone or buprenorphine, may result in alteration of physiological reactivity to stimuli associated with drugs by reducing craving and attenuating withdrawal symptoms, most likely through a modification of the reward response.[99,113] The moderating mechanism underlying the predicted reduction of craving and negative affect in neurofeedback therapy is different because it may be ascribed to a cognitive remediation and behavioral shift toward other types of positive reward, and through discouragement of the perpetuation of maladaptive dysphoric states.

Rationale of Strategy of Intervention That Combines Replacement Therapy and Neurofeedback in Opiate Addicts

The approach that we suggest fits with the model of addiction and strategies of intervention proposed by Volkow et al.[75] Those authors suggested that the treatment of drug dependence should focus on reducing the reward value of drugs while increasing saliency and motivational values for natural rewards. The approach considers strategies to reduce conditioned drug behaviors and increase frontal executive functions as potential moderators. Furthermore, to achieve more prolonged results, the strategy of biobehavioral intervention in the field of addiction must incorporate techniques aimed to re-educate patients to control and self-regulate their emotional and motivational states, and train them to relearn the induction of positive affect in an attempt to try to re-establish the normal biological, cognitive, behavioral and hedonic homeostasis distorted by drug abuse.[77,78] In the "allostatic model of addiction" Koob and LeMoal[77] suggested that continued drug use may gradually deteriorate natural hedonic homeostasis and result in the higher threshold for the amount of emotionally positive stimulation needed to experience reward and positive affect states.[114–116] Active drug use and withdrawal-related alterations in neural structures involved in the stress response are well known,[79] and according to Li and Sinha,[117] these neuroadaptive changes in stress circuits may contribute to the increased salience of drug and drug-related stimuli in a variety of challenge or "stress" contexts.[69,93,106,107] This may contribute to a reduced coping ability, poor behavioral flexibility and deficient problem-solving capacity under stress or emotional challenges in substance abusers.[70,117,118] As was proposed in our conceptual paper,[34] drug abusers may develop hypersensitivity not only to drug-related stimuli, but also to stress stimuli, thus presenting similar psychophysiological reactivity to both drug- and stress-related cues. This may partially explain the high rate of comorbidity between substance use and anxiety disorders.[119,120] Neurofeedback with emotion self-regulation training elements, combined with opiate substitution therapy, is a potentially beneficial strategy to significantly change extent of implicit reactivity to drug cues, promote resilience to stress and increase positive emotionality during experimental exposures and real-life situations.

We propose that craving, anhedonia, negative affect and excessive reactivity to drug-related cues and environments are core mediating mechanisms. These mechanisms precede the drug-seeking and drug-taking behaviors in drug dependence and are major factors in liability to relapse. Comparing the qEEG profiles and correlates of craving, drug-cue responsiveness and more general emotional processes may provide more knowledge of the interaction between craving, affect-related states and motivational processes. Combining measures of EEG variables and autonomic responses with subjective reports offers an innovative and possibly very useful technique for assessing motivational relevance and the emotional value of drug-related and naturally affective stimuli. This technique may provide further understanding of craving and motivation to seek drugs in opiate dependency.

The conceptual framework of the proposed treatment model includes the realization that attenuated reactivity of the reward system to natural reinforcers (e.g., anhedonia) might itself be a consequence both of drug withdrawal and chronic intoxication, resulting in disruption of dopamine and endorphin turnover. Another important point of the proposal is an emphasis on the possible role of excessive stress responsiveness to the habit-forming properties of opiates. The addictive processes have been examined from multiple perspectives; however, there have been no studies examining the *experience* of the emotions in clinical populations of drug-dependent users in substitute treatment, especially with regard to everyday stimuli not related to situations of drug use.

Such studies might contribute by adding more emotion-specific physiological data to complement recent neuroimaging studies that have detected a lower activation of the emotional response of drug users to stimuli whose content generally is perceived as pleasant by the non-addicted population.[81,82] Among the possible therapeutic recommendations for the treatment of addictions, Volkow et al.[75] propose the need to carry out interventions designed to increase the value of natural reinforcers not related to drugs, for the purposes of increasing the sensitivity of addicts to these natural stimuli and re-establishing new sources of reinforcement.

RATIONALE FOR NEUROFEEDBACK APPLICATION IN ADOLESCENT SUBSTANCE ABUSERS WITH COMORBID DISRUPTIVE BEHAVIORAL DISORDERS

Characteristics of SUD, ADHD and Other Disruptive Behavioral Disorders in Adolescents

The high prevalence of drug and alcohol use, and the incidence of substance abuse in children and adolescents, has become a major public health concern in the United States. According to the Substance Abuse and Mental Health Services Administration,[40] about 28.2% of children and adolescents aged 12–20 reported drinking alcohol, and rates of reported illicit drug use were 17% among 16–17-year-olds, and as high as 22.3% among 18–20-year-olds. More alarmingly, the rate of substance dependence or abuse in 12–17-year-olds has been reported to be as high as 8.0%. Epidemiological statistics point to the widespread use of alcohol and illegal substances by underage persons in the United States, and the development of SUD in children and adolescents under 21 should be of public concern. Couwenbergh et al.[121] analyzed the prevalence of comorbid psychiatric disorders in nontreated adolescents and young adults with SUD in the general population. The prevalence of comorbid psychiatric disorders varied from 61% to 88%. Externalizing disorders, especially ADHD, conduct disorder (CD) and oppositional defiant disorder (ODD), were most consistently linked to SUD in treatment-seeking adolescent males.[122] Childhood behavioral problems are important risk factors for the development of SUD.[123–128] It has been suggested that common genetic risk factors may underlie both childhood behavioral disorders and adulthood alcohol and drug dependence.[129]

ADHD is one of the most common psychiatric conditions of childhood, affecting between 5% and 6% of school-aged children.[130,131] Some studies cite an even higher rate (up to 7.5%) among 6–17-year-olds.[132] Some primary symptoms of ADHD are distractibility, impulsivity and hyperactivity.[133] ADHD is a risk factor predisposing children to psychiatric and social pathology in later life. Even though several controlled studies indicate that up to 80% of ADHD children have beneficial clinical effects from stimulant medications,[134] the majority of parents with an ADHD child either do not seek treatment or discontinue treatment because of the fear of adverse medication effects.[135–137] Reluctance regarding medication usage is a significant impediment to treatment, and therefore the development of non-pharmacological approaches to ADHD are needed. The most common comorbid disorders in ADHD are disruptive behavioral disorders, with studies reporting that between 42% and 93% of children with ADHD have CD or ODD.[131,138–143] Disruptive behavioral disorders (i.e., CD and ODD) are characterized by a recurring pattern of antisocial behavior involving the violation of others' rights and societal norms.[144–147] Young persons exhibiting various forms of CD victimize others, disrupt families, fail at school, commit crimes in the community, and often abuse alcohol and illicit drugs. ADHD symptoms predicted increases in oppositional defiant behavior and conduct problems over time and were uniquely related to future academic difficulties. Although EEG studies have found consistent differences between children with and without ADHD, attention deficit is often a highly comorbid disorder, being found especially in conjunction with CD or ODD.[148]

Behavioral and Neurobiological Factors of Substance Abuse in Adolescents

There is substantial evidence to suggest that adolescents diagnosed with ADHD and comorbid disruptive behaviors are more likely to develop problems related to substance use than those without these comorbidities.[140,150] Therefore, although behavioral problems may explain substance use in adolescents with ADHD, ADHD may be a stronger predictor of substance use in adulthood. The so-called "self-medication theory of addiction"[151,152] may explain the relationship between ADHD and substance abuse, proposing that persistent ADHD symptoms may lead to impairments in academic, family and social functioning, and these impairments in turn may lead to a propensity to use alcohol or drugs to cope with functional deficits.[152,153] One of the important characteristics of adolescent drug users is that they belong to a so-called "opportunistic users" category, because they have not yet formed a preferred substance choice compared to adult drug addicts. Furthermore, high impulsivity and low behavior inhibition control, typical in ADHD, may drive them to try a novel substance without thinking about the consequences. Adolescents represent a vulnerable group at heightened risk for experimentation with narcotic substances, and the early experimentation is known to be associated with higher rates of substance dependence in adulthood.[154]

There are also several neurobiological factors involved in the etiology of adolescent addiction, and various neural and behavioral mechanisms are implicated in its development. Some of these neurobiological developmental factors, such as immature frontal–limbic connections, immature frontal lobe development, lesser myelination and lesser pruning than in adults, lowered serotoninergic function, and abnormal hypothalamopituitary–adrenal axis function, are capable of predisposing adolescents to a heightened risk for SUD. These neurobiological liabilities may correspond with and translate into impairment in decision-making, keeping company with behaviorally deviant peers, and various undesirable externalizing behaviors. As has been noted by others, these and other cognitive and behavioral traits can converge with neurobiological factors to increase the risk of SUD.[108,154]

It has been shown that emotional abnormalities are typical for addicts[72,82] and may also occur in adolescents, making them vulnerable to experimentation with drugs. ADHD is also often characterized by emotional disturbances, such as mood lability, dysphoria, and temper outbursts.[133] CD has even more extreme emotional deficiency manifestations, often owing to an inability to correctly "read" the emotions of peers. Thus, it seems reasonable to pay attention to affective abnormalities in SUD, ADHD and other disruptive behavioral disorders, and, perhaps especially, to examine disturbances in emotion recognition and processing in adolescents with dual diagnoses.

TREATMENT STRATEGIES FOR ADHD AND SUBSTANCE ABUSE IN ADOLESCENTS

For a more effective clinical outcome and reliable prevention of relapse in adolescents and young adults using alcohol and drugs, a long-term treatment for SUD is usually necessary.[155,156] Although effective agonist/antagonist pharmacotherapies as well as symptomatic treatments exist for opioid dependence (e.g., methadone or Suboxone maintenance), neither agonists nor antagonists have been approved as uniquely effective for the treatment of stimulant dependence.[157] Because no proven effective pharmacological interventions are available for cocaine or methamphetamine addiction, treatment of stimulant addiction has to rely on existing CBTs or other behavioral approaches.[158] The best current intervention for cannabis abuse also is oriented to behavioral approaches rather than pharmacotherapy.

Treatment of a comorbid mental condition may require concurrent treatment of drug addiction.[159] In some cases comorbid drug addiction results from attempts to alleviate a psychiatric disorder through self-medication.[150,151] Furthermore, in some cases the severity of comorbid psychiatric symptoms then increases as a consequence of drug abuse.[75,89] In patients with drug abuse arising from an attempt to self-medicate, treatment of the comorbid mental disorder might have prevented the abuse. For instance, treatment of a pre-existing condition of ADHD in childhood and adolescence may prevent psychostimulant abuse in adulthood.[108,160–162] Pharmacotherapy, primarily in the form of psychostimulants such as methylphenidate, remains the mainstream treatment for ADHD.[163–165] However, many clinicians are very reluctant to prescribe stimulants to adolescents with a drug abuse record, especially those with a history of prescription medication misuse and diversions.[166,167]

Neurofeedback training-based neurotherapy is one of the potentially efficacious nonpharmacological treatment options for SUD.[30,34,108,168] Neurofeedback is promising as a treatment modality for adolescents, especially those with stimulant abuse and attention and conduct problems.[108,169] There is practically no literature on the use of neurofeedback in adolescent addictions, and the only information available comes from studies published on adult addiction treatment. Neurofeedback has been studied as a method for treatment of addictive disorders in adults over the past 20 years or so, with a slowly accumulating body of evidence supporting its use in different circumstances. Several recent reviews[30,34,108,159,168–171] have detailed the literature regarding its use and the development of neurofeed-back for SUD.

Neurofeedback techniques for SUD may be of special interest for adolescent medicine because of the high comorbidity of SUD and ADHD in adolescents.[169] Among alternative treatment approaches, neurofeedback has gained promising empirical support in recent years.[136,172–177] Short-term effects were shown to be comparable to those of stimulant medication at the behavioral and neuropsychological level, leading to significant decreases in inattention, hyperactivity and impulsivity.[135,178–181] Techniques that combine classic ADHD neurofeedback approaches with addiction neurofeedback approaches hold special interest for adolescents with SUD. Such techniques are medication free and thus minimize opportunities for medication abuse, either by inappropriate self-overdosing or by trading medication for other substances. Neurofeedback techniques may be especially applicable in attempting to treat the constellation of CD, non-alcohol SUD and ADHD in already stimulant-abusing teens. Trudeau[170] reported on the high incidence of childhood ADHD in a sample of chronic SUD adults and found that childhood ADHD status in this population predicted adult stimulant abuse. This research sample supports other literature finding a significant overrepresentation of adults and adolescents with comorbid ADHD and SUD, and also of children with ADHD who eventually develop SUD.[160,184–188] By providing low-risk and medication-free therapy for both ADHD and SUD, neurofeedback becomes another treatment option open to practitioners reluctant to prescribe controlled substances to ADHD adolescents at risk for, or already having, SUD.

Based on our earlier pilot research on neurofeedback therapy in addiction,[28,30,34,168,189] and on studies of behavioral interventions based on effects of motivational interviewing[116] in cocaine-dependent subjects and in ADHD,[106,108–110,189] we propose that combining neurofeedback with an appropriate CBT technique will result in an effective biobehavioral intervention for adolescent addicts with ADHD and/or CD comorbidity. There are currently several CBT programs that can be used in community mental health services for adolescents,[190] for example the Seven Challenges.[191]

Adolescent patients with a co-occurring mental disorder and drug addiction are more resistant to treatment than those without dual diagnoses and are reluctant to enter either inpatient or outpatient treatment programs.[192–195] CBT may enhance remediation of behavioral problems that complicate the engagement of dually diagnosed adolescents in treatment. Treatment of adolescent patients with SUD using neurofeedback may become more complicated when they present with various psychiatric conditions. When addiction is comorbid with ADHD, it is suggested that in many cases SMR or beta increase and theta decrease training should be conducted first, to address the ADHD symptoms.[161] More research needs to be done to determine the clinical outcome and efficacy of neurotherapy based on EEG self-regulation in SUD comorbid with disruptive behavioral disorders. This also needs to be done first in SUD co-occurring with ADHD, because ADHD very often is accompanied by comorbid CD and ODD.

Although there is little work available on the prevention and treatment of SUD in adolescents and children using neurofeedback, there is no reason to suspect that the applicability of the approaches used in adults would not be applicable in SUD adolescents.[169] There has been only one unpublished report of brainwave biofeedback used to treat co-occurring ADHD and conduct problems in adolescents with SUD.[196] That study did not address the issue of SUD per se, and outcome data regarding long-term follow-up of substance use status are not available. One study of behavioral control in adult offenders using EEG biofeedback techniques has been published,[197] again suggesting the utility of neurofeedback in settings where conduct/behavior problems are of concern.

Neurofeedback for ADHD in children and adolescents has been extensively reviewed.[136,172,174,177,199] To date, several controlled-group studies[135,178–181,183,1100] have been reported in peer-reviewed journals. However, so far there have been no reported studies of the effect of neurofeedback treatment on the prevention of SUD in adolescents.

Neurofeedback for ADHD may be medication free, or combined adjunctively with medication. It may be a preferred approach for child and adolescent ADHD when stimulant medication abuse is suspected, or if side effects of medication are not tolerated, or if medication is not fully effective. It also may be the choice of patients and therapists who prefer nonmedication treatments. Side effects commonly associated with medication (such as growth retardation, poor appetite, sleep disturbances, etc.) have not been reported with neurofeedback. Furthermore, self-regulation of brain electrical activity may have even more potential in adolescence than in adulthood, because of the greater plasticity of neural systems at that age.

NEUROFEEDBACK-BASED INTERVENTION IN DRUG ABUSING ADOLESCENTS WITH ADHD

In this section we present various details of proposed research concerning neurofeedback-based treatment for drug-abusing adolescents with a concurrent diagnosis of ADHD. We propose the utility of such clinical research in the development and implementation of substance use and ADHD in adolescence that specifically target the development and strengthening of executive functions using operant conditioning of specific EEG frequencies, along with cognitive–behavioral remediation of the social functioning domain using CBT techniques. Pre- and post-treatment and later follow-up assessments using clinical, behavioral, and specific executive and emotional functioning tests should be used to provide insight into possible mediators and moderators of the integrated intervention outcome. We propose that behavioral, cognitive and emotional functions should be considered among the possible mediators of effects on substance abuse outcomes. Our proposed integrated treatment promotes neurocognitive efficiency by providing adolescents with the opportunity to practice skills related to frontal lobe development and executive function through EEG training, and through behavioral skills training, which has been found to be significantly related to decreases in substance abuse and aberrant behaviors. Few, if any, other substance abuse interventions explicitly intend to promote the development of neurocognitive abilities using intensive and specific training based on real-time EEG analysis. We advocate an integrated intervention to promote skills such as conscious strategies for self-control, attention, concentration and problem-solving, which may ultimately aid further in the development of adolescents' neurocognitive capabilities.

Current theoretical models of ADHD suggest that a core deficit is not attention as such, but rather disruption of executive functions, and in particular behavioral inhibition deficit. Converging evidence supports the view that ADHD is related to the atypical development of cognitive control along frontostriatal networks. The same self-regulation deficits occur in SUD, and, of course, in CD. Whereas qEEG studies present well-documented differences between adolescents with ADHD and controls, it is very likely that more differences among EEG markers will be manifested during the performance of specific tests, e.g., executive function tests, and electrocortical abnormalities in both ADHD and SUD patients will become apparent. In addition to attentional and cognitive impairment, there are disruptions in processing emotion and mood abnormalities in many individuals with ADHD,[200] CD, ODD and substance abuse, but little is known about the neural basis or EEG correlates of these affective impairments.

Methods of self-regulation of executive functions in vulnerable adolescents should be based on specific protocols that set training goals resulting in improvement in attention, vigilance, activity level and the development of skills to inhibit impulsive behavioral responses. The neurobiological nature of vulnerabilities for addiction,[75,85,88,89] the high rate of comorbid ADHD/SUD, and the negative impact of drugs on the brain and behavior of youth make it extremely important to apply efforts to develop theoretically and practically sound early intervention methods. Neurofeedback, qEEG evaluations and neurocognitive tests should constitute an important part of treatment and outcome assessment. Because untreated ADHD is a risk factor for SUD, neurofeedback treatment of ADHD may be an especially important intervention for adolescents at risk for developing SUD. Future studies combining CBT and neurofeedback in adolescent drug and alcohol abuse treatment settings, where SUD and ADHD often co-occur, should be conducted to assess the clinical effectiveness and outcomes of this promising technique. A crucial point about neurofeedback is that it acts directly on the brain oscillations that are altered in SUD and ADHD. Neurofeedback-induced modifications must be treated as a manifestation of neural plasticity, which we consider to be a basic mechanism for behavioral modifications. And, as noted earlier, self-regulation of brain activity may have even more potential in adolescence because of the greater plasticity of neural systems at this age compared to the adult population.

FURTHER RESEARCH

It was not the aim of this chapter to be an exhaustive treatise on the state of research into neurofeedback and addictive disorders. Neurotherapy is a new and rapidly developing field, and substantially more information is needed about many aspects of neurofeedback and SUD to validate its clinical utility and efficacy. In this section we mention several areas we consider especially promising for future research.

For example, more information is needed regarding qEEG-guided biofeedback and addictive disorder. Specific patterns of qEEG abnormality associated with substance use toxicity, such as those found in stimulant abuse or alcohol abuse, or with comorbidities such as ADHD, PTSD or TBI, suggest underlying brain pathologies that might be especially amenable to individualized EEG biofeedback. These approaches would likely be individualized rather than protocol based and could be used independently or in conjunction with, for example, classic alpha/theta or theta/beta training. qEEG patterns and abnormalities depend significantly on factors such as whether the subject is still currently using, the chronicity of use, and the current stage of withdrawal or protracted abstinence. A neurofeedback protocol selected for an individual client with SUD should be directly related to the level of current substance use or abstinence, especially in drugs such as heroin, where withdrawal syndrome results in substantial physiological manifestations, including transient qEEG changes. Even though there are no reported systematic studies of EEG biofeedback treatment of commonly occurring comorbidities of SUDs, it makes sense that clinical EEG biofeedback treatment and research protocols consider the presence of ADHD, TBI, PTSD, depression and drug-associated neurotoxicity. This approach may improve outcome, especially in participants resistant to conventional treatments.

A very important objective for future neurofeedback treatment for SUD should be to integrate neurotherapy with other well-known behavioral interventions for drug abuse, such as CBT,[155] motivation enhancement therapy[109,116] and maintenance pharmacotherapy (e.g., methadone[111]). As a population, drug addicts are very difficult to treat, characterized by low motivation to change their drug habit and reluctance to enter inpatient treatment. CBT and MET are powerful psychotherapeutic interventions to bring about rapid commitment to change addictive behaviors. These behavioral therapies are especially useful to enhance compliance in the drug-dependent individual and facilitate their engagement in neurofeedback treatment. Suboxone-based substitute therapy in opiate addicts also usually requires compliance with program requirements and may facilitate patients' engagement in the neurofeedback program.

EEG biofeedback treatment of ADHD may be especially important for children and adolescents at risk for developing SUD and therefore should be a focus of future research. It may be possible that EEG biofeedback therapy of childhood ADHD will result in a decrease in later life SUD.[201] So far there have been no reported studies of the effect of neurofeedback treatment on the prevention of SUD, but we propose that this could be one of the most promising approaches to preventing the progression of drug abuse to drug dependence in adolescents with disruptive behaviors (ADHD, ODD, CD).

Drugs of abuse can impair cognitive, emotional and motivational processes. More qEEG and cognitive ERP research is needed to characterize the chronic and residual effects of drugs on attention, emotion, memory and overall behavioral performance. More research also is needed to relate cognitive functionality measures to clinical outcome (e.g., relapse rate, drug screens, psychiatric status, etc.). Such qEEG/ERP studies may facilitate the translation of clinical neurophysiology research data into routine practical tools for the assessment of functional recovery, both in alcoholism and addiction treatment clinics. We believe that some of the above-described qEEG assessments at the pretreatment baseline might be useful as predictors of clinical outcome and relapse risk. Incorporation of cognitive tests with EEG and ERP measures into cognitive–behavioral and neurofeedback-based interventions may have significant potential for identifying whether certain qEEG/ERP measures can be used as psychophysiological markers of treatment progress (and/or relapse vulnerability), and also whether they may provide useful information in planning cognitive–behavioral and neurotherapy treatment in substance abuse comorbid with mental disorder.

With the advances made over the past several years, it is hoped that continued interest will be generated to further study brainwave biofeedback treatment of addictive disorders. Effectiveness with certain hard-to-treat populations (conventional treatment-resistant alcoholics, crack cocaine addicts, cognitively impaired substance abusers) is especially promising. The prospect of an effective medication-free neurophysiologic and self-actualizing treatment for a substance-based brain-impairing and self-defeating disorder such as SUD is very attractive.

REFERENCES

1. Gloor P, ed. Hans Berger on the electroencephalogram of man. *Electroencephalography and Clinical Neurophysiology* (suppl 28). Amsterdam, The Netherlands: Elsevier, 1969:95–132.
2. Peniston EG, Kulkosky PJ. Alpha/theta brainwave training and beta endorphin levels in alcoholics. *Alcohol: Clin Exp Res.* 1989;13:271–279.
3. Peniston EG, Kulkosky PJ. Alcoholic personality and alpha/theta brainwave training. *Med Psychother.* 1990;2:37–55.
4. Peniston EG, Kulkosky PG. Alpha/theta brain wave neurofeedback for Vietnam veterans with combat related post traumatic stress disorder. *Med Psychother.* 1991;4:1–14.
5. Scott W, Kaiser D. Augmenting chemical dependency treatment with neurofeedback training. *J Neurotherapy.* 1998;3:66.
6. Scott WC, Kaiser D, Othmer S, Sideroff SI. Effects of an EEG biofeedback protocol on a mixed substance abusing population. *Am J Drug Alcohol Abuse.* 2005;31:455–469.
7. Nowlis DP, Kamiya J. The control of electroencephalograhic alpha rhythms through auditory feedback and the associated mental activity. *Psychophysiology.* 1970;6:476–484.
8. Brinkman DN. Biofeedback application to drug addiction in the University of Colorado drug rehabilitation program. *Int J Addict.* 1978;13:817–830.

9.   DeGood DE, Valle RS. Self-reported alcohol and nicotine use and the ability to control occipital EEG in a biofeedback situation. *Addict Behav*. 1978;1:13–18.

10. Denney MR, Baugh JL, Hardt HD. Sobriety outcome after alcoholism treatment with biofeedback participation: a pilot inpatient study. *Int J Addict*. 1991;26:335–341.

11. Goldberg RJ, Greenwood JC, Taintor Z. Alpha conditioning as an adjunct treatment for drug dependence: part I. *Int J Addict*. 1976;11:1085–1089.

12. Goldberg RJ, Greenwood JC, Taintor Z. Alpha conditioning as an adjunct treatment for drug dependence: part II. *Int J Addict*. 1977;12:195–204.

13. Goslinga JJ. Biofeedback for chemical problem patients: a developmental process. *J Biofeedback*. 1975;2:17–27.

14. Jones FW, Holmes DS. Alcoholism, alpha production, and biofeedback. *J Consult Clin Psychol*. 1976;44:224–228.

15. Passini FT, Watson CG, Dehnel L, Herder J, Watkins B. Alpha wave biofeedback training therapy in alcoholics. *J Clin Psychol*. 1977;33:292–299.

16. Tarbox AR. Alcoholism, biofeedback and internal scanning. *J Stud Alcohol*. 1983;44:246–261.

17. Watson CG, Herder J, Passini FT. Alpha biofeedback therapy in alcoholics: an 18-month follow-up. *J Clin Psychol*. 1978;34:765–769.

18. Green EE, Green AM, Walters ED. Alpha/theta biofeedback training. *J Biofeedback*. 1974;2:7–13.

19. White N. The transformational power of the Peniston protocol: a therapist's experiences. *J Neurotherapy*. 2008;12:251–265.

20. Twemlow SW, Bowen WT. Sociocultural predictors of self actualization in EEG biofeedback treated alcoholics. *Psychol Rep*. 1977;40:591–598.

21. Twemlow SW, Sizemore DG, Bowen WT. Biofeedback induced energy redistribution in the alcoholic EEG. *J Biofeedback*. 1977;3:14–19.

22. Peniston EG, Marriman DA, Deming WA, Kulkosky PG. EEG alpha/theta brain wave synchronization in Vietnam theater veterans with combat related post traumatic stress disorder and alcohol abuse. *Med Adv Med Psychother*. 1993;6:37–50.

23. Saxby E, Peniston EG. Alpha/theta brainwave neurofeedback training: an effective treatment for male and female alcoholics with depressive symptoms. *J Clin Psychol*. 1995;51:685–693.

24. Bodenhamer-Davis E, Callaway T. Extended follow-up of Peniston protocol results with chemical dependency. *J Neurotherapy*. 2004;8:135.

25. Callaway TG, Bodenhamer-Davis E. Long-term follow-up of a clinical replication of the Peniston protocol for chemical dependency. *J Neurotherapy*. 2008;12:243–259.

26. DeBeus R, Prinzel H, Ryder-Cook A, Allen L. QEEG-Based versus research-based EEG biofeedback treatment with chemically dependent outpatients: preliminary results. *J Neurotherapy*. 2002;6:64–66.

27. Fahrion SL, Walters D, Coyne L, Allen T. Alterations in EEG amplitude, personality factors and brain electrical mapping after alpha/theta brainwave training: a controlled case study of an alcoholic in recovery. *Alcohol: Clin Exp Res*. 1992;16:547–551.

28. Finkelberg A, Sokhadze E, Lopatin A, et al. The application of alpha/theta EEG biofeedback training for psychological improvement in the process of rehabilitation of the patients with pathological addictions. *Biofeedback Self Regul*. 1996;21:364.

29. Kelley MJ. Native Americans, neurofeedback, and substance abuse theory: three year outcome of alpha/theta neurofeedback training in the treatment of problem drinking among Diné (Navajo) People. *J Neurotherapy*. 1997;2:24–60.

30. Sokhadze EM, Cannon R, Trudeau DL. EEG biofeedback as a treatment for substance use disorders: review, rating of efficacy and recommendations for future research. *Appl Psychophysiol Biofeedback*. 2008;33:1–28.

31. Kaiser DA, Othmer S. Effect of neurofeedback on variables of attention in a large multi-center trial. *J Neurotherapy*. 2000;4:5–15.

32. Prichep LS, Alper KA, Sverdlov L, et al. Outcome related electrophysiological subtypes of cocaine dependence. *Clin Electroencephalogr*. 2002;33:8–20.

33. Burkett SV, Cummins JM, Dickson R, Skolnick MH. An open clinical trial utilizing real-time EEG operant conditioning as an adjunctive therapy in the treatment of crack cocaine dependence. *J Neurotherapy*. 2005;9:27–47.

34. Sokhadze E, Stewart C, Hollifield M. Integrating cognitive neuroscience research and cognitive behavioral treatment with neurofeedback therapy in drug addiction comorbid with posttraumatic stress disorder: a conceptual review. *J Neurotherapy*. 2007;11:13–44.

35. Gurnee R. Subtypes of alcoholism and CNS depressant abuse. In: *Abstracts of the Winter Brain, Optimal Functioning, and Positive Psychology Meeting*. Palm Springs, CA. <http://www.brainmeeting.com/2004_abstracts.htm> ; 2004.

36. Grabowski J, Shearer J, Merrill J, Negus SS. Agonist-like, replacement pharmacotherapy for stimulant abuse and dependence. *Addict Behav*. 2004;29:1439–1464.

37. De Lima MS, de Oliveira Soares BG, Reisser AA, Farrell M. Pharmacological treatment of cocaine dependence: a systematic review. *Addiction*. 2002;97:931–949.

38. Venneman S, Leuchter A, Bartzokis G, et al. Variation in neurophysiological function and evidence of quantitative electroencephalogram discordance: predicting cocaine-dependent treatment attrition. *J Neuropsychiatry Clin Neurosci*. 2006;18:208–216.

39. Mendelson J, Flower K, Pletcher MJ, Galloway GP. Addiction to prescription opioids: characteristics of the emerging epidemic and treatment with buprenorphine. *Exp Clin Psychopharmacol*. 2008;16:435–441.

40. Substance Abuse and Mental Health Services Administration. Results from the 2006 National Survey on Drug Use and Health: National findings (Office of Applied Studies, NSDUH Series H-32, DHHS Publication No. SMA 07–4293). Rockville, MD: 2007.

41. Centers for Disease Control Prevention [CDC]. Unintentional and undetermined poisoning deaths—11 states, 1990–2001. MMWR. 2004; 53: 233–238.

42. Center for Substance Abuse Treatment. Clinical Guidelines for the Use of Buprenorphine in the Treatment of Opioid Addiction. Treatment Improvement Protocol (TIP) Series 40. DHS Publication No. (SMA) 04–3939. Rockville, MD: Substance Abuse and Mental Health Services Administration, 2004.

43. Hser YI, Hoffman V, Grella CE, Anglin MD. A 33-year follow-up of narcotics addicts. *Arch Gen Psychiatry*. 2001;58:503–508.

44. Daulouede J-P, Caer Y, Galland R, et al. Preference for buprenorphine/naloxone and buprenorphine among patients receiving buprenorphine maintenance therapy in France: a prospective, multicenter study. *J Subst Abuse Treat*. 2010;38:83–89.

45. Chiang CN, Hawks RL. Pharmacokinetics of the combination tablet of buprenorphine and naloxone. *Drug Alcohol Depend*. 2003;70:S39–S47.

46. Collins GB, McAllister MS. Buprenorphine maintenance: a new treatment for opioid dependence. *Cleve Clin J Med*. 2007;74:514–520.

47. Gerra G, Baldaro B, Zaimovic A, et al. Neuroendocrine responses to experimentally-induced emotions among abstinent opioid-dependent subjects. *Drug Alcohol Depend*. 2003;71:25–35.

48. Gerra G, Leonardi C, D'Amore A, et al. Buprenorphine treatment outcome in dually diagnosed heroin dependent patients: a retrospective study. *Prog Neuro-Psychopharmacol Biol Psychiatry*. 2006;30:265–272.

49. Gerra G, Maremmani I, Capovani B, et al. Long-acting opioid-agonists in the treatment of heroin addiction: Why should we call them 'Substitution'? *Subst Use Misuse*. 2009;44:663–671.

50. Gowing L, Ali R, White J. Buprenorphine for the management of opioid with-
    drawal. *Cochrane Database Syst Rev.* 2006:2.
51. Kakko J, Svanborg KD, Kreek MJ, Heilig M. 1- year retention and social function
    after buprenorphine – assisted relapse prevention treatment for heroin dependence
    in Sweden: a randomized, placebo-controlled trial. *Lancet.* 2003;361:662–668.
52. Kakko J, von Wachenfeldt J, Svanborg KD, Lidstrom J, Barr CS, Heilig M. Mood
    and neuroendocrine response to a chemical stressor, metyrapone, in buprenorphine-
    maintained heroin dependence. *Biol Psychiatry.* 2008;63:172–177.
53. Aharonovich E, Nguyen HT, Nunes EV. Anger and depressive states among treat-
    ment-seeking drug abusers: Testing the psychopharmacological specificity hypoth-
    esis. *Am J Addict.* 2001;10:327–334.
54. Everitt BJ, Dickinson A, Robbins TW. The neuropsychological basis of addictive
    behaviour. *Brain Res Rev.* 2001;36:129–138.
55. Hyman SE. Addiction: a disease of learning and memory. *Am J Psychiatry.*
    2005;162:1414–1422.
56. Nunes EV, Sullivan MA, Levin FR. Treatment of depression in patients with opiate
    dependence. *Biol Psychiatry.* 2004;56:793–802.
57. Pani PP, Maremmani I, Trogu E, Gessa GL, Ruiz P, Akiskal HS. Delineating the psy-
    chic structure of substance abuse and addictions: should anxiety, mood and impulse-
    control dysregulation be included? *J Affect Disord.* 2010;122:185–197.
58. Drummond D. Theories of drug craving, ancient and modern. *Addiction.*
    2001;96:33–46.
59. Rosenberg H. Clinical and laboratory assessment of the subjective experience of
    drug craving. *Clin Psychol Rev.* 2009;29:519–534.
60. Skinner MD, Aubin H-J. Craving's place in addiction theory: contribution of the
    major models. *Neurosci Biobehav Rev.* 2010;34:606–623.
61. Weiss F, Ciccocioppo R, Parsons LH, et al. Compulsive drug-seeking behavior
    and relapse. Neuroadaptation, stress, and conditioning factors. *Ann N Y Acad Sci.*
    2001;937:1–26.
62. Wilson SJ, Sayette MA, Fiez JA. Prefrontal responses to drug cues: a neurocognitive
    analysis. *Nat Neurosci.* 2004;7:211–214.
63. Robinson TE, Berridge KC. The neural basis of drug craving: an incentive-sensitiza-
    tion theory of addiction. *Brain Res Rev.* 1993;18:247–291.
64. Wise RA, Leone P, Rivest R, Leeb K. Elevations of nucleus accumbens dopa-
    mine and DOPAC levels during intravenous heroin self-administration. *Synapse.*
    1995;97:140–148.
65. Wise RA, Rompre PP. Brain dopamine and reward. *Annu Rev Psychol.*
    1989;97:191–225.
66. Wise RA. Neurobiology of addiction. *Curr Opin Neurobiol.* 1996;6:243–251.
67. Franken IHA. Drug craving and addiction: integrating psychological and psy-
    chopharmacological approaches. *Prog Neuro-Psychopharmacol Biol Psychiatry.*
    2003;27:563–579.
68. Franken IHA, Kroon LY, Hendriks VM. Influence of individual differences in
    craving and obsessive cocaine thoughts on attentional processes in cocaine abuse
    patients. *Addict Behav.* 2000;25:99–102.
69. Sinha R, Catapano D, O'Malley S. Stress-induced craving and stress response in
    cocaine dependent individuals. *Psychopharmacology (Berl).* 1999;142:343–351.
70. Sinha R, Garcia P, Paliwal M, Kreek MJ, Rounsaville BJ. Stress-induced cocaine
    craving and hypothalamic-pituitary-adrenal responses are predictive of cocaine
    relapse outcomes. *Arch Gen Psychiatry.* 2006;63:324–331.
71. Aguilar de Arcos F, Verdejo-Garcia AJ, Peralta-Ramirez MI, Sanchez-Barrera M,
    Perez-Garcia M. Experience of emotions in substance abusers exposed to images

containing neutral, positive, and negative affective stimuli. *Drug Alcohol Depend.* 2005;78:159–167.

72. Fukunishi I. Alexithymia in substance abuse: relationship to depression. *Psychol Rep.* 1996;78:641–642.

73. Handelsman L, Stein JA, Bernstein DP, Oppenheim SE, Rosenblum A, Magura S. A latent variable analysis of coexisting emotional deficits in substance abusers: alexithymia, hostility, and PTSD. *Addict Behav.* 2000;25:423–428.

74. Panksepp J, Knutson B, Burgdorf J. The role of brain emotional systems in addictions: a neuro-evolutionary perspective and new 'self-report' animal model. *Addiction.* 2002;97:459–469.

75. Volkow ND, Fowler JS, Wang GJ. The addicted human brain: insights from imaging studies. *J Clin Investig.* 2003;111:1444–1451.

76. Koob GF. Stress, corticotropin-releasing factor, and drug addiction. *Ann NY Acad Sci.* 1999;897:27–45.

77. Koob GF, Le Moal M. Drug addiction, dysregulation of reward, and allostasis. *Neuropsychopharmacology.* 2001;24:97–129.

78. Koob GF, Le Moal M. *Neurobiology of Addiction.* London, UK: Academic Press; 2006.

79. Koob GF, Ahmed SH, Boutrel B, et al. Neurobiological mechanisms in the transition from drug use to drug dependence. *Neurosci Biobehav Rev.* 2004;27:739–749.

80. Zijlstra F, Veltman DJ, Booij D, Brink W, Franken IHA. Neurobiological substrates of cue-elicited craving and anhedonia in recently abstinent opioid-dependent males. *Drug Alcohol Depend.* 2009;99:183–192.

81. Garavan H, Pankiewicz J, Bloom A, et al. Cue-induced cocaine craving: neuroanatomical specificity for drug users and drug stimuli. *Am J Psychiatry.* 2000;157:789–1798.

82. Wexler BE, Gottschalk CH, Fulbright RK, et al. Functional magnetic resonance imaging of cocaine craving. *Am J Psychiatry.* 2001;158:86–95.

83. Sell LA, Morris JS, Bearn J, Frackowiak RS, Friston KJ, Dolan RJ. Neural responses associated with cue evoked emotional states and heroin in opiate addicts. *Drug Alcohol Depend.* 2000;60:207–216.

84. Davidson RJ. Cognitive neuroscience needs affective neuroscience (and vice versa). *Brain Cogn.* 2000;42:89–92.

85. Goldstein RZ, Volkow ND. Drug addiction and its underlying neurobiological basis: neuroimaging evidence for the involvement of the frontal cortex. *Am J Psychiatry.* 2002;159:1642–1652.

86. Jaffe JH, Jaffe AB. Neurobiology of opioids. In: Galanter M, Kleber HD, eds. *Textbook of Substance Abuse Treatment.* 3rd ed. Washington, DC: American Psychiatric Press; 2004:17–30.

87. Self DW. Regulation of drug-taking and -seeking behaviors by neuro-adaptations in the mesolimbic dopamine system. *Neuropharmacology.* 2004;47:242–255.

88. Volkow ND, Fowler JS. Addiction, a disease of compulsion and drive: involvement of the orbitofrontal cortex. *Cereb Cortex.* 2000;10:318–325.

89. Volkow ND, Fowler JS, Wang GJ. The addicted human brain viewed in the light of imaging studies: brain circuits and treatment strategies. *Neuropharmacology.* 2004;47:3–13.

90. Berridge KC, Robinson TE. What is the role of dopamine in reward: hedonic impact, reward learning, or incentive salience? *Brain Res Rev.* 1998;28:309–369.

91. Everitt BJ, Parkinson JA, Olmstead MC, Arroyo M, Robledo P, Robbins TW. Associative processes in addiction and reward. The role of amygdala-ventral striatal subsystems. *Ann NY Acad Sci.* 1999;877:412–438.

92. Everitt BJ, Belin D, Economidou D, Pelloux Y, Dalley JW, Robbins TW. Neural mechanisms underlying the vulnerability to develop compulsive drug-seeking habits and addiction. *Philos Trans R Soc Lond B Biol Sci.* 2008;363:3125–3135.

93. Robinson TE, Berridge KC. The psychology and neurobiology of addiction: an incentive–sensitization view. *Addiction.* 2000;95:91–117.

94. Robinson TE, Berridge KC. Incentive-sensitization and addiction. *Addiction.* 2001;96:103–114.

95. Bonson KR, Grant SJ, Contoreggi CS, et al. Neural systems and cue-induced cocaine craving. *Neuropsychopharmacology.* 2002;26:376–386.

96. Grant S, London ED, Newlin DB, et al. Activation of memory circuits during cue-elicited cocaine craving. *Proc Natl Acad Sci U S A.* 1996;93:12040–12045.

97. London ED, Ernst M, Grant S, Bonson K, Weinstein A. Orbitofrontal cortex and human drug abuse: functional imaging. *Cereb Cortex.* 2000;10:334–342.

98. Daglish MR, Weinstein A, Wilson S, et al. Changes in regional cerebral blood flow elicited by craving memories in abstinent opiate-dependent subjects. *Am J Psychiatry.* 2001;158:1680–1686.

99. Daglish MR, Lingford-Hughes A, Williams T, et al. Brain opioid receptor changes in early abstinence from methadone. *Addict Biol.* 2002;7:334–335.

100. Cuthbert BN, Schupp HT, Bradley MM, Birbaumer N, Lang PJ. Brain potentials in affective picture processing: covariation with autonomic arousal and affective report. *Biol Psychology.* 2000;52:95–111.

101. Schupp HT, Cuthbert BN, Bradley MM, Cacioppo JT, Ito T, Lang PJ. Affective picture processing: the late positive potential is modulated by motivational relevance. *Psychophysiology.* 2000;37:57–261.

102. Kouri EM, Lukas SE, Mendelson JH. P300 assessment of opiate and cocaine users: effects of detoxification and buprenorphine treatment. *Biol Psychiatry.* 1996;60:617–628.

103. Hyman SE, Malenka RC. Addiction and the brain: the neurobiology of compulsion and its persistence. *Nat Rev Neurosci.* 2001;2:695–703.

104. Lee JL, Milton AL, Everitt BJ. Cue-induced cocaine seeking and relapse are reduced by disruption of drug memory reconsolidation. *J Neurosci.* 2006;26:5881–5887.

105. Sokhadze E, Stewart C, Hollifield M, Tasman A. Event-related study of executive dysfunctions in a speeded reaction task in cocaine addiction. *J Neurotherapy.* 2008;12:185–204.

106. Sokhadze E, Stewart C, Sokhadze G, Husk M, Tasman A. Effects of neurofeedback-based behavioral therapy on ERP measures of executive functions in drug abuse. *J Neurotherapy.* 2009;13:260–262.

107. Sokhadze E, Stewart C, El-Baz A, Ramaswamy R, Hollifield M, Tasman A. Induced EEG gamma oscillations in response to drug- and stress-related cues in cocaine addicts and patients with dual diagnosis. *J Neurotherapy.* 2009;13:270–271.

108. Sokhadze E, Stewart CM, Tasman A, Daniels R, Trudeau D. Review of rationale for neurofeedback application in adolescent substance abusers with comorbid disruptive behavioral disorders. *J Neurotherapy.* 2011;15:232–261.

109. Sokhadze E, Cowan J, Horrell T, Tasman A, Sokhadze G, Stewart C. Effects of gamma neurofeedback training on perceived positive emotional state and cognitive functions. *J Neurotherapy.* 2010;14:343–345.

110. Horrell T, Sokhadze E, Stewart C, El-Baz A, Tasman A. Evoked and induced gamma EEG response to drug cues in cocaine addicts after neurofeedback treatment. *J Neurotherapy.* 2010;14:195–216.

111. Arani FD, Rostami R, Nostratabadi M. Effectiveness of neurofeedback training as a treatment for opioid-dependent patients. *Clin Electroencephalogr Neurosci.* 2010;41:170–177.

112. Lubman DI, Yucel M, Kettle JWL, et al. Responsiveness to drug cues and natural rewards in opiate addiction: associations with later heroin use. *Arch Gen Psychiatry.* 2009;66:205–212.

113. Bodkin JA, Zornberg GL, Lukas SE, Cole JO. Buprenorphine treatment of refractory depression. *J Clin Psychopharmacol.* 1995;15:49–57.

114. Franken IHA, Rassin E, Muris P. The assessment of anhedonia in clinical and non-clinical populations: further validation of the Snaith-Hamilton Pleasure Scale (SHAPS). *J Affect Disord.* 2007;99:83–89.

115. Koob GF, Weiss F. Neuropharmacology of cocaine and ethanol dependence. *Recent Dev Alcohol.* 1992;10:201–233.

116. Miller W, Rollnick S. *Motivational Interviewing.* NY: Guilford Press; 2002.

117. Li CR, Sinha R. Inhibitory control and emotional stress regulation: Neuroimaging evidence for frontal–limbic dysfunction in psycho-stimulant addiction. *Neurosci Biobehav Rev.* 2008;32:581–597.

118. Peters J, Kalivas PW, Quirk GJ. Extinction circuits for fear and addiction overlap in prefrontal cortex. *Learn Mem.* 2009;16:279–288.

119. Breslau N, Davis GC, Andreski P, Peterson E. Traumatic events and posttraumatic stress disorder in an urban population of young adults. *Arch Gen Psychiatry.* 1991;48:216–222.

120. Triffleman E, Carroll K, Kellogg S. Substance dependence posttraumatic stress therapy: an integrated cognitive-behavioral approach. *J Subst Abuse Treat.* 1999;17:3–14.

121. Couwenbergh C, Brink W, Zwart K, Vreugdenhil C, Wijngaarden-Cremers P, Gaag RJ. Comorbid psychopathology in adolescents and young adults treated for substance use disorders. *Eur Child Adolesc Psychiatry.* 2006;15:319–328.

122. Chan Y-F, Dennis ML, Funk RR. Prevalence and comorbidity of major internalizing and externalizing problems among adolescents and adults presenting to substance abuse treatment. *J Subst Abuse Treat.* 2008;34:14–24.

123. Cadoret RJ, Troughton E, O'Gorman W. Genetic and environmental factors in alcohol abuse and antisocial personality disorder. *J Stud Alcohol.* 1987;48:1–8.

124. Horner BR, Scheibe KE. Prevalence and implications of attention-deficit hyperactivity disorder among adolescents in treatment for substance abuse. *J Am Acad Child Adolesc Psychiatry.* 1997;36:30–36.

125. Simkin DR. Adolescent substance use disorders and comorbidity. *Pediatr Clin North Am.* 2002;49:463–477.

126. Swanson JM, Sergeant JA, Taylor E, Sonuga-Barke EJ, Jensen PS, Cantwell DP. Attention-deficit hyperactivity disorder and hyperkinetic disorder. *Lancet.* 1998;351:429–433.

127. Tarter RE, Kirisci L, Mezzich A, et al. Neurobehavior disinhibition in childhood predicts early age at onset of substance disorder. *Am J Psychiatry.* 2003;160:1078–1085.

128. Tarter RE, Kirisci L, Habeych M, Reynolds M, Vanyukov MM. Neurobehavior disinhibition in childhood predisposes boys to substance use disorder by young adulthood. Direct and mediated etiologic pathways. *Drug Alcohol Depend.* 2004;73:121–132.

129. Bauer LO, Hesselbrock VM. CSD/BEM localization of P300 sources in adolescents 'at risk': Evidence of frontal cortex dysfunction in conduct disorder. *Biol Psychiatry.* 2001;50:600–608.

130. Clarke A, Barry RJ, McCarthy R, Selikowitz M. EEG-defined subtypes of children with attention-deficit/hyperactivity disorder. *Clin Neurophysiol.* 2001;112:2098–2105.

131. Clarke AR, Barry RJ, McCarthy R, Selikowitz M. Children with attention-deficit/hyperactivity disorder and comorbid oppositional defiant disorder: an EEG analysis. *Psychiatry Res.* 2002;111:181–190.

132. Graetz BW, Sawyer MG, Hazell PL, Arney F, Baghurst P. Validity of DSM-IVADHD subtypes in a nationally representative sample of Australian children and adolescents. *J Am Acad Child Adolesc Psychiatry.* 2001;40:1410–1417.

133. *Diagnostic and Statistical Manual of Mental Disorders.* 4th ed. [DSM-IV-TR]. Washington, DC: American Psychiatric Association, 2000.
134. Swanson JM, Kinsbourne M, Nigg J, et al. Etiologic subtypes of attention-deficit/hyperactivity disorder: brain imaging, molecular genetic and environmental factors and the dopamine hypothesis. *Neuropsychol Rev.* 2007;17:39–59.
135. Monastra VJ, Monastra DM, George S. The effects of stimulant therapy, EEG biofeedback, and parenting style on the primary symptoms of attention-deficit/hyperactivity disorder. *Appl Psychophysiol Biofeedback.* 2002;27:231–249.
136. Monastra VJ. Clinical applications of electroencephalographic biofeedback. In: Schwartz MS, Andrasik F, eds. *Biofeedback: A Practitioner's Guide.* 3rd ed. New York, NY: Guilford Press; 2003:438–463.
137. Monastra VJ, Lynn S, Linden M, Lubar JF, Gruzelier J, LaVaque TJ. Electroencephalographic biofeedback in the treatment of attention-deficit/hyperactivity disorder. *Appl Psychophysiol Biofeedback.* 2005;30:95–114.
138. Aron AR, Poldrack RA. The cognitive neuroscience of response inhibition: relevance for genetic research in attention-deficit/hyperactivity disorder. *Biol Psychiatry.* 2005;57:1285–1292.
139. Barry RJ, Clarke AR, McCarthy R, Selikowitz M. EEG coherence in children with attention-deficit/hyperactivity disorder and comorbid oppositional defiant disorder. *Clin Neurophysiol.* 2007;118:356–362.
140. Biederman J, Spencer TJ, Newcorn JH, et al. Effect of comorbid symptoms of oppositional defiant disorder on responses to atomoxetine in children with ADHD: a meta-analysis of controlled clinical trial data. *Psychopharmacology (Berl).* 2006;190:31–41.
141. Bird H, Gould M, Staghezza B. Patterns of diagnostic comorbidity in a community sample of children aged 9 through 16 years. *J Am Acad Child Adolesc Psychiatry.* 1993;32:361–368.
142. Clarke AR, Barry RJ, McCarthy R, Selikowitz M, Brown CR. EEG evidence for a new conceptualization of attention deficit hyperactivity disorder. *Clin Neurophysiol.* 2002;113:1036–1044.
143. Pliszka S. Comorbidity of attention-deficit/hyperactivity disorder with psychiatric disorder: an overview. *J Clin Psychiatry.* 1998;59:S50–S58.
144. Lahey BB, Loeber R, Quay HC, Frick PJ, Grimm J. Oppositional defiant and conduct disorders: issues to be resolved for DSM-IV. *J Am Acad Child Adolesc Psychiatry.* 1992;31:539–546.
145. Loeber R, Burke JD, Lahey BB, Winters A, Zera M. Oppositional defiant and conduct disorder: A review of the past 10 years. *J Am Acad Child Adolesc Psychiatry.* 2000;39:1468–1484.
146. Pardini DA, Frick PJ, Moffitt TE. Building an evidence base for DSM-5 conceptualizations of oppositional defiant disorder and conduct disorder: introduction to the special section. *J Abnorm Psychol.* 2010;119:683–688.
147. Pardini DA, Fite PJ. Symptoms of conduct disorder, oppositional defiant disorder, attention-deficit/hyperactivity disorder, and callous-unemotional traits as unique predictors of psychosocial maladjustment in boys: advancing an evidence base for DSM-V. *J Am Acad Child Adolesc Psychiatry.* 2010;49:1134–1144.
148. Jensen P, Martin D, Cantwell D. Comorbidity in ADHD: implications for research, practice, and DSM-V. *J Am Acad Child Adolesc Psychiatry.* 1997;36:1065–1079.
149. Mannuzza S, Klein RG, Moulton JL. Does stimulant treatment place children at risk for adult substance abuse? A controlled, prospective follow-up study. *J Child Adolesc Psychopharmacol.* 2003;13:273–282.
150. Khantzian EJ. The self-medication hypothesis of addictive disorders: focus on heroin and cocaine dependence. *Am J Psychiatry.* 1985;142:1259–1264.

151. Khantzian EJ. The self-medication hypothesis of substance use disorders: a reconsiderations and recent applications. *Harv Rev Psychiatry*. 1997;4:231–244.
152. Cyders MA, Smith GT. Emotion-based dispositions to rash action: positive and negative urgency. *Psychol Bull*. 2008;134:807–828.
153. Kalbag AS, Levin FR. Adult ADHD and substance abuse: diagnostic and treatment issues. *Subst Use Misuse*. 2005;40:1955–1981.
154. Schepis S, Adinoff B, Rao U. Neurobiological processes in adolescent addictive disorders. *Am J Addict*. 2008;17:6–23.
155. Crits-Christoph P, Siqueland L, Blaine J, et al. Psychosocial treatments for cocaine dependence: National Institute On drug abuse collaborative cocaine treatment study. *Arch Gen Psychiatry*. 1999;56:493–502.
156. Crits-Christoph P, Siqueland L, Blaine J, et al. The National Institute on drug abuse collaborative cocaine treatment study. Rationale and methods. *Arch Gen Psychiatry*. 1997;54:721–726.
157. Grabowski J, Shearer J, Merrill J, Negus SS. Agonist-like, replacement pharmacotherapy for stimulant abuse and dependence. *Addict Behav*. 2004;29:1439–1464.
158. Van den Brink W, van Ree JM. Pharmacological treatments for heroin and cocaine addictions. *Eur Neuropsychopharmacol*. 2003;13:476–487.
159. Trudeau DL. EEG biofeedback for addictive disorders – the state of the art in 2004. *J Adult Dev*. 2005;12:139–146.
160. Biederman J, Wilens T, Mick E, Milberger S, Spencer TJ, Faraone SV. Psychoactive substance use disorders in adults with attention deficit hyperactivity disorder (ADHD): effects of ADHD and psychiatric comorbidity. *Am J Psychiatry*. 1995;152:1652–1658.
161. Biederman J, Wilens T, Mick E, et al. Is ADHD a risk factor for psychoactive substance use disorders? Findings from a four-year prospective follow-up study. *J Am Acad Child Adolesc Psychiatry*. 1997;36:21–29.
162. Trudeau DL, Thuras P, Stockley H. Quantitative EEG findings associated with chronic stimulant and cannabis abuse and ADHD in an adult male substance use disorder population. *Clin Electroencephalogr*. 1999;30:165–174.
163. Levin FR, Evans SM, Brooks DJ, Garawi F. Treatment of cocaine dependent treatment seekers with adult ADHD: double-blind comparison of methylphenidate and placebo. *Drug Alcohol Depend*. 2007;87:20–29.
164. Mariani JJ, Levin FR. Treatment strategies for co-occurring ADHD and substance use disorders. *Am J Addict*. 2007;16:S45–S56.
165. Riggs PD, Jellinek MS. Clinical approach to treatment of ADHD in adolescents with substance use disorders and conduct disorder. *J Am Acad Child Adolesc Psychiatry*. 1998;37:331–332.
166. Kollins SH. A qualitative review of issues arising in the use of psychostimulant medications in patients with ADHD and co-morbid substance use disorders. *Curr Med Res Opin*. 2008;24:1345–1357.
167. Wilens TE, Adler LA, Weiss MD, et al. Atomoxetine treatment of adults with ADHD and comorbid alcohol use disorders. *Drug Alcohol Depend*. 2008;96:145–154.
168. Trudeau DL, Sokhadze TM, Cannon R. Neurofeedback in alcohol and drug dependency. In: Budzynski T, Evans J, Budzynski H, eds. *Advanced QEEG and Neurofeedback*. Amsterdam, The Netherlands: Elsevier; 2008:239–267.
169. Trudeau DL. Applicability of brain wave biofeedback to substance use disorder in adolescents. *Child Adolesc Clin North Am*. 2005;14:125–136.
170. Trudeau DL. A review of the treatment of addictive disorders by EEG biofeedback. *Clin Electroencephalogr*. 2000;31:13–26.
171. Trudeau DL. Individualizing EEG biofeedback in addictive disorders. *Biofeedback*. 2000;28:22–26.

172. Arns M, de Ridder S, Strehl U, Breteler M, Coenen A. Efficacy of neurofeedback treatment in ADHD: the effects of inattention, impulsivity and hyperactivity: a meta-analysis. *Clin EEG Neurosci.* 2009;40:180–189.

173. Fox DJ, Tharp DF, Fox LC. Neurofeedback: an alternative and efficacious treatment for attention deficit hyperactivity disorder. *Appl Psychophysiol Biofeedback.* 2005;30:365–373.

174. Lubar JF. Neurofeedback for the management of attention deficit disorders. In: Schwartz MS, Andrasik F, eds. *Biofeedback: A Practitioner's Guide.* 3rd ed. New York, NY: Guilford Press; 2003:409–437.

175. Monastra VJ, Lubar JF, Linden M. The development of a quantitative electroencephalographic scanning process for attention deficit-hyperactivity disorder: reliability and validity studies. *Neuropsychology.* 2001;15:136–144.

176. Van den Bergh W. (English translation by S. Clark) *Neurofeedback and State Regulation in ADHD: A Therapy Without Medication.* Texas: BMED Press; 2010.

177. Williams JM. Does neurofeedback help reduce attention-deficit hyperactivity disorder? *J Neurotherapy.* 2010;14:261–279.

178. Fuchs T, Birbaumer N, Lutzenberger W, Gruzelier JH, Kaiser J. Neurofeedback treatment for attention-deficit/hyperactivity disorder in children: a comparison with methylphenidate. *Appl Psychophysiol Biofeedback.* 2003;28:1–12.

179. Gevensleben H, Holl B, Albrecht B, et al. Is neurofeedback an efficacious treatment for ADHD? A randomised controlled clinical trial. *Child Psychol Psychiatry.* 2009;50:780–789.

180. Gevensleben H, Holl B, Albrecht B, et al. Distinct EEG effects related to neurofeedback training in children with ADHD: a randomized controlled trial. *Int J Psychophysiol.* 2009;74:149–157.

181. Gevensleben H, Holl B, Albrecht B, et al. Neurofeedback training in children with ADHD: 6-month follow-up of a randomised controlled trial. *Eur Child Adolesc Psychiatry.* 2010;19:715–724.

182. Levesque J, Beauregard M, Mensour B. Effects of neurofeedback training on the neural substrates of selective attention in children with attention-deficit/hyperactivity disorder: a functional magnetic resonance imaging study. *Neurosci Lett.* 2006;394:216–221.

183. Linden M, Habib T, Radojevic V. A controlled study of the effects of EEG biofeedback on cognition and behavior of children with attention deficit disorder and learning disabilities. *Biofeedback Self Regul.* 1996;21:35–49.

184. Barkley RA, Fischer M, Edelbrock CS, Smallish L. The adolescent outcome of hyperactive children diagnosed by research criteria: I. An 8-year prospective follow-up study. *J Am Acad Child Adolesc Psychiatry.* 1990;29:546–557.

185. Biederman J. Pharmacotherapy for attention-deficit/hyperactivity disorder (ADHD) decreases the risk for substance abuse: findings from a longitudinal follow-up of youths with and without ADHD. *J Clin Psychiatry.* 2003;64:3–8.

186. Carroll KM, Rounsaville BJ. History and significance of childhood attention deficit disorder in treatment-seeking cocaine abusers. *Compr Psychiatry.* 1993;34:75–82.

187. Gittleman R, Mannuzza S, Shenker R, Bonagura N. Hyperactive boys almost grown up. *Arch Gen Psychiatry.* 1985;42:937–947.

188. Manuzza JS, Klein RG, Bessler A, Malloy P, LaPadula M. Adult psychiatric status of hyperactive boys grown up. *Am J Psychiatry.* 1998;155:493–498.

189. Sokhadze EM. Neurofeedback and cognitive-behavioral therapy based intervention in dual diagnosis: a neurobiological model. *J Neurotherapy.* 2005;9:123–124.

190. Becker SJ, Curry JF. Outpatient interventions for adolescent substance abuse: a quality of evidence review. *J Consult Clin Psychol.* 2006;76:531–543.

191. Schwebel R. *The Seven Challenges Manual.* Tucson, AZ: Viva Press; 2004.
192. Brown PJ, Recupero PR, Stout R. PTSD-substance abuse comorbidity and treatment utilization. *Addict Behav.* 1995;20:251–254.
193. O'Brien CP, Charney DS, Lewis L, et al. Priority actions to improve the care of persons with co-occurring substance abuse and other mental disorders: a call to action. *Biol Psychiatry.* 2004;56:703–713.
194. Schubiner H, Tzelepis A, Milberger S, et al. Prevalence of attention-deficit/hyperactivity disorder and conduct disorder among substance abusers. *J Clin Psychiatry.* 2000;61:244–251.
195. Swartz JA, Lurigio AJ. Psychiatric illness and comorbidity among adult male jail detainees in drug treatment. *Psychiatry Serv.* 1999;50:1628–1630.
196. Martin G. EEG biofeedback with incarcerated adolescent felons. *J Neurotherapy.* 2003;7:66–67.
197. Quirk DA. Composite biofeedback conditioning and dangerous offenders: III. *J Neurotherapy.* 1995;1:44–54.
198. Sherlin L, Arns M, Lubar J, Sokhadze E. A position paper on neurofeedback for the treatment of ADHD. *J Neurotherapy.* 2010;14:66–78.
199. Rossiter TR, LaVaque TJ. A comparison of EEG biofeedback and psychostimulants in treating attention deficit/hyperactivity disorders. *J Neurotherapy.* 1995;1:48–59.
200. Williams LM, Hermens DF, Palmer D, et al. Misinterpreting emotional expressions in attention-deficit/hyperactivity disorder: evidence for a neural marker and stimulant effects. *Biol Psychiatry.* 2008;63:917–926.
201. Wilens TE, Biederman J, Mick E. Does ADHD affect the course of substance abuse? Findings from a sample of adults with and without ADHD. *Am J Addict.* 1998;7:156–163.

CHAPTER TWELVE

Neurofeedback for Seizure Disorders

Origins, Mechanisms and Best Practices

M.B. Sterman and Lynda M. Thompson

MG was a 32-year-old woman starting a new career as an author and journalist in Los Angeles. During the summer of 1992, she became aware of brief episodes of sudden nausea, dizziness and the presence of a foul odor. She attributed these experiences to intestinal issues because of bad food or the flu. She barely noticed that they were becoming more frequent and were associated with some trembling and unexplained fear. Finally, in the fall of 1993, while sitting on the carpet drinking coffee and reading the newspaper, she suddenly fell backwards, spilling the coffee and dropping into unconsciousness for several minutes. The next day she was referred to a neurologist, who ordered computed tomography and magnetic resonance imaging (MRI) studies. A right anterior temporal lobe astrocytoma was revealed, and this was confirmed by electroencephalographic (EEG) studies showing abnormal slow activity in this region. She was placed on an anticonvulsant drug regimen of depakote, tegretol and neurontin. In early 1994 the tumor was surgically removed.

Following surgery, MG was seizure free for about 1 week. However, she again began having the same brief episodes of nausea and confusion, but now the foul odor was gone. While she was having at least one of these episodes per day, her medication was changed to a single drug, Kepra, 250 mg twice daily. During the next 4 years she reported averaging some 10 events per month. In 1998 she was married and wanted to have children but feared the well-documented pathological influence of anticonvulsant medication on the unborn fetus. At this point the prospect of an anterior temporal lobectomy led her to research treatment alternatives. Through an article in *Psychology Today*, she became aware of the non-invasive EEG biofeedback treatment for epilepsy that might allow her to terminate her medication. With the grudging approval of her neurologist,

Clinical Neurotherapy.
Doi: http://dx.doi.org/10.1016/B978-0-12-396988-0.00012-X

who was aware of the published work in this area, she sought treatment in the office of one of the authors of this chapter, Dr Sterman. A quantitative EEG study confirmed significant slowing along the lateral frontotemporal plane in the right hemisphere. During 36 1-hour weekly sessions directed toward suppressing this slow frontotemporal activity, together with reinforcement of a 12–15 Hz rhythm in the adjacent medial sensorimotor cortex (C4), her seizures gradually ceased and she was ultimately able to withdraw from her medication. She later became pregnant and gave birth to healthy twin boys. A dozen years later, with only two periods of additional booster sessions, her seizures continue to be well controlled.

ORIGINS OF NEUROFEEDBACK IN THE TREATMENT OF SEIZURE DISORDERS

The origins of neurofeedback in the treatment of seizure disorders can be traced directly to the first systematic demonstration of confirmed and valid EEG operant conditioning, initially in animals (for an in-depth review, see Sterman[1]). In the context of sleep research, Sterman and associates conducted a series of studies investigating learned suppression of a previously rewarded cup-press response for food in cats.[2–5] Cats were trained with operant conditioning to inhibit the cup-press response during the intermittent presentation of a tone. A unique EEG rhythm gradually appeared over the sensorimotor cortex at a voltage above the nonrhythmic low-voltage background activity. The anatomically based term "sensorimotor rhythm", or SMR, was coined to describe this pattern.[3] The rhythm occurred at a peak frequency of 13 Hz, with a modal spectral range of 12–15 Hz, not unlike mammalian EEG sleep spindles. An earlier study had defined a greater range of 11–19 Hz, depending on the accompanying level of arousal, the frequency increasing or decreasing in more or less aroused waking states.[2] This fact could help explain the apparent confusion between the terms SMR and mu rhythm in humans. Distinguishing among alpha, SMR, mu and beta when measuring electrical activity in the 12–15 Hz range is challenging but can be done based on morphology, location, amplitude and reactivity.

These investigators decided to study this clearly visible and distinct EEG rhythm directly, first attempting to apply the principles of operant conditioning to see whether cats with indwelling cortical EEG electrodes could be trained to reliably produce SMR activity voluntarily. A food reward was delivered in a special experimental chamber contingent

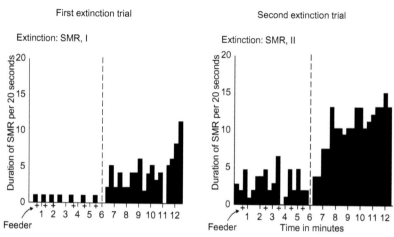

Figure 12.1 Bar graph showing cumulative seconds of 12–15 Hz SMR responses per minute for the first 6 minutes of rewarded responses, followed by an abrupt withholding of reward (vertical line) and a subsequent 7-minute extinction trial. The first extinction trial occurred after 6 weeks of thrice-weekly 1-hour feedback sessions, and the second extinction trial was obtained after a second identical 6-week training period. Comparison of SMR output during feedback and extinction trials between 6 and 12 weeks of training demonstrates a clearly increased substrate for this EEG frequency. (*Modified from Wyrwicka and Sterman.[4]*)

upon SMR production (a 500 ms train of 12–15 Hz rhythmic activity at an amplitude 100% above mean EEG baseline voltage in the sensorimotor cortex). The cats easily learned this EEG self-regulation task, even more quickly than the bar-press. Further, after 18 sessions of training (1 hour three times per week for 6 weeks), when food reward was withheld in these studies, using a procedure called "extinction" in operant conditioning parlance, a remarkable elevation of SMR output and associated quiescent behavior was observed. This confirmed that the SMR response was, indeed, operantly conditioned.

Extended feedback training of the SMR for an additional 18 sessions in these cats led both to increased amplitude and duration of SMR responses during training and to further increases during a follow-up extinction trial, where food was again withheld, as seen in Figure 12.1.[4] This training had clearly altered neural circuitry. The observed behavior associated with SMR production was one of immobility, with 12–15 Hz SMR bursts over the somatosensory cortex regularly preceded by a drop in muscle tone.[4–6] In a serendipitous twist, Sterman's laboratory was soon afterwards commissioned to establish the dose–response functions of a highly epileptogenic hydrazine fuel compound. It was found that a dose of 9 mg/kg typically produced generalized convulsions at approximately 60 minutes after injection. When using the cats that had previously taken part in SMR conditioning as experimental animals, the cats were found to display significantly prolonged resistance to convulsions. Some animals showed no seizures for over 4 hours of observation.[5] This finding suggested that SMR training had somehow inoculated the cats against experiencing seizures. Other studies replicated these earlier cat findings in rhesus monkeys.[7] Subsequently, this research was successfully extrapolated to humans, where it was repeatedly documented that seizure incidence and severity could be significantly reduced. Patients reported that their quality of life had also improved. Occasionally seizures appeared to be totally controlled, allowing at least one client to obtain a California driver's license. This work was followed by numerous other studies examining the effects of SMR EEG feedback training on seizure frequency in people with epilepsy.

Part of the success of using neurofeedback for seizure disorders stems from the relationship between training to increase SMR and a concomitant increase in sleep spindle density at night. Seizures often occur at night, as the brain shifts patterns of firing from one stage of sleep to another. Increasing sleep spindle density is associated with smoother transitions in sleep, fewer awakenings, and feeling more refreshed in the morning. Patients with epilepsy have fewer night-time seizures. Figure 12.2 shows how 18 weeks of twice-weekly training reduced excess 4–7 Hz activity while increasing 12–15 Hz activity in a patient with epilepsy.

The data from these studies have been reviewed in meta-analyses by Sterman[8] and Tan et al.[9] In the Sterman review of 18 studies done between 1972 and 1996,[8] 5% of the 174 patients became seizure free (followed for up to 1 year), and 82% showed seizure reduction >30% and an average reduction in seizure frequency of 50%. Tan and his colleagues[9] reviewed 63 studies performed between 1970 and 2005 that reported a reduction in seizure frequency in response to feedback training, and 10 of these met the criteria for inclusion in a meta-analysis. Nine studies increased SMR and one trained slow cortical potentials (SCPs). In 64 out of 87 patients (74%), there was a significant decrease of >50% in seizure incidence. In all of these studies the subjects were treatment resistant and had not been able to achieve seizure control using medications.

The application of established criteria for treatment efficacy indicates that neurofeedback for seizure disorders can be termed "efficacious", which is Level 4 on a scale of 1–5 for efficacy.[10]

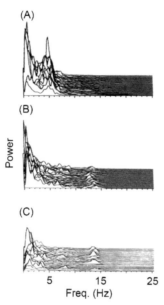

Figure 12.2 Compressed power spectral arrays computed during stage 2 sleep in an adult epileptic undergoing twice-weekly SMR feedback training are compared here at approximately 6-week intervals. At the start of training (A) a typical pattern of abnormal slow 4–7 Hz (theta) peaks is seen, together with little or no 12–15 Hz sleep spindle (sigma) activity. After 6 weeks (B) the slow peaks are significantly reduced and germinal sleep spindle peaks became apparent. By the end of 18 weeks (C) there is little or no evidence of abnormal 4–7 Hz activity, together with prominent evidence of 12–15 Hz sleep spindles. *(From Sterman and Shouse.[49])*

MECHANISMS

Because it was originally observed and correlated with intracranial recordings in animals, the neurogenesis of SMR is fairly well understood. A model based on neurophysiological findings from this work is presented in Figure 12.3. The SMR was found to emanate from the ventrobasal nuclei (nVB) of the thalamus,[11] which are generally concerned with relaying afferent somatosensory information. During the learned enhancement of the SMR rhythm, firing patterns in the lateral VB nucleus shift from fast and nonrhythmic (tonic) discharges to systematic, rhythmic bursts of discharge,[12] which in turn are associated with the suppression of somatosensory information transmission[13] and reduction in muscle tone.[4,6] Upon reduction of afferent somatosensory input, the nVB cells hyperpolarize. Instead of remaining at a stable level of inhibition, however, a gradual depolarization, mediated

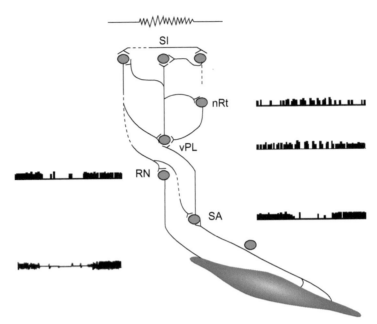

Figure 12.3 Pathways between muscle (with a muscle spindle within) shown in red and the sensory area of the cortex (S1), including sensory afferents (SA), red nucleus (RN), ventralis posterior lateralis nucleus (VPL), and thalamic reticular nucleus (nucleus reticularis thalimi or nRT). SMR 12–15 Hz activity is generated by membrane polarity changes in the ventrobasal nucleus of the thalamus (VPL), which is generally concerned with relaying afferent somatosensory information. Inhibitory influences associated with decreases in efferent motor excitability (seen here in unit recordings from the red nucleus, RN) and associated muscle tone result in decreased discharge in somatic afferent (SA) pathways projecting to the dorsal columns and thalamus. The resulting decrease in excitation of thalamic VPL relay cells initiates a slow membrane hyperpolarization leading to a unique bursting discharge, which is relayed to the sensorimotor cortex and simultaneously to the thalamic reticular nucleus (nRT). Stimulation of neurons in this nucleus results in a corresponding burst discharge, in this case of GABAergic neurons, imposing reciprocal inhibition on the original pool of VPL relay cells, thereby returning them to a hyperpolarized state. A new cycle of oscillatory cellular bursting is thus initiated. In this way, the interplay between neuronal populations in VPL, nRt and the sensorimotor cortex results in rhythmic thalamocortical volleys and cortical EEG oscillations which, in the quiet but alert state, appear as a 12–15 Hz EEG rhythm (SMR). *(From Sterman and Bowersox.[14])*

by a slow calcium influx, causes the nVB neurons to discharge a unique burst of spikes, which is relayed to the sensorimotor cortex and simultaneously to neurons of the thalamic reticular nucleus (nRT). Stimulation of the latter in turn leads to a burst discharge of gamma-aminobutyric acid (GABA) neurons, imposing reciprocal inhibition on the original pool of VB relay cells, thereby returning them to a hyperpolarized state and initiating a new cycle of slow depolarization. Thus, as modeled in Figure 12.3, the interplay between neuronal populations in nVB, nRT and the sensorimotor cortex results in reciprocal rhythmic thalamocortical volleys and consequent cortical EEG oscillations which in the quiet state under normal circumstances appear as 12–15 Hz SMR rhythms.[1,14] Convincing evidence suggests that all normal rhythmic patterns in the EEG may arise from a similar process but may be expressed at different frequencies based on anatomical differences in thalamocortical projection pathways.[15]

Frequencies also vary as a function of background arousal[16,17] and consequent degrees of thalamic neuronal hyperpolarization.[18] The neural networks of the mammalian forebrain, however, are highly interconnected and can generate a wide variety of synchronized activities. These can include normal brain rhythms as well as those underlying epileptic seizures. The cerebral cortex and hippocampus are particularly prone to the generation of the large, synchronized bursts of activity that underlie many forms of seizures. This is because of multiple factors that influence these circuits, including strong recurrent excitatory connections, the presence of intrinsically burst-generating neurons, the interactions among closely spaced neuronal axons, and synaptic plasticity. Accordingly, the propensity for seizures could be reduced by inhibitory influences reducing abnormal excitation, cellular bursting and ephaptic interactions (a form of neuronal transmission involving axon–axon interactions). Influences promoting thalamocortical inhibition and consequent normal rhythmic patterns might achieve this goal. Support for this possibility was in fact obtained in an early pilot study in Sterman's laboratory. They were providing SMR neurofeedback training to several presurgical patients with partial complex seizures, who were implanted with bilateral fine wire subcortical electrodes in the hippocampus and amygdala in order to locate abnormal interictal (between seizures) foci. Preliminary evidence was obtained, suggesting a reciprocal relationship between learned SMR EEG trains and this abnormal discharge (Figure 12.4).

The simplest form of epileptiform activity in the amygdala and hippocampus is the interictal spike, a synchronized burst of action potentials in a localized pool of pyramidal neurons. These are generated by phasic hyperexcitability in these cells and are associated with strong axonal efferent activation. This activation leads to a subsequent period of feedback hyperpolarization resulting from the excitation of collateral recurrent

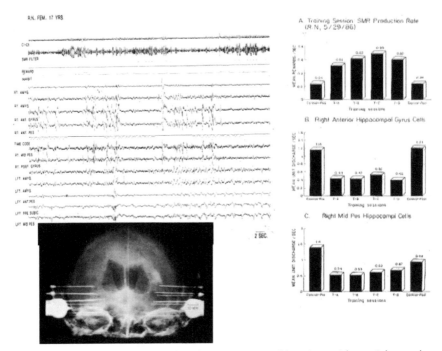

Figure 12.4 This collage shows data from a 17-year-old patient with partial complex epilepsy in phase 2 of the seizure surgery program at UCLA. The X-ray at bottom presents a frontal view of the calvarium revealing the bilateral implantation of electrodes into the amygdala and hippocampus of this patient. The central image shows the EEG recording montage used to simultaneously monitor subcortical and cortical activity during neurofeedback training to facilitate the 12–15 Hz SMR in the sensorimotor cortex. A reward channel is shown below the cortical recording. Note that during recurrent trains of rewarded SMR activity, subcortical interictal discharge was suppressed. The graph on the right presents a plot of pre- and post-feedback SMR incidence compared with output across four 5-minute training trials (top) and corresponding mean abnormal interictal discharges at two hippocampal recording sites. This quantitative display confirms a suppression of abnormal subcortical activity during SMR production, which was partially sustained after training (bottom plot). *(From Sterman and Bloomfield.[56])*

interneurons, which impose transient inhibition on the pyramidal neurons of origin. This inhibition gives rise to the "wave" component of spike–wave patterns. However, even in the absence of spike discharges, cortical hyperexcitability and resulting inhibition produce a slowed EEG rhythm, typically in the 4–8 Hz range.[19] Accordingly, patterns of prominent 4–8 Hz theta slow waves can serve as a signature for focal epileptogenic sites in the cerebral cortex.

Seizure activity also can be generated in response to a loss of balance between excitatory and inhibitory influences, and can take the form of either tonic depolarization or repetitive rhythmic burst discharges, either as clonic or as spike–wave activity, again mediated both by intrinsic membrane properties and synaptic interactions. As reviewed above, the interaction of the cerebral cortex and the thalamus, in conjunction with abnormally enhanced GABA-induced thalamic oscillations, can also generate spike waves similar to those occurring during absence seizure discharges. Although epileptic syndromes and their causes are diverse, the cellular mechanisms of seizure generation appear to fall into only two categories: rhythmic or tonic "runaway" excitation, or the synchronized and rhythmic interplay between excitatory and inhibitory neurons and membrane conductance.[20]

Clinical epilepsy is a diverse disorder of which there are over 40 recognized types, segregated into distinct syndromes (Commission on Classification and Terminology of the International League Against Epilepsy: Proposal for revised classification of epilepsies and epileptic syndromes, 1989). This diversity arises from both the numerous underlying cellular and molecular mechanisms and the spatial and temporal characteristics of the seizure.

Most epileptic syndromes are grouped into two basic categories: partial and generalized. Partial seizures occur within a localized area of the brain, whereas generalized seizures, in terms of their EEG manifestations, appear throughout the forebrain from the outset. If the partial seizure does not cause a disruption of consciousness or cognitive abilities, it is said to be simple; if it does, it is referred to as complex.

There is great diversity in the pathologies leading to, and clinical manifestations of, the epileptic syndrome. It is thought, however, that the actual generation of many of the different types of seizure may occur through common cellular mechanisms and networks. Although practically every part of the brain may generate an epileptic seizure, the investigation of the cellular and network mechanisms of epilepsy over the last several decades has focused largely on three structures: the cerebral cortex, the hippocampus and the thalamus. As mentioned above, there are multiple factors contributing to the epileptogenicity of these structures, including the presence of massive recurrent excitatory connections, reliance upon inhibition for the regulation of excitability of this recurrent network, the ability of synaptic connections to strengthen or weaken with repetitive activation, and the presence of intrinsically burst-generating cells.

Investigation of the possible mechanisms for generation of partial, complex partial and generalized seizures in these structures has demonstrated that every aspect of neuronal and glial function, from genes to synapses to networks, has at least a modulatory influence. Extensive and informative reviews of many of these aspects are available.[20–22] A detailed discussion of these mechanisms, however, is beyond the scope of this review. Suffice it to say that the loss of regulating inhibitory modulation is clearly involved. There is convergent evidence that neurofeedback therapy can affect this deficit.

Although attenuation of efferent motor and afferent somatosensory activity can initiate SMR, the oscillatory activity is also largely influenced by nonspecific cholinergic and monoaminergic neuromodulation, which can affect excitability levels both in thalamic relay nuclei and in the cortical areas receiving the relayed signals. During waking activity, these neuromodulatory influences, as well as cortical projections, normally keep VB cells depolarized and thus suppress rhythmic bursting patterns, whereas during behavioral stillness oscillations at SMR frequency may be observed. Because SMR constitutes the dominant "standby" frequency of the integrated thalamocortical, somatosensory and somatomotor pathways, learned regulation of the SMR is assumed to result in improved control over excitation in this system. Raised thresholds for excitation, in turn, are thought to underlie the clinical benefits of SMR training in epilepsy and other disorders characterized by cortical and/or thalamocortical hyperexcitability. For instance, SMR training has been shown to be an effective treatment for attention deficit hyperactivity disorder (ADHD). For recent reviews see Monastra et al.[23,24] Furthermore, this training has been documented to result in a reduction of impulsive response tendencies in healthy volunteers.[25,26]

More recently, functional MRI (fMRI) studies in human subjects have shown that the SMR EEG pattern is clearly associated with an increase in metabolic activity in the striatum of the basal ganglia nuclear complex.[27] Further, examining fMRI changes in children with ADHD who improved significantly in cognitive tests after SMR neurofeedback training, Levesque and Beauregard[28] observed a specific and significant increase in metabolic activity in the striatum and substantia nigra of the basal ganglia complex. Collectively, these findings support the notion that the neuronal state changes mediating the SMR are associated with functional changes in the striatum. The striatum, which is the anterior component of the basal ganglia, has been characterized anatomically as a system of fiber connections that form a loop from cerebral cortex and back to cerebral cortex via thalamic

relays.[29] The two major components of the striatum include the putamen/
globus pallidus complex and the caudate nucleus. The striatum has been
attributed a role in managing background motor tone and the planning
phase of movements.[30] Although many different neurotransmitters are used
within the basal ganglia (principally acetylcholine [ACh], GABA, and dopamine), the overall effect on thalamus and premotor networks in the mesen-
cephalic tegmentum and superior colliculus is inhibitory.[31] This inhibitory
influence upon thalamic relays to motor cortex and brain-stem involuntary motor circuits may reduce muscle tone and the intention to move.
Consistent with an activation of striatal inhibitory mechanisms, the studies
mentioned earlier have documented this possibility, confirming a reduction
in background motor tone, reflex excitability and activity in extrapyramidal
motor pathways during SMR bursts.[3,5,6,12,32] It is also evident that both animals and humans suppress the intention to move.[1] This convergence of findings suggests that facilitation of the SMR component of the EEG through
positive feedback reward favors reduced motor excitability and disrupted
afferent input to the thalamus, thereby reducing the propensity to seizures.

An especially important fact here may be that this reorganization of
motor and thalamic status is accompanied by volleys of strong oscillatory
discharges to the cortex with each trained SMR response. The relevance
of this derives from a different and highly significant area of investigation.
Findings from the study of synaptic mechanisms mediating experience-
based neuronal reorganization, and hence learning, provide an appealing
theoretical basis for a potentially unique consequence of SMR training.[33]
Many studies have shown that strong, repetitive afferent input to cortical
and other forebrain neurons can promote increased synaptic strength in
relevant circuits (see reviews by Abel & Lattal,[34] Malenka & Nicoll,[35] and
Soderling & Derkach[36]). These changes, produced over time by protein
synthesis and the insertion of new excitatory transmitter channels at postsynaptic receptor sites, result in a synaptic state called "long-term potentiation", or LTP. Under appropriate circumstances, LTP increases synaptic
sensitivity and the probability of future activation in affected neuronal circuits. The normal thalamocortical oscillatory volleys underlying the SMR
constitute recurrent bursts of afferent discharge to the sensorimotor cortex. This recurrent discharge arrives at the base of cortical pyramidal cell
apical dendrites (layer 4). The unique timing and location of these strong
recurrent afferent bursts appears to be particularly significant. Activation
of distal portions of these same pyramidal neurons must accompany this
input because of the attention required for SMR operant conditioning.

This convergence of thalamocortical bursting and background activation provides a potentially ideal milieu for LTP and synaptic reorganization, consistent with recent concepts of "coincidence detection" and synaptic plasticity.[37] That is, the coincidence of strong thalamic afferent input near the pyramidal cell body and back-depolarization from cognitively based distal excitation of the same cell magnifies local depolarization and subsequent LTP.

Thus, the functional changes in sensorimotor circuits mediating the discrete and recurrent onset of SMR activity in the EEG may be specifically strengthened over time during feedback training through a progressive potentiation process, resulting in a lasting decrease in sensorimotor excitability. There is abundant indirect evidence that such changes can indeed occur with SMR operant conditioning. For example, when cats were provided with several weeks of SMR training and then subjected to an extinction trial with the reward withheld, there was a marked increase in the expression of SMR activity during the initial period of the extinction trial, as described earlier (Figure 12.2). Such an increase is a marker for valid operant conditioning. However, when an identical test was performed after several more months of training, both the output of SMR during rewarded trials and the response to the extinction procedure were significantly – and dramatically – increased. Additionally, studies in both animals and humans have found that sleep recordings obtained after several months of SMR training were characterized by a lasting increase in sleep spindle density compared to pretraining recordings.[38–41] Control feedback conditions had no such effect. When the effect of SMR neurofeedback was studied in epileptics over time, patients with characteristic focal slowing and deficient sleep spindles in the sensorimotor cortex displayed a gradual reduction in slow activity and increase in 12–15 Hz sleep spindles (Figure 12.3). Of course epileptic patients differ in their seizure pathology, seizure history and medication regimens. Because of these factors, results have varied from profound to mild.

Virtually all patients studied, however, have demonstrated some clinical benefits from this training. Consistent with the concept of neuroplasticity, this behavioral treatment must significantly affect both structural and biochemical status, resulting in improved regulation of abnormal processes.

CLINICAL CONSIDERATIONS

About 30% of people with epilepsy have seizures that are not well controlled by medication. Some 60% of poorly controlled seizure disorder patients suffer from partial complex seizures. EEG characteristics in this population have been carefully compared statistically to a nonepileptic control group during stage 2 sleep.[42] Findings included a significant elevation in 0–3 and 4–8 Hz slow frequencies together with a significant reduction in 12–15 Hz spindle frequency activity. These findings, as well as the animal studies described earlier, provided guidance for the initial application of SMR EEG feedback treatment to human epileptic research subjects and clinical patients.

The earliest studies were carried out with volunteer epileptic subjects who were poorly controlled by medication.[43,44] Most were partial complex seizure disorders of moderate to long duration. One electrode site was used exclusively, always placed in the left medial central (sensorimotor) cortex at C3. In later studies, when quantitative EEG assessment became available, a second electrode was added and placed over areas of abnormal slow activity, typically but not always at frontotemporal sites.[41,45–48] In these cases the central electrode was placed at the medial central site in the same hemisphere as the most prominent slow activity (usually in the 4–8 Hz range): for example, increased reward for 12–15 Hz at medial central sites C3 or C4, and inhibition of 4–8 Hz activity at corresponding hemispheric temporal cortex sites T3 or T4 (T7 and T8 using the revised nomenclature). Later studies added simultaneous negative reward for spike discharges, eye movement and muscle artifacts.

The initial theoretical goal was to strengthen an inhibitory standby state in efferent motor pathways. If a focus for abnormal activity was identified, this was combined with an effort to suppress the focal cortical hyperexcitability. Variations on this general protocol have been used in most of the studies that followed this work and remain prominent today.[8,9] In some of the later studies, robust experimental controls were introduced, such as double-crossover ABA designs and multiple treatment comparisons.

Interestingly, similar functional objectives were sought by Rockstroh and colleagues by rewarding positive SCPs instead of SMR.[49–51] Based on the measurement of SCPs, this kind of feedback trains the direct current (DC) shifts between positive and negative polarities in the cortex that underlie the alternating current (AC) of the EEG. SCP training to increase positivity (less arousal) has also proved successful in the treatment of epilepsy. Conceptually, SCP and SMR neurofeedback share the same goal of reducing cortical excitability. Negative slow potentials are reflective of increased excitation (through depolarization) in the apical dendrites of cortical pyramidal neurons, whereas positive slow potentials represent decreased excitation. Thus, SCP training in epileptics is aimed at enabling the patient to voluntarily produce cortical inhibition (i.e., positive SCPs) and thus interrupt the onset of seizures (for a review, see Birbaumer[52]). Interestingly, Birbaumer[27] also reports that both the SMR pattern in the EEG and learned increases in positive SCPs were associated with increased metabolic activity in the striatum of the basal ganglia, suggesting a convergent effect of SMR and SCP training.

We have focused on SMR neurofeedback in the treatment of epilepsy, primarily because this treatment has now been so well documented that the American Academy of Child and Adolescent Psychiatry considers neurofeedback for seizure disorders to meet the criteria for evidence-based treatments, a recommendation stating that a particular practice should always be considered by the clinician. As a comparison example, the same criterion is met by stimulant medication treatment for ADHD and for neurofeedback training for ADHD.[53]

It should be noted, however, that regardless of conceptual and experimental objectives, and despite adequate controls, valid outcomes in neurofeedback training depend critically on the proper technical and methodological application of EEG operant conditioning.[54] Those attempting clinical application of this treatment for epilepsy are therefore obliged to acquire a competent understanding of this methodology and the technological specifications of the hardware and software they use. Further, it is important to again point out that the treatment of seizure disorders by any approach is made challenging by the diversity of their etiologies, developmental histories, resulting clinical manifestations and severity. Equally important is the variability of such contextual factors as family sophistication and support, social interactions, intellectual capacity and comorbidity with other neurological pathologies. Thus, it is not surprising that some patients may not respond to any intervention, neither medications nor EEG biofeedback training. However, most patients with epilepsy who have participated in neurofeedback research studies, and many who seek this treatment today, represent unquestionable failures of anticonvulsant drug therapies, particularly with complex partial seizure disorders. What is particularly impressive is that, even in treatment–refractory drug nonresponders, positive outcomes have often been obtained. It may be tempting to attribute these outcomes to alternative explanations, such as placebo effects or changes in medication compliance. However, it should be recalled that this work has its roots in studies of cats and monkeys, who also evidenced raised seizure thresholds but were in no way affected by expectation or secondary gain influences. Additionally, early clinical research documenting significant reductions in seizure rate and severity in human epileptic subjects, specifically after SMR EEG feedback training, closely monitored anticonvulsant blood levels at each stage of a controlled double-crossover design, and found no significant changes in levels of medication.[41]

Considering the noninvasive and relatively benign nature of EEG feedback therapy, as opposed to the common side effects and costs associated with lifelong use of antiseizure medication, we do not view neurofeedback treatment as a "last resort" option for drug-resistant cases only, but rather as a generally viable adjunctive treatment for any patient suffering from seizures.

Furthermore, in contrast to drug-dependent symptom management, the altered modulation of thalamocortical and brain-stem motor excitability through neurofeedback training may raise seizure thresholds sufficiently to greatly improve the prospects for the long-term management of seizures using less medication, thereby also reducing the risk of progressive cognitive and neurobehavioral decline.[55] We therefore conclude that when clinicians with training in essential clinical skills carry out a careful assessment and then apply appropriate operant conditioning methodology to training their clients, EEG feedback therapy can indeed recruit neuroplasticity to provide a meaningful pathway toward altered neural circuitry and normalization of function.

REFERENCES

1. Sterman MB. Physiological origins and functional correlates of EEG rhythmic activities: implications for self-regulation. *Biofeedback Self Reg.* 1996;21:3–33.
2. Roth SR, Sterman MB, Clemente CC. Comparison of EEG correlates of reinforcement, internal inhibition, and sleep. *Electroencephalogr Clin Neurophysiol.* 1967;23:509–520.
3. Sterman MB, Wyrwicka W. EEG correlates of sleep: evidence for separate forebrain substrates. *Brain Res.* 1967;6:143–163.
4. Wyrwicka W, Sterman MB. Instrumental conditioning of sensorimotor cortex EEG spindles in the waking cat. *Physiol Behav.* 1968;3:703–707.
5. Sterman MB, Wyrwicka W, Roth SR. Electrophysiological correlates and neural substrates of alimentary behavior in the cat. *Ann NY Acad Sci.* 1969;157:723–739.
6. Chase MH, Harper RM. Somatomotor and visceromotor correlates of operantly conditioned 12–14 c/s sensorimotor cortical activity. *Electroencephalogr Clin Neurophysiol.* 1971;31:85–92.

7. Sterman MB, Goodman SJ, Kovalesky RA. Effects of sensorimotor EEG feedback training on seizure susceptibility in the rhesus monkey. *Exp Neurol.* 1978;62(3):73S–747.

8. Sterman MB. Basic concepts and clinical findings in the treatment of seizure disorders with EEG operant conditioning. *Clin Electroenceph.* 2000;31(1):45–55.

9. Tan G, Thomby DC, Hammond U, Strehl B, et al. Meta-analysis of EEG biofeedback in treating epilepsy. *Clin EEG & Neurosci.* 2009;40(3):173–179.

10. Yucha, C, Montgomery, D, eds. *Evidence-Based Practice in Biofeedback and Neurofeedback.* Wheat Ridge, CO, Association for Applied Psychophysiology and Biofeedback; 2008.

11. Howe RC, Sterman MB. Cortical-subcortical EEG correlates of suppressed motor behavior during sleep and waking in the cat. *Electroencephalogr Clin Neurophysiol.* 1972;32:681–695.

12. Harper RM, Sterman MB. Subcortical unit activity during a conditioned 12–14 Hz sensorimotor EEG rhythm in the cat. *Fed Proc.* 1972;31:404.

13. Howe RC, Sterman MB. Somatosensory system evoked potentials during waking behaviour and sleep in the cat. *Electroencephalogr Clin Neurophysiol.* 1973;34:605–618.

14. Sterman MB, Bowersox SS. Sensorimotor EEG rhythmic activity: a functional gate mechanism. *Sleep.* 1981;4(4):408–422.

15. Hughes S, Crunelli V. Just a phase they're going through: the complex interaction of intrinsic high-threshold bursting and gap junctions in the generation of thalamic alpha and theta rhythms. *Int J Psychophysiol.* 2007;64:3–17.

16. Bouyer JJ, Detet L, Konya A, Rougeul A. Convergence de trios systems rythmiques thalamo-corticaux sur l'aire somesthesique du chat et du babouin normaux. *Rev Electroenceph Clin Neurophysiol.* 1974;4:397–406.

17. Rougeul A, Letalle A, Corvisier J. Activite rythmique du cortex somesthesique primair in relation avec l'immobilite chez le chat libre eveille. *Electroencephalogr Clin Neurophysiol.* 1972;33:23–39.

18. McCormick DA, Huguenard JR. A model of the electrophysiological properties of thalamocortical relay neurons. *J Neurophysiol.* 1992;68:1384–1400.

19. Gloor P, Pellegrini A, Kostopoulos GK. Effects of changes in cortical excitability upon the epileptic bursts in generalized penicillin epilepsy of the cat. *Electroencephalogr Clin Neurophysiol.* 1979;46(3):274–289.

20. McCormick DA, Contreras D. On the cellular and network bases of epileptic seizures. *Annual Rev Physiol.* 2001;63:815–846.

21. Dichter MA, Ayala GF. Cellular mechanisms of epilepsy: a status report. *Science.* 1987;237:157–164.

22. Steriade M, McCormick DA, Sejnowski TJ. Thalamocortical oscillations in the sleeping and aroused brain. *Science.* 1993;262:679–685.

23. Monastra VJ, Lynn S, Linden M, Lubar JF, Gruzelier J, LaVaque TJ. Electroencephalographic biofeedback in the treatment of attention-deficit/hyperactivity disorder. *Appl Psychophysiol Biofeedback.* 2005;30:95–114.

24. Arns M, de Ridder S, Strehl U, et al. Efficacy of neurofeedback treatment in ADHD: the effects of inattention, impulsivity and hyperactivity: a meta-analysis. *Clin EEG and Neurosci.* 2009;40(3):180–188.

25. Egner T, Gruzelier JH. Learned self-regulation of EEG frequency components affects attention and event-related brain potentials in humans. *Neuro Report.* 2001;12(18):4155–4160.

26. Egner T, Gruzelier JH. EEG Biofeedback of low beta band components: frequency-specific effects on variables of attention and event-related brain potentials. *Clin Neurophysiol.* 2004;115:131–139.

27. Birbaumer N. Breaking the silence: brain-computer interfaces in paralysis. Proceedings of the Annual Conference, *Int Soc for Neuronal Reg.* 2005;13:2.
28. Levesque J, Beauregard M. Effect of neurofeedback training on the neural substrates of selective attention in children with attention-deficit/hyperactivity disorder: a functional magnetic resonance imaging study. *Neurosci Letters.* 2005;8:27–34.
29. Brodal P. The basal ganglia. In: Brodal P, ed. *The Central Nervous System: Structure and Function.* New York, NY: Oxford University Press; 1992:246–261.
30. DeLong MR. Primate models of movement disorders of basal ganglia origin. *TINS.* 1990;13(7):281–285.
31. Chevalier G, Deniau JM. Disinhibition as a basic process in the expression of striatal functions. *Trends Neurosci.* 1990;13:277–280.
32. Babb MI, Chase MH. Masseteric and digastric reflex during conditioned sensorimotor rhythm. *Electroencephalogr Clin Neurophysiol.* 1974;36:357–365.
33. Sterman MB. Principles of Neurotherapy. Proceedings of the Annual Conference, *Int. Soc. for Neuronal Reg.* 2005;13:23–28.
34. Abel T, Lattal KM. Molecular mechanisms of memory acquisition, consolidation and retrieval. *Curr Opin Neurobiol.* 2001;11:180–187.
35. Malenka RC, Nicoll RA. Long-term potentiation–a decade of progress? *Science.* 1999;285:1870–1874.
36. Soderling TR, Derkach VA. Postsynaptic protein phosphorylation and LTP. *Trends Neurosci.* 2000;23:75–80.
37. Froemke RC, Poo MM, Dan Y. Spike-timing-dependent synaptic plasticity depends on dendritic location. *Nature.* 2005;434:221–225.
38. Hauri P. Treating psychophysiologic insomnia with biofeedback. *Arch Gen Psychiatry.* 1981;38:752–758.
39. Hoedlmoser K, Pecherstorfer T, Gruber G, et al. Instrumental conditioning of human sensorimotor rhythm (12-15 Hz) and its impact on sleep as well as declarative learning. *Sleep.* 2008;31(10):1401–1408.
40. Sterman MB, Howe RD, Macdonald LR. Facilitation of spindle-burst sleep by conditioning of electroencephalographic activity while awake. *Science.* 1970;167:1146–1148.
41. Sterman MB, MacDonald LR. Effects of central cortical EEG feedback training on incidence of poorly controlled seizures. *Epilepsia.* 1978;19:207–222.
42. Sterman MB. Power spectral analysis of EEG characteristics during sleep in epileptics. *Epilepsia.* 1981;22:95–106.
43. Sterman MB, Friar L. Suppression of seizures in an epileptic following sensorimotor EEG feedback training. *Electroencephalogr Clin Neurophysiol.* 1972;33:89–95.
44. Sterman MB. Neurophysiologic and clinical studies of sensorimotor EEG biofeedback training: some effects on epilepsy. *Semin Psychiatry.* 1973;5(4):507–525.
45. Lubar JF, Bahler WW. Behavioral management of epileptic seizures following EEG biofeedback training of the sensorimotor rhythm. *Biofeedback Self Regul.* 1976;1:77–104.
46. Lubar JF, Shabsin HS, Natelson SE, et al. EEG operant conditioning in intractable epileptics. *Arch Neurol.* 1981;38:700–704.
47. Sterman MB, MacDonald LR, Stone RK. Biofeedback training of the sensorimotor EEG rhythm in man: effects on epilepsy. *Epilepsia.* 1974;15:395–417.
48. Sterman MB, Shouse MN. Quantitative analysis of training, sleep EEG and clinical response to EEG operant conditioning in epileptics. Electroenceph. *Clin Neurophysiol.* 1980;49:558–576.
49. Rockstroh B, Elbert T, Birbaume N, et al. Cortical self-regulation in patients with epilepsies. *Epilepsy Res.* 1993;14:63–72.

50. Kotchoubey B, Strehl U, Holzapfel S, Blankenhorn V, Froscher W, Birbaumer N. Negative potential shifts and the prediction of the outcome of neurofeedback therapy in epilepsy. *Clin Neurophysiol.* 1999;110(4):683–686.

51. Kotchoubey B, Strehl U, Uhlmann C, et al. Modification of slow cortical potentials in patients with refractory epilepsy: a controlled outcome study. *Epilepsia.* 2001;42:406–416.

52. Birbaumer N. Slow cortical potentials: their origin, meaning, and clinical use. In: Boxtel GJM, von Böcker KBE, eds. *Brain and Behaviour–Past, Present and Future.* Tilborg: University Press; 1997:25–39.

53. Hirshberg LM, Chiu S, Frazier JA. Emerging brain-based interventions for children and adolescents: overview and clinical perspective. *Child Adolesc Psychiatr Clin N Am.* 2005;14:1–19.

54. Sherlin LH, Arns M, Lubar J, et al. Neurofeedback and basic learning theory: implications for research and practice. *J Neurotherapy.* 2011;15(4):292–304.

55. Lin JJ, Mula M, Hermann BP. Uncovering the neurobehavioural comorbidities of epilepsy over the lifespan. *The Lancet.* 2012;380:1180–1192.

56. Sterman MB, Bloomfield S. Limbic neuronal discharge correlates of sensorimotor EEG feedback training in pre-surgical patients with intractable epilepsy. *Proceedings of the 18th annual meeting of the Biofeedback Society of America.* 1987: 102.

FURTHER READING

Andrews DJ, Schonfeld WH. Predictive factors for controlling seizures using a behavioral approach. *Seizure.* 1992;1(2):111–116.

Bal T, Debay D, Destexhe A. Cortical feedback controls the frequency and synchrony of oscillations in the visual thalamus. *J Neurosci.* 2000;20:7478–7488.

Blumenfeld H, McCormick DA. Corticothalamic inputs control the pattern of activity generated in thalamocortical networks. *J Neurosci.* 2000;20:5153–5162.

Brogden WJ. Animal studies of learning. In: Stevens SS, ed. *Handbook of Experimental Psychology.* New York, NY: John Wiley & Sons; 1951:568–612.

Contreras D, Destexhe A, Sejnowski TJ, Steriade M. Control of spatiotemporal coherence of a thalamic oscillation by corticothalamic feedback. *Science.* 1996;274:771–774.

Destexhe A. Spike-and-wave oscillations based on the properties of GABAB receptors. *J Neurosci.* 1998;18:9099–9111.

Destexhe A, Contreras D, Steriade M. Mechanisms underlying the synchronizing action of corticothalamic feedback through inhibition of thalamic relay cells. *J Neurophysiol.* 1998;79:999–1016.

Fuchs T, Birbaumer N, Lutzenberger W, Gruzelier JH, Kaiser J. Neurofeedback treatment for attention-deficit/hyperactivity disorder in children: A comparison with methylphenidate. *Appl Psychophysiol Biofeedback.* 2003;28:1–12.

Kuhlman WN, Allison T. EEG feedback training in the treatment of epilepsy: some questions and some answers. *Pav J Biol Sci.* 1978;12(2):112–122.

Lantz D, Sterman MB. Neuropsychological assessment of subjects with uncontrolled epilepsy: effects of EEG biofeedback training. *Epilepsia.* 1988;29(2):163–171.

Sanchez-Vives MV, McCormick DA. Cellular and network mechanisms of rhythmic recurrent activity in neocortex. *Nat Neurosci.* 2000;3:1027–1034.

Steriade M, Contreras D. Relations between cortical and thalamic cellular events during transition from sleep patterns to paroxysmal activity. *J Neurosci.* 1995;15:623–642.

Steriade M, Contreras D, Amzica F. Synchronized sleep oscillations and their paroxysmal developments. *Trends Neurosci.* 1994;17:199–208.

Steriade M, Jones EG, McCormick DA, eds. *Organisation and Function,* vol. 1. New York, NY: Elsevier; 1997.

Sterman MB, LoPresti RW, Fairchild MD. Electroencephalographic and behavioral studies of monomethyl Hydrazine toxicity in the cat. *Historical Archives: J Neurotherapy.* 2010;14:293–300.

Sterman MB, Mann CA, Kaiser DA, Suyenobu BY. Multiband topographic EEG analysis of a simulated visuomotor aviation task. *Int J Psychophysiol.* 1994;16:49–56.

CHAPTER THIRTEEN

Diagnosing and Treating Developmental Disorders with qEEG and Neurotherapy

Teresa Bailey

INTRODUCTION

The topic of neurotherapy treatment using neurofeedback for developmental disorders covers a vast range of diagnoses and syndromes with overlapping symptoms. Developmental disorders, by definition, are those disorders that are caused by suboptimal developmental trajectories in any developmental domain or combination of domains. There are many known and unknown etiologies, some of which are more amenable to improvement than others. The primary distinction between developmental disorders and other disorders of childhood is that developmental disorders are not acquired by infection or injury, or caused primarily by social factors. All of these factors, however, may act together in varying degrees with the primary underlying developmental disorders and cannot be neatly separated from them. Increasingly, developmental disorders have been shown to have significant genetic components. The genetics of developmental disorders are proving to be much more complex than previously expected.[1–3] Although biopsychosocial factors can have a significant effect on the trajectory of developmental disorders throughout a life course, it is becoming recognized that developmental disorders are brain based and often have a genetic component. As longitudinal studies are demonstrating, even with optimal parenting, medical treatment, educational and social supports, children with developmental disorders in any single domain or combination of the neuropsychological domains (i.e., attention and concentration, language, memory, visuospatial orientation, sensorimotor functioning, executive functioning and emotion) are unlikely to have as good a developmental outcome as those who do not have a developmental disorder.[2–4]

Clinical Neurotherapy.
Doi: http://dx.doi.org/10.1016/B978-0-12-396988-0.00013-1

Confounding the diagnostic picture, some aspects of developmental disorders do not manifest until the child enters school and must learn more complex tasks, such as reading, writing, math, and ever more complex cognitive and motor organization, and self-management. Secondary difficulties in learning are often misattributed to nonspecific factors such as poor motivation, not trying hard enough, or insufficient parental involvement.

Recent work has demonstrated that attention deficits, impulsivity, reading disorders, and some aspects of auditory processing and language disorders are as highly heritable as type 1 diabetes.[1–3] With approximately 70% of a disorder's manifestation caused by genetic factors, neurofeedback practitioners need to keep in mind that when discussing outcomes, we are often intervening in the approximately 30% window that is amenable to change through therapeutic interventions. It is extremely rare to cure a developmental disorder. As a result, many children will eventually develop secondary emotional symptoms as a result of the unyielding challenges,[5] some of which, such as anxiety,[6,7] also respond to neurofeedback intervention.

Children's brains are still developing, so that even fairly well defined behavioral syndromes may have multiple sources of disruption. Because of the greater plasticity of children's brains, individuals may develop one or more pathway accommodations that result in inefficient functioning, but not the kind of localizable lesion that is characteristic of many adult-onset neurobehavioral difficulties.[8]

Instead of discrete lesions or areas of injury, developmental disorders often involve disruptions in distributed networks. This is an emerging area of research that promises to free clinicians, teachers and families from overly simplistic explanations for failures to develop according to age expectations. Electroencephalography (EEG) has experienced a resurgence as a cost-effective, noninvasive way to image brain function with millisecond functional accuracy. The arrival of quantitative methods of analyzing digital EEG signals creates additional opportunities for refining the data produced by EEG sampling. EEG does not, however, lend itself to defining the direction of signals within a network. Because it is a sample of cortical signals that are subject to great variation throughout development, and which are only rarely directly accessible, for example during tumor or epilepsy surgery, many unverifiable assumptions are made in modeling the hypothesized sources of these signals.[9] Even more assumptions are made when a neurotherapy such as neurofeedback is claimed to be affecting a single particular brain structure as the source of a complex behavioral presentation.[10,11]

THE ROLE OF qEEG IN THE DESCRIPTION AND CLASSIFICATION OF DEVELOPMENTAL DISORDERS

Quantitative electroencephalography (qEEG) contributes to the description and classification of functional neurodevelopmental disorders. Currently, it is not advisable to diagnose a specific neurodevelopmental disorder or cluster of disorders based solely on qEEG. Because of this, a child with a developmental disorder should be evaluated by a team consisting of a physician to rule out physical causes of a disorder and a psychologist or neuropsychologist to assess other developmental, cognitive and emotional contributors to the symptom picture. School-based or psycho-educational testing alone is rarely enough to make a thorough evaluation of a child's constellation of developmental difficulties. Part of the differential diagnostic problem lies in the significant overlap in symptoms among developmental disorders. School-based evaluations and psycho-educational assessments focus on classifying a child according to educational services criteria, which vary greatly among school districts. The current nosology of the Diagnostic and Statistical Manuals is based solely on behavioral symptoms rather than more objective tests and measures.[12,13] The anticipated DSM-5 revision does not rely on advances in developmental neuroscience. As a result, DSM-5 perpetuates the situation that if a person meets the criteria for one DSM diagnosis, it is likely that the diagnostic criteria for additional diagnoses will be met. Although it is important to document the behavioral constellation associated with a developmental disorder, behavior is a final common pathway for multiple, mutually influencing factors that rarely point to a single cause with a single treatment solution.

qEEG provides an objective, replicable measure of brain function that is less dependent on observational behavioral reports that may vary across settings and informants. The accuracy and reliability of a qEEG assessment does not rely on a client's motivation or a therapeutic alliance with the person acquiring the qEEG. As neurofeedback research progresses, the use of full 19 or more channel pre- and posttreatment qEEG data will advance the description of and treatment planning for neurodevelopmental syndromes. As developmental neuroscience continues to demonstrate, most developmental disorders are not a result of discrete lesions or malfunctions in isolated brain structures; they arise from multiple causes and result in dysfunctional brain networks.[14–19]

Full cap simultaneous qEEG data acquisition in both resting and task conditions appears to offer the best option among current technologies to document the functional state of these networks. If we think of behavioral and emotional symptoms as final common pathways that can have a wide variety of causes and sources, a purely symptom-based approach that assumes a one-to-one behavior- or emotion-to-location correspondence no longer suffices if we are to optimize treatment in terms of both outcome and time- and cost-effectiveness.

SINGLE-SITE TRAINING AND EMERGING NEUROSCIENTIFIC FINDINGS ABOUT NEURAL NETWORKS

Partly as a matter of ease and simplicity, and partly from outdated theories about localization of brain functions, many neurofeedback practitioners focus on training one site at a time, and often several individual sites serially. Sites would often be chosen by relating symptoms to scalp sites in a more or less 1:1 ratio.[20] If one site did not produce the expected results, there were secondary and tertiary sites that could be tried, and there has been enough success with clinical case series,[6,7] and to a lesser extent comparison-controlled research,[21–24] while working with both children and adults, that this model continues to be used today.

This model is based on site of lesion studies in adults, where specific deficits or clusters of deficits are verifiably present. In intact, normally developed adults without lesions, these sites are reasonably reliable indicators of localized dysfunctions. In children, however, there is less direct correspondence because the neural network is still developing. In children with developmental disorders, even the networks do not develop reliably according to intact normal adult models. In developmental disabilities, some portion(s) of a network or networks do(es) not function sufficiently for developmentally expected thoughts, feelings and behaviors to manifest. Sites of lesions in adults can be informative about where to start thinking about where a problem may lie, but in children they are insufficient to guide clinical diagnosis and intervention.[25] Increasingly, and particularly as research on attention disorders, autism spectrum disorders (ASDs) and language-based learning disorders progresses, the role of networks in brain functioning continues to challenge our thinking about diagnosis and treatment targets. The research on networks increases our understanding about why developmental disorders are so resistant to monomodal treatment interventions, including single-site neurofeedback training.

What this means for neurofeedback in those with developmental disorders is that theory and research about the best forms of treatment and diagnosis are going to continue to evolve based on research findings. Treatment protocols that show less robust findings in controlled research settings may do so because the research findings actually reflect less success than some clinicians claim, or it may be that, as the result of a researcher's necessary attempt to control as many possibly confounding factors as possible, the research treatment protocols exclude or overlook important factors that should be included. These include factors that practitioners have noted for some time, and which, researchers are acknowledging, need to be included in future research.[21] Among these factors are treatment protocols based on each individual's qEEG findings, providing more intensive treatment at the beginning of therapy and continuing in treatment long enough to consolidate gains. Many research protocols use only a single site or two sites to train all participants, regardless of whether they have different qEEG profiles and/or symptom presentations. Without full cap simultaneous recording, there is no comprehensive way to understand coherence,[19,26] co-modulation[27] and other connectivity dysfunction issues in a client.[10,14–16,25,28–32] With sequential recording multiple sites may be sampled, but because the samplings are not simultaneous there is no way to compare performance accurately and validly between one area or set of sites and another.

SPECIAL CONSIDERATIONS OF qEEG ASSESSMENT AND PERSONS WITH DEVELOPMENTAL DISORDERS

Some practitioners forgo full cap qEEG because it can be difficult to obtain sufficient cooperation from a child, especially a child with hyperactivity and/or an ASD. If a practitioner is not able to gather the data reliably, he or she can refer the child to a qEEG specialist or to an EEG technician who is experienced in working with children and specify that the data are to be gathered in a format that will allow comparison with the database the practitioner will be using to plan treatment. Magnetic resonance imaging (MRI) centers have recognized that many children cannot tolerate the conditions for acquiring an MRI without prior exposure to the machines and procedures. They schedule practice sessions in which the child is exposed to the equipment and procedures, but no data are gathered at that time. Some children require several sessions to become acclimated to the situation and to be able to cooperate sufficiently with the evaluation procedures so that reliable data can be acquired.

A useful technique for children with hyperactivity includes working quickly for brief periods, followed by giving the child the chance to move, wriggle and shift position. Parents can be educated about the length of time needed for a particular set of data to be gathered and can have a child practice sitting still at home until he or she can sit quietly for 3–5 minutes, followed by the chance to move. They will also need to be able to do this to do neurofeedback training, so it can only support treatment efficiency to train them toward this goal as part of getting baseline measurements. Some children who fidget excessively or who have core truncal instability may be able to sit in a beanbag chair or on a parent's lap. If the child sits on the parent's lap, the parent can stabilize the child by wrapping his or her arms around the child, so long as the child is positioned so that the parent's breathing and heartbeat do not contaminate the EEG recording. This can be addressed by placing a thin pillow or thick towel between the parent and the child. It is not advisable to have a child lie down for the EEG recording if the database being used for comparison was gathered on persons who were sitting. Changes in position such as these affect EEG signals to the extent that erroneous interpretations of the data will result.[33,34] These findings raise the question about the advisability of training persons in a position different from the one in which the training program data norms were gathered. Information about the position used to acquire the data for the reference database sample may not be easily found in the training program's manual but should be ascertained from the publisher.

Children with sensory sensitivities can be desensitized through work with the parent(s) and/or an occupational therapist experienced in working with such children. Different EEG caps provide different amounts of pressure on the head. Some are elasticized and may feel more like a swim cap; others are looser and require stabilization with chin straps, chest straps and/ or loop openings for the ears. Some children find the elasticized caps more comfortable, and some like the caps with less pressure, even if it means having to wear a chin or chest strap to stabilize them. Having options available can help give the child a choice and more of a feeling of control in the situation, provided the qEEG recording device can accept the various kinds of connectors associated with the different caps.

Sensor placement and impedance adjustment processes can be quite uncomfortable for children with sensory sensitivities and may cause some anxiety for many children, even those without sensory sensitivities, because the process is outside their usual experience. The opportunity to see and touch the materials, to be shown that the syringe used to deliver conductive gel to the sensors does not break the skin, that they will not be receiving a shot even though the syringe looks like the needles in a doctor's office, and that the gels and pastes come off easily with water can go a long way toward reducing anxiety and promoting cooperation. During setup, children can be distracted with a book, video games they bring in on their mobile devices or that the practitioner has available in the office, or by playing games with a parent. Having something to focus on during setup can make the time go more quickly for the child, distract him or her from sensory overload, and keep some kinds of disruptive movements to a minimum.

When gathering qEEG data, it is important to replicate the findings within the acquisition session and to include task conditions. Replication is easily accomplished by acquiring the data in a fixed sequence that allows for at least two acquisitions of each of the resting conditions. An example would be acquiring data in the order: eyes closed, eyes open, task 1, task 2, eyes open, eyes closed. Because qEEG for treatment planning purposes is different from neurological diagnostic encephalography, there is no need – and it may even be counterproductive – for a client to become sleepy. Usually 3–4 minutes of data acquisition for each condition is sufficient to obtain enough artifact free data for processing. Thus, once setup is complete, less than half an hour is needed to gather replicated data sets that will provide strong reliability for the findings.

Sitting quietly with eyes open and eyes closed is part of many standard qEEG gathering protocols. qEEG acquisition with relevant tasks (such as reading, math, spelling, and for some studies auditory and visual continuous performance tests, and/or facial emotion recognition) provides important information about how the brain activates or fails to activate during important tasks that are often impaired in persons with developmental disabilities. In some cases relatively normal eyes open and eyes closed findings become significantly and specifically abnormal during one or more task conditions. Because different cortical networks are involved in different tasks, integrity in one task does not necessarily predict integrity in another, or between tasks and different resting conditions.[31] Although tasks will generate additional artifacts from eye movement, possible muscle tension and body adjustment, instructions to the client to remain as still as possible and to allow up to 5 or 6 minutes per task condition for gathering the data sets, usually results in sufficient interpretable data. Databases that include norms for specific task conditions allow for additional clinically relevant comparisons to normally developing age-matched persons.

During qEEG data acquisition and during the initial treatment sessions, it may be helpful to schedule somewhat longer sessions to accommodate the developmentally disordered person's longer learning curve, so that he or she can become familiar and comfortable with the process. This prevents the practitioner and the family from feeling rushed and puts less stress on the client. Preventing frustration and potentially a sense of failure or futility may mean the client is more likely to continue with treatment. As the client becomes more accustomed to the procedures, less time may be needed to complete the setup and accomplish the training within a session.

Working with persons with developmental disabilities requires both empathy and clinical skills. It is important to acknowledge to clients that the practitioner is aware that they might be uncomfortable with the set-up procedures, and to remind them that the discomfort is temporary. It is important for practitioners or their EEG technicians to respond with empathy while still achieving the necessary impedance levels to provide a valid recording and valid training.

Not every practitioner or technician will have or develop the skills needed to achieve this with particularly sensitive individuals. If this is the case, then the practitioner should refer to a colleague who has these skills. When setting up a full-cap qEEG data acquisition, especially if the practitioner or technician does not have experience in working with wriggly or sensory-sensitive children, having a pediatric EEG technician come to the office to do the setup and acquire the data, or to have this done at the technician's office in a format compatible with the practitioner's database, may be the best solution.

A special consideration for working with children on the autism spectrum is that approximately 30% or more may have a comorbid seizure disorder. Many more may be susceptible to seizures that have not yet manifested or have areas of poor stabilization[35,36] that may be detected through a full-cap qEEG. Although neurofeedback practitioners are not doing qEEG for neurological diagnostic purposes, at times a qEEG evaluation of a client may produce incidental information indicating that further referral and evaluation by a neurologist is necessary. The patients in whom this is more likely to occur are those with ASDs and those with a history of concussion or head injury, where there is increased vulnerability to paroxysmal events that do not necessarily result in overt seizures. If abnormalities in the raw qEEG are observed,[37] the client should be referred to his or her physician for further evaluation to determine the clinical significance of the finding.

GENERAL CONSIDERATIONS IN TREATMENT PLANNING AND TREATMENT FOR DEVELOPMENTAL DISORDERS

Evidence-based treatment planning for persons with developmental disorders continues to evolve. Findings for different diagnostic groups will be discussed in more detail below. In general, there are no research-based findings that result in a symptom-to-single-site-location guideline. Even the most rigorous research reports acknowledge that a "one site fits most" model is unlikely to result in optimal outcomes, even for behaviorally similar children with developmental disorders of attention.[31,38,39]

Training persons with developmental disabilities requires additional attention to motivation and rewards. Persons known to have difficulty with the acquisition of new skills may or may not find that learning to self-regulate through neurofeedback presents the same challenges as learning in other domains and situations. Some persons with developmental disabilities find neurofeedback easier than learning at school; others find it presents similar challenges, and some find it more difficult. It is therefore even more important to set training parameters to optimal reinforcement levels to keep the client engaged and motivated. It is here that the practitioner's knowledge of the theory and practice of operant conditioning, along with clinical skills in behavioral and emotional management, come together to make neurofeedback a rewarding experience for the person being trained. For persons with developmental disabilities, it is sometimes helpful to have a parent or caretaker remain in the room during training, so long as that person does not interfere by talking too much, either to the client or to the practitioner, or by passing judgment on how the trainee is doing. In my practice, parents are often present while I train children, but they sit behind and to the side of their child so that they can observe what is happening, be available for behavioral management issues, but not distract the child while the child is training. This is especially true when working with autistic children, who may take a long time to feel comfortable being left with a practitioner they see only once or twice a week. Some children like their parents to be present to interact with them during setup by playing games with them; the parent may then leave during the training. This is also a time when the practitioner can gain information from both the parent and the child about how the child has been doing between sessions. Sometimes there are conversations that need to take place between the practitioner and the parent without the child present. If the child cannot wait quietly while unattended in the reception area, a separate time should be scheduled for this discussion with the parent(s) so that it does not interfere with the scheduled training.

Persons with developmental disabilities are often sensitive to failure and resist participating in activities where they will be challenged too much or too frequently. It is important to remind them that no one performs perfectly every time. Whatever the reward structure is during the training, it should be at a level that reassures clients that their efforts are allowing them to reach a goal, while setting the goal just far enough beyond their current ability that they have to remain engaged with the process to reach it.

One of the problems with automated threshold setting is that it is more likely to reward suboptimal effort in ways that are contrary to operant conditioning principles. If a person is rewarded for where he or she is on average, there is little incentive for change. When specific benchmarks are set and are rewarded only when met or exceeded, the goal is clear, as is whether the person achieved that goal or not. Effort will vary within and between sessions. Fatigue, time of day, health, diet, emotional state, medications and other factors will affect an individual's performance on a given day. A skilled practitioner will be able to observe these things, and, in interaction with the client, provide motivation to expend effort while setting goals that are achievable on that day, keeping in mind the context of past performance and ultimate training goals.

Successive approximation is one part of operant conditioning techniques that forms the basis of neurofeedback work. Successive approximation in neurofeedback is used when training one site is stepped in a series of three to four levels. The first level is easily achievable with little or no effort. The next level requires somewhat more work to achieve, and the subsequent level(s) require even more work. This way, training can proceed based on carefully calibrated changes in effort while allowing for client success in the context of optimal, motivating frustration.[40] This kind of stepped training can also give the clinician valuable insight into adjusting thresholds to optimal levels when it appears that a plateau has been reached. Commercial video game manufacturers and casino gaming developers have studied the phenomena around frustration tolerance and reward structures more than have clinical practitioners. As a result, individuals, even those with significant attention deficits and developmental delays, become engaged in otherwise nonproductive gaming activities for hours and days at a time. Auto-thresholding is not the optimal solution to this problem, because it does not provide optimal frustration combined with a desirable goal, and may, in the end, reinforce suboptimal effort by adjusting too soon to too little effort.

When adding a second, third or fourth site in simultaneous networked training, it is often necessary to reset thresholds to levels that are easier than the client can achieve when training at a single site. What was achievable with self-regulation of one site often requires more effort to coordinate achieving thresholds for multiple sites. Once a client is able to achieve the treatment goals for the minimum period of time, it is then possible to set the goal of holding the goal state for a longer period. When this parameter is changed, it will usually be necessary to relax the threshold levels again while the client learns simultaneously to regulate an additional factor.

Care must be taken in setting time goals not to set the time so long that sites hypersynchronize and possibly kindle seizure activity. One well-researched technique to guard against hypersynchronization is to incorporate sensorimotor rhythm (SMR) training into the training protocols. SMR training has been shown in various studies to raise seizure thresholds in vulnerable individuals. A description of Sterman's approach to SMR training with multiple sites can be found in the Open Source publication the *Cleveland Clinic Journal of Medicine*, which can be accessed free of charge on the internet. SMR training has shown additional benefits of improving attention, optimizing the amount of time for on-task behavior, improving some motor skills and improving sleep.[28,40,41]

Multiple-site training, although used in many clinical practices, is only now starting to appear in research designs. Many research protocols, in an attempt to reduce confounding information and to be able to point to verifiable, replicable treatment effects, limit the number of sites trained at a time, usually to one, such as CZ. In addition, to keep everything as constant as possible for research consistency, even when full-cap qEEGs have been gathered and complex analyses of the data have been made, participants in the study still received the same treatment at the same scalp site, regardless of what other sites or treatment strategies may have been indicated by the qEEG analysis. By reducing the number of variables, the researchers have been able to establish that even in a one-strategy-fits-most model, neurofeedback has shown to be efficacious for the disordered attention aspects of complex developmental disorders.[7,17,22,23] Other recent studies have noted that within these models there are individuals who respond well to this approach and others who do not respond as predicted.[21,23,24,38,39,42,43] Given the constraints of the research protocol, however, there was no opportunity to adjust the treatment scalp site(s) in order to optimize outcome. This is in contrast to what happens in most clinical practices, where better rates of response to treatment with customized site selection are reported.[6,15,16,21,26,31,32,40,44–46]

Collateral information about frustration tolerance and what kinds of rewards motivate the client can help in setting up a reward structure. The more severe the developmental disorder, especially with intellectual disabilities, the more important role behavioral shaping will play in the training. It may be necessary to start with one site, and through successive approximations bring the trainee to the point where that one site can reliably be trained to achieve a goal. This is accomplished by the successive approximation technique of setting a series of stepped goals that are easier to attain than the target. The easiest goal would require little or no effort, the next one a bit more, and so on until the actual goal for that session segment is being achieved between 30% and 50% of the time. If the goal is either too easy or too difficult to reach, motivation quickly fades.[47] In addition, little attention has been paid to postreinforcement synchronization, an electrophysiological correlate of the SMR that appears to be correlated with motivation for reward-seeking behavior and learning rate.[32,48] Auto-thresholding programs, despite having the advantage of providing a kind of auto-tracking of the client, are susceptible to rewarding suboptimal effort by adjusting the thresholds too frequently. Unskilled setting of goals, whether manually or through auto-thresholding, which are too easy or too difficult to achieve can reduce effort altogether. Continuous training can deprive both the practitioner and the trainee of needed breaks to assess and adjust goals to keep the learning curve optimal for both motivation and achievement, and goes against the rules of operant conditioning using discrete trials.[49] When working with persons with developmental disabilities, the question of additional rewards beyond the computer program being used arises, whether the program displays points, or pictures, produces sounds, or provides mixed rewards, such as a video with sound and motion. For some clients food rewards are motivating, especially if the food is one that is available only on special occasions or. for extra effort. Some families and practitioners object to the use of food rewards on principle, so alternative reward structures should be offered. Other rewards may be used, such as tokens that can be exchanged for trinkets, stickers, or various kinds of prizes, including money or credits toward a desired item or activity. Any reward that is not provided by the practitioner, such as money, credits toward a desired item, or participation in activities that take place outside the office, should be discussed and agreed on between the practitioner and the parent before being offered to the child. Some parents may disapprove of a reward structure altogether. This issue needs to be resolved so that the family is comfortable with the reward structure, and so that the structure provides adequate motivation in the client. Some clients are content to work with whatever rewards the computer program provides and do not need additional rewards, so there may be nothing to be gained by introducing additional incentives into the training situation.

Whatever the reward structure is, it should follow operant conditioning principles. It should be further understood that the structure of the neurofeedback training will involve moving the goalposts as training progresses, so that what was rewarded at the beginning will eventually require increased performance to achieve rewards over the course of training. Persons with developmental disabilities may have stronger emotional responses whenever the demands increase. The practitioner should be prepared to respond with empathy yet clarity about the structure of sessions and remind the client about agreed incentives and rewards to keep the client moving forward toward goals.

At times the client may plateau in training, or, because of fatigue or illness, regress in his or her ability to meet goals. If this occurs, it is permissible to relax the goal temporarily, but the practitioner must be vigilant to ensure that the principles of operant conditioning continue to be met, while adjusting for intra-individual differences within a session as well as over time.

PRINCIPLES OF PLANNING NEUROFEEDBACK TREATMENT OF DEVELOPMENTAL DISORDERS

The application, both clinically and in research, of neurofeedback treatment for developmental disorders has historically focused on a localization theory for guiding treatment decisions, more or less on a one-to-one symptom-to-location cookbook model of treatment. Until recently the lack of rigorous clinical trials to test this approach has left practitioners and clients reliant mostly on anecdotal reports and small case series for evidence of efficacy. As research design has improved in this field, and controlled clinical trials along with larger case series designs are now being published for various developmental disorders, strong evidence is emerging that single-site training based on oversimplified localization theory-driven models is not returning optimal or even experimentally predicted results.[21–24,50] It is to the field's credit that this is being discussed openly in the research literature. Based on these failures to produce expected results, modifications in treatment protocols and research design, based on emerging network models of neuroscience and developmental neuroscience, are likely to be incorporated into future experiments.[11,21,22,32,37,51]

It is becoming increasingly clear that single-site training based solely on symptoms will give way to training of one or more sites based on various analyses of full-cap qEEG data compared to a normative database.[16] Except in cases of highly focal seizures or tumors, full-cap simultaneous recordings rarely identify only one area of difficulty. Beyond scalp electrode site data, functional network data for co-modulation,[18] coherence[19,26] and other emerging connectivity analyses[10,14–16,25,28–32] demonstrate that connectivity contributes to the total symptom picture in addition to local dysfunction. This argues even more strongly that databases should include various connectivity analyses for task conditions as well as resting states.

The adage that "neurons that fire together wire together" is especially important in order to conceptualize and plan treatment for developmental disorders. Children and adolescents with developmental disorders have brains that are not wiring and firing within normal limits. Neurofeedback based on full-cap simultaneous recordings with eyes open, eyes closed and task conditions that can be compared to normative databases appears to offer the best opportunity to evaluate the functioning not just of individual sites, but also of various connectivity difficulties. These opportunities then direct the practitioner's ability to normalize dysfunctional connectivity as well as to improve functioning at individual sites.

Training networks is not simply a matter of connecting dysfunctional sites together. As clients learn how to interact with the user interfaces, training a single site at the start makes for easier learning, supports success, and builds motivation for being able to stay with more complex and difficult challenges when training two or more sites simultaneously. This is especially important for clients with developmental disabilities, who often have significant histories of failures regardless of the amount of effort expended, and who may have poor coping skills and low frustration tolerance.

RESEARCH ON NEUROFEEDBACK TREATMENT OF SPECIFIC DEVELOPMENTAL DISABILITIES

General Findings and Learning Disorders

Cantor and Chabot[38] reviewed qEEG studies in assessment and treatment of various childhood disorders and noted that cortical, subcortical, brainstem and cerebellar processes contribute to complex manifestations of childhood disorders. They further noted that between 76% and 89% of the variance found in EEG frequency bands is accounted for by genetics, and about 60% of the variance found in coherence. This is in line with other findings of heritable conditions, such as type I diabetes, attention deficit hyperactivity disorder (ADHD) and dyslexia.[3]

Cantor and Chabot's review of the literature on EEG and learning disorders concluded that the EEG abnormalities found in children with learning disabilities are so heterogeneous that no conclusion can be drawn about what to expect for an individual, and that no specific treatment guidelines can be given without having the qEEG data for the individual. The best that can be said at this point is that children with learning disorders are six to seven times more likely to have abnormal qEEG findings than children without learning disorders.

Cantor and Chabot reported that there are maturational factors that must be considered when discussing qEEG and developmental disorders in children. The qEEG may range from grossly abnormal, to appearing grossly normal, but not for the child's age. This raises the often-discussed question of the extent to which some learning disabilities and attention disorders reflect a disorder or simply a lag in maturation. To the extent that a lag in maturation affects future development, however, it makes sense to document and understand the lag, and to provide intervention aimed at normalizing the abnormal functioning.

Another important issue raised by Cantor and Chabot is that even though some general statements are made about frequency bands and ratios, it is not possible to apply them to all children with developmental disorders.[25,31,38] These findings argue strongly for individualized assessment and treatment planning, based on data gained from full-cap simultaneous qEEG recording and analysis. In addition, the data analysis should consider individual frequencies and base training on individualized bands when abnormalities fall outside typically reported frequency band ranges, which are not always consistent across studies, data analyses or training software. Cantor and Chabot reported studies that demonstrated discriminant ability to distinguish between normal and low-IQ children with attention deficits, between children with attention disorders and normal children without attention disorders, and children with learning disorders with and without attention disorders. In clinical practice these conditions are often comorbid and are further complicated by emotional disorders brought on by the stress of having to attend school and cope with the educational and social consequences of their developmental disorders.[5]

The heterogeneity of learning disorders and their frequent comorbidity with attention disorders complicates treatment planning, because most research has focused on children with attention disorders but without comorbid learning problems or other diagnosed developmental and emotional disorders. The other major focus of qEEG and neurofeedback studies has been with autism.

Mental Retardation/Intellectual Disabilities with and without Seizure Disorders

As the incidence of ASDs has increased, the incidence of primary diagnoses of intellectual disabilities has decreased. There is an association between ASDs, poor cognitive abilities and developmental language disorders. As awareness of the range of symptom and syndrome presentations of ASDs has increased, it has become less common to see serious generalized intellectual disabilities diagnosed in the absence of comorbid developmental disorders.

Although clinicians report that some of their clients improve intelligence test scores and academic performance, the research literature in this area is sparse.[6,7,10,26,50] So far, there have been no studies that meet psychometric standards for measuring reliable change with an intelligence test that have been conducted with properly matched controls to compare claims of increased intelligence scores as a result of neurofeedback training.

Surmeli and Ertem[6] published a clinical case series study of 23 participants aged 7–16 years old with mild to moderate mental retardation/intellectual disability, with IQ scores of 40 to 68 on the Wechsler Intelligence Scale for Children – Revised (WISC-R). The study included 14 participants who were previously nonresponders to various medications, including stimulants, antidepressants and both typical and atypical antipsychotics. During the study only two students, both with epilepsy, received medication. The other 21 participants were medication free. All participants received a full-cap qEEG evaluation with customized treatment based on individual qEEG findings. qEEG findings varied across subjects, so that no general treatment protocol for training sites and bands could be recommended for clients with intellectual disabilities. The authors noted that most children needed 20–40 30-minute training sessions before changes were observed by parents and researchers. Participants received one or two 30-minute sessions per day, and the average number of sessions completed was 120 within 90–180 days. The maximum number of sessions for a participant was 200. Surmeli and Ertem reported that 19 of the participants showed increased IQ scores, two showed a decline and two showed no change. Although pre/post index transformed score changes were found to be statistically significant using paired samples and Wilcoxon's signed ranks tests, none of the averaged absolute changes in scores changed by >0.5 standard deviations (SDs), possibly owing to the large SDs. This means that there was not enough of an increase in score improvement to be considered psychometrically significant. WISC-R subtests, which have an SD of three points, showed that two subtests, Picture Completion and Coding, approached an SD of change with improvements at 2.3 and 2.7 points of improvement, respectively. Because there are no alternate forms of the WISC-R, practice effects cannot be ruled out as an explanation for the improvements observed at the 6-month re-administration of the test. It was not reported whether corrections for multiple comparisons were used, which raises the possibility that even the reported significant trends could have occurred by chance.

The participants also were tested in both the visual and auditory modes of the Test of Variables of Attention (TOVA), a test that is relatively immune to practice effects. Significant improvements were demonstrated, with fewer errors of omission, errors of commission and a reduction in response time variability. The scores for the TOVA, which have an average of 100 with an SD of 15, showed statistically and psychometrically significant improvements of at least 1 SD between pre- and post-measures, although the SD remained wide across participants.

The authors reported improved behavior in all participants, with a wide range of reported improved behaviors, including better control of continence and digestive problems, aggression and sleep, as well as improvements in attention, language and social behaviors. Because no behavioral pre- and post-data are reported in forms that allow for statistical comparison, these findings are more difficult to interpret scientifically.

The two intellectually disabled participants with comorbid seizure disorders reported significant decreases in seizure activity. The protocols for these students were not described in detail. One reduced seizures from a range of 240–300 per month to a range of three to six per month at 2-year follow-up. A second participant who had been seizure free on medication for the 2 years prior to the study reported a 50% reduction in medication dosage after 60 sessions and a reduction in pre/post-sleep EEG from 21 to 6 spike–wave events during 70 minutes of sleep recording.

Follow-up of all participants was conducted by telephone every 3 months over 2 years. Of the 22 subjects who reported behavioral and/or intelligence gains at the conclusion of the training period, their families reported that their gains remained stable.

This is an example of a study with children having serious developmental disorders who presented with a wide range of symptoms, all of whom had intellectual disabilities in the mild to moderate range. The heterogeneity of their symptoms – and supposedly a wide range of unknown etiologies – make it difficult to draw either diagnostic or treatment conclusions from this study. Nevertheless, the heterogeneity of the studied population and the heterogeneity of reported improvements, the report of stability of gains over the course of 2 years, and the decrease in seizure activity in the two children with seizures give reason to pursue additional research with individuals who have intellectual disability as part of their diagnostic and symptom profile.

Because the individualized therapy plans were based on full-cap EEG data, no recommendations were made about which sites and bands to train to increase intellectual capacity. The initial range of IQ scores was almost 2 SD. There was too much variability to make scientifically meaningful statements about what the aggregate IQ scores meant, especially when the IQ scores are themselves in the lower limits of what the test can reliably measure. Without reporting the individual changes in scores for each subject, it was impossible to know whether there were any individuals who made psychometrically meaningful changes in IQ scores.

The conclusions that can be drawn from this study are that it is possible to do neurofeedback with intellectually disabled persons, and that at 2-year follow-up the reported gains appeared to hold. The statistical significance of those gains cannot be known from the reported data, but the findings suggest that this is an area that should receive further investigation. The two participants with documented seizure disorders appear to have reliably reduced their seizures and maintained that reduction over the course of 2 years. These findings are consistent with earlier reports of the efficacy of neurofeedback with seizure disorders in adults.[40,51,52]

Reading and Spelling Disorders

Thornton and Carmody[26] reported improved reading and memory in a case series study that did not involve a comparison group. The treatment plan was based on qEEG evaluations that included eyes closed, eyes open and relevant task conditions, as well as training the children while they were engaged in reading and memory tasks. Their training approach, i.e., using reading and memorization tasks during neurofeedback, has strong ecological validity that has not yet been addressed in other research models. It may be that their strong findings were produced in part by reinforcing the deficient abilities simultaneously with reinforcing the normalization of the network coherence through feedback.

Not until 2010 was there a randomized controlled study for language-based developmental disabilities for reading and spelling.[21] Treatment protocols were customized based on qEEG data gathered only in an eyes open condition. After training, a significant effect was found only for improved spelling, and no significant improvement in reading or hypothesized frontocentral changes in qEEG power and coherence. Consistent with changes reported by Thornton and Carmody,[26] Butler and colleagues[2] reported improvements in alpha coherence and attributed the positive changes to improved attention. Note was made that this study did not differentiate the students based on the individual's type or severity of dyslexia. One of the strengths of this study was using qEEG to customize the treatment protocols. In their review of the literature, they noted the heterogeneity of findings among various studies and concluded that individualized treatment based on the child's actual qEEG would more likely benefit the child because the general research findings are not specific enough to guide treatment for the individual.

Autism Spectrum Disorders

Autism is a group of developmental syndromes that likely have multiple etiologies. There is no single gene or set of genes that identify autistic individuals, although various genetic disorders result in autism syndrome symptoms.[2] Most etiologies of autism are, however, unknown.

Pineda et al.[17] provide an introduction to recent theoretical and neuroscientific investigations of neuroanatomical aberrations and connectivity dysfunctions in children with autism. Because of the wide range of presenting symptoms that manifest at different ages in different individuals, no reliable qEEG markers have been found that allow for definitive differential diagnosis of ASDs from other developmental disorders. One area of promise, however, is consistent findings of local areas of hyperconnectivity in the presence of hypoconnectivity between distant parts of the brain.[17,29,44]

Thompson et al.[46] published a detailed review of the functional neuroanatomy and rationale for qEEG-based neurofeedback in ASDs, with a focus on the higher-functioning Asperger's disorder clients who had no significant history of early speech delays, although they may have had difficulties in social pragmatic language. The authors noted the overlap of symptoms among Asperger's disorder, autism, ADHD, other developmental language disorders, dyspraxias and learning disorders.

They performed both CZ and full-cap simultaneous qEEG evaluation, and treatment with both neurofeedback and biofeedback in a case series of 150 Asperger's disorder and nine autism disorder patients seen over the course of 15 years. Their review revealed patterns that were similar to those found in ADHD, as well as differences in coherence patterns from normative databases.

As part of their evaluations, the authors used low-resolution electromagnetic tomography analysis (LORETA). LORETA is an enticing technology fraught with still unproven assumptions[9,33,34,53] for estimating the localization of dysfunctional sources based on the scalp recording of cortical surface signals.[11] LORETA is further based on the Talairach digital brain atlas, mapped from the smaller than average brain of one adult woman, analyzed with uneven slices.[52] As a result, all imaging and localization studies based on Talairach's atlas, including MRI and functional MRI, require considerable manipulation of client data to fit a model based only on one nonstandard person's data. To date there have been no published reports of a digital atlas or developmental series of digital atlases for children. An additional concern regarding children and LORETA is brain-to-skull conductivity ratios, because children are still growing.[54] Skull circumference and brain size differences in persons with autism compared to those of normally developing children are another concern.[55,56] Most peer-reviewed studies using LORETA with children are about localization of seizure foci in epilepsy. One study used LORETA to examine and train executive attention in normally developing young adults.[10] The authors cautioned that their findings, using a spherical three-concentric shell brain model, provide only a "reasonable approximation" of signal sources. Therefore, if a practitioner uses LORETA methods in the evaluation and treatment of developmentally disabled clients, it is important to describe findings and treatment goals with appropriate limitations on the method's precision, so that realistic expectations are maintained with regard to the approximate nature of the reported localization(s) apart from the scalp sensor locations.

Contrary to DSM-IV-TR diagnostic criteria, which prohibit the diagnosis of ADHD in the presence of a pervasive developmental disorder,[12] Thompson et al.[7] frequently demonstrated attention deficit and executive function EEG patterns among their patient population. Other studies have made similar observations on the comorbidity of autism spectrum and attention disorders.[43,57] An analysis of core diagnostic factors in autism did not include attention deficits,[58] but this does not mean that they are not found in persons with autism. The extent to which disordered attention can be parceled out is unclear at this time.[7,23,24,55,57] Clinical trials of neurofeedback for ASDs that involve control groups are finding that whereas the tightly defined, highly restricted treatment protocols are not resulting in improvements in core ASD symptoms, improvements are being seen in attention. Researchers currently hypothesize that improved attention likely accounts for some of the reported improvements on behavioral rating scales.[22–24,43]

Chan and Sze[42] reported that they were able to differentiate autistic children from normal controls when they used eyes open 24-electrode simultaneous recordings gathered in a visual task condition. The task was to watch a computer screen display of colored fish swimming. Consistent with claims made by Dennis et al.[30] that intelligence should not be considered a covariant when studying developmental disorders, Chan and Sze found that intelligence, as measured by a test of nonverbal intelligence, did not appear to be a significant factor, even though the mean scores differed almost 2 SD, with p < .001.

In a comparison reanalysis of symptom-based treatment[20] and EEG connectivity-guided neurofeedback treatment for autism,[44] Coben and Meyers[15] concluded that although both approaches resulted in symptom improvement, the connectivity-guided approach resulted in greater improvement on the Autism Treatment Evaluation Checklist (ATEC),[59] resulting from the individualized treatment based on qEEG findings. Their review of qEEG findings in autism further revealed strong heterogeneity in findings across studies. For the most effective outcome, no specific guidelines for treatment could be given based on symptoms alone. They noted the congruity between white matter tractography and MRI studies, and their findings of dysfunctional coherence based on qEEG analysis. One problem with this and other studies that used the ATEC for measuring change as the result of treatment is that ATEC scores are not standardized. The result is that there is no ability to measure effect sizes of the treatment. Although a percentage change in symptoms is calculated, there is no way to know whether the change is statistically significant based on the psychometric properties of the scales.

Several researchers have begun to test basic neuroscience findings about network disruptions by designing neurofeedback training based on a combination of behavioral symptoms and functional neuroanatomy.

Pineda et al.[24] conducted two studies in which they trained 10–13 Hz at C4. In both studies no improvement in social imitation was found, although this frequency band is known to be associated with mirror neuron functioning. They observed increases in sustained attention, decreased impulsivity, and improvement in some ATEC scores, but no specific improvement in imitation behavior.

An alternative interpretation for their findings may be that the improvement in sustained attention is likely a result of the training of the overlapping frequencies of the SMR over the sensorimotor strip at C4. This has been well documented in the literature, beginning with Sterman.[32,40,41,51] When Pineda's group observed attenuation of 10–13 Hz over the central sites near the sensorimotor area, it was likely not caused as much by the hypothesized suppression in the mirror neuron system, as it was the result of the band frequency overlap with the SMR (on average 12–15 Hz, but as wide as 12–20 Hz),[60] which also attenuates during attentiveness. Furthermore, if, as Pineda et al. have documented,[17] mirror neuron functionality at 10–13 Hz is a frontoparietal network involving imitative behaviors, it does not make sense that single-site training at C4 alone will be sufficient to strengthen this clinically underdeveloped network. An experimental simultaneous training between at least two frontal and parietal sites makes more sense in terms of both the neuroanatomy of mirror neurons and the documented poor connectivity between these areas.

A brief look at a qEEG evaluation of an 8-year-old client of this author's brings together many of the themes addressed thus far in this chapter. The client was independently diagnosed with autism. The client has speech delays but is verbal. There are no reported academic difficulties. There are some classic autism symptoms and comorbid ADHD, but no significant behavior problems in a quiet, ordered environment. No seizures or absence phenomena have been observed by the parents. Although there are abnormal findings in other frequencies, especially 3–7 Hz, because of space concerns only data from the alpha 8–12 Hz range are presented here. Figures 13.1–13.5 show deviations from a normative child database,[61] under resting eyes open (Figure 13.1), and task conditions for reading (Figure 13.2), and math (Figure 13.3). Connectivity analyses, contrary to the literature, show no significant deviations in coherence values (Figure 13.4), but co-modulation analysis shows several significant deviations (Figure 13.5). Several events were recorded during qEEG acquisition that could be either artifacts or paroxysms and require a qEEG specialist to interpret.

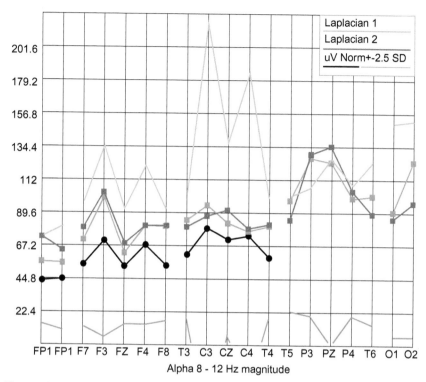

Figure 13.1 8–12 Hz resting eyes open replicated qEEG findings in an 8-year-old diagnosed with autism and ADHD.

Two examples are shown in resting with eyes open (Figure 13.6) and during reading (Figure 13.7). Case examples such as this support the adage that when a clinician has seen one child with autism, the clinician has seen one child with autism. Regardless of what research findings based on group average statistics suggest, in the end clinicians evaluate and treat individuals. For ASDs, as for all developmental disorders, individualized evaluation and treatment are necessary.

The following sections on sleep and elimination disorders may also be relevant to clients with a primary diagnosis of autism.

Developmental Disabilities, Sleep Disorders and SMR Training

Sleep disturbances are more common in children than previously suspected.[50] Among school-aged children and adolescents, sleep disorders were more likely to be diagnosed in boys, children with high body mass

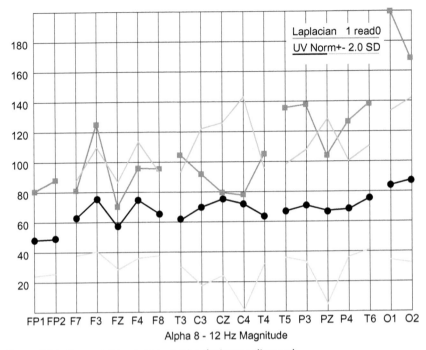

Figure 13.2 Same child as in Figure 13.1 during reading task.

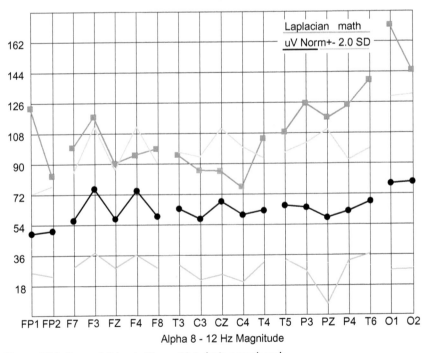

Figure 13.3 Same child as in Figure 13.1 during math task.

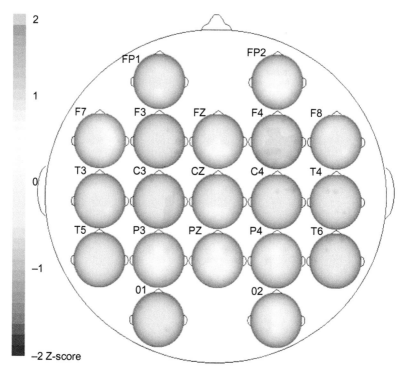

Figure 13.4 Same child as in Figure 13.1, coherence. Note no significant deviations from the normative child database.

indices, some minorities and income groups, as well as children with ADHD or an ASD. The authors noted that there is no medication that has been approved by the Food and Drug Administration for children with sleep disorders, although some physicians prescribe a melatonin supplement or adult sleep medication off-label.

In a study that investigated pathogenic components in ASDs, circadian rhythm dysfunction was identified. Taken together with the other three identified components, immune dysfunction, neurodevelopmental delay and sterotypic behaviors, circadian rhythm dysfunction constituted 74.5% of the phenotypic variance in a sample of 245 autistic patients and their first-degree relatives.[55]

Two studies address neurofeedback therapy for sleep disorders. Arns and Kenemans[28] reviewed sleep disorders and comorbid ADHD. They reported that for a subset of ADHD patients with sleep-onset insomnia, both SMR and slow cortical potential (SCP) training improved sleep spindle function by increasing sleep spindle density. Increasing sleep

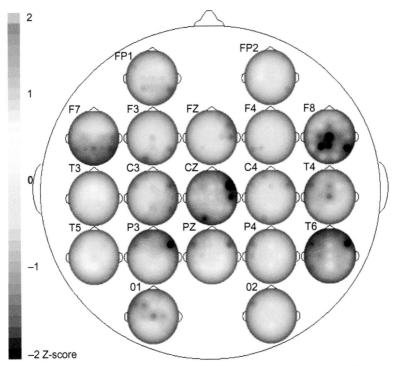

Figure 13.5 Same child as in Figure 13.1, co-modulation. Note several significant deviations from the normative child database.

spindle density into the normative range normalized sleep-onset insomnia. When the insomnia was resolved, ADHD symptoms improved as part of a delayed effect of having treated the insomnia. They speculated that the resolution of sleep-onset insomnia may be an indication that neurofeedback treatment might be able to be stopped at that clinical marker, and that the patient could expect eventual improved attention after some unspecified time delay. They further suggested that follow-up of the extent to which these effects occur and are maintained should be considered the endpoint in treatment, and not just the cessation of the training sessions. These speculations have yet to be demonstrated experimentally.

In a small study in which eight adults with insomnia completed a single-blind randomized treatment protocol trial, Hammer et al.[62] compared modified SMR training[27] and sequential qEEG-guided individualized SCP protocols based on qEEG pretreatment evaluations. Using pre- and posttreatment qEEG, they found that both approaches, which

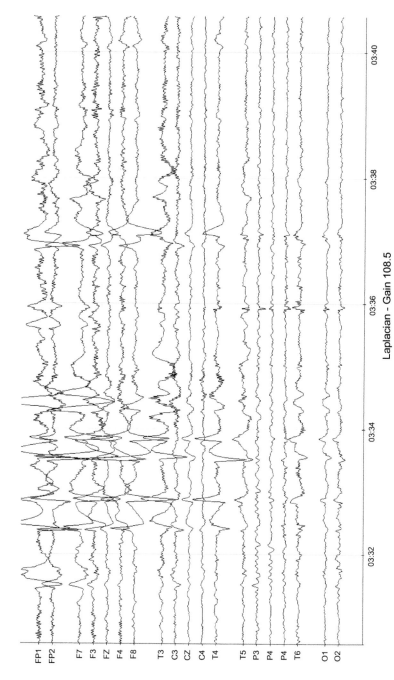

Laplacian - Gain 108.5

Figure 13.6 Event that could be either artifact or paroxysm, should be interpreted by a diagnostic EEG expert.

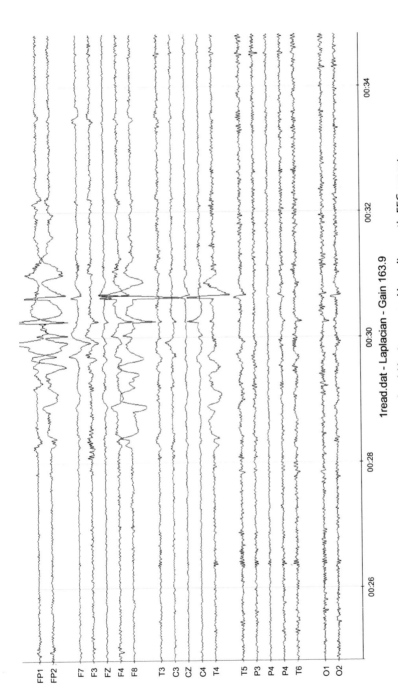

Figure 13.7 Event that could be either artifact or paroxysm, should be interpreted by a diagnostic EEG expert.

used 15 20-minute sessions of Z-score training, resulted in normalized sleep. They used the presence of excessive delta band frequencies to infer daytime sleepiness, and inferred hyperarousal from excessive beta band power findings. Both of these band frequencies normalized during the training. The structure of their protocols led them to conclude that the modified SMR approach was easier to administer and produced similar results to SCP training. Based on this small trial, a larger investigation was reported to have been planned.

Enuresis, Encopresis and Constipation

Elimination disorders may present as single disorders or as comorbidities in various developmental disorders. Constipation is a common problem in persons with ASDs. Enuresis is linked to sleep disorders, including sleep enuresis and sleep-disordered breathing.[63] This includes (but is not limited to) obstructive sleep apnea, which is often associated with obesity, even in children.[62] Enuresis also occurs during the day for some children. Although Surmeli and Ertem did not hypothesize that they would find improvements in elimination problems in their sample of intellectually disabled children and adolescents, they reported incidental findings of improved bladder and bowel control using neurofeedback treatment alone.[6] Thompson et al. did not report any findings about elimination problems that their clients may have experienced but did use a combination of neurofeedback and biofeedback techniques in their clients with a range of ASDs and anxiety disorders, demonstrating that it is feasible to combine the two treatment modalities.[46] Because elimination disorders are common comorbidities in persons with an ASD, neurofeedback practitioners who treat individuals with developmental disorders may wish to consider becoming proficient in biofeedback techniques relevant to these disorders as a logical and empirically validated extension of their work.

Electromyographic pelvic floor biofeedback has been used to treat enuresis in both children and adults. Treatment with biofeedback in a group of 78 children 5–14 years old had positive effects, ranging from 70% improvement for daytime wetting and 86% for nocturnal enuresis at 6-months' follow-up.[64] Biofeedback has been used to treat paradoxical pelvic floor muscle dysfunction in children with enuresis, constipation or both.[65] In another study with 2- and 4-year follow-up after achieving bladder control with perineal floor electromyography biofeedback, 87% maintained control at 2 years and 80% at 4 years.[66] Other studies have found a difference in success depending on whether there was primary or secondary incontinence, with secondary incontinence having a better overall outcome than primary incontinence in a protocol that was limited to only 10 training sessions. At a 21-month follow-up, they concluded that additional training sessions would likely have resulted in maintaining gains of 96% for daytime and 83% for nighttime incontinence observed at the conclusion of the therapy. During the follow-up period, there was 8% relapse for daytime and 33% relapse for nighttime incontinence. The main difference in maintaining success was whether the problem was primary or secondary incontinence.[67]

Constipation is a commonly reported dysfunction in children with autism. Croffie et al.[68] investigated encopresis and constipation in children who had failed at least 6 months of conventional treatments. They found that the children had paradoxical pelvic floor muscle movements, such that they would push to eliminate when they should have been contracting muscles to retain urine and feces. These children responded well to pelvic floor muscle biofeedback training. One neurofeedback study on children with intellectual disabilities reported an incidental improvement in constipation and unspecified digestive symptoms, although these were not a specific focus of the treatment.[6]

CONCLUSIONS

Although the reader may be disappointed that there is no simple decision tree for treatment planning in persons with developmental disorders, there are nevertheless specific guidelines for understanding the complexity of presentations, and important caveats of which to be mindful when doing planning treatment and neurofeedback therapy with this diverse population. Developmental disorders, by definition, begin in childhood and often have a strong genetic component. This is true even for common disorders such as ADHD, dyslexia and anxiety. When developing a treatment plan, it is important to be honest with oneself and with the client and the family about how much change can be expected. Clinicians are often working in the 30% theoretical window of a genetically influenced disorder's susceptibility to alteration by outside factors. It is best not to give false hope to a family that an intervention will restore an individual to a state of wellness, as if the individual did not have the genetic loading to have a developmental disorder and its accompanying challenges.

Developmental disorders rarely present in pure form. Rather, they often appear in clusters within the same person, or with aspects of other disorders, even if the full diagnostic criteria for the other disorders are not met.

If a person has one developmental disorder, he or she likely meets the diagnostic criteria for more than one disorder. Learning disorders have neurodevelopmental components that may be genetic, psychosocial or both.

The strongest current evidence from neurofeedback research with good designs and control comparison groups is that most of the observed positive treatment effects in developmental disorders appear to be a result of improved attention and, to a lesser extent, a decrease in impulsivity and hyperactivity, regardless of the primary developmental diagnosis or treatment approach. Because many behavioral problems stem from inadequate attention and concentration, it is possible that observed behavioral improvements are related to improvements in attention. Because many research designs trained participants at single central sites, such as C3, C4 or CZ, it is not surprising that sites located near the sensorimotor strip produced results consistent with well-documented benefits of sensorimotor training, especially improved attention and on-task behaviors. It is also possible that there are other training benefits that experimental designs did not measure and therefore could not report as results.

There is no specific treatment approach that can be applied based solely on behavioral diagnosis or symptom reports. Research is beginning to converge on the need for full-cap simultaneous recording of the EEG to understand developmental connectivity differences in persons with developmental disorders, as well as the need to train the networks involved, rather than single sites. The techniques for doing so have not so far been published in detail. A general rule is to use the findings from qEEG analysis to guide which sites and networks need to be inhibited or rewarded, and at which specific frequencies, not necessarily semi-standardized bands.[31] Because qEEG data analyses report deviations from the norm in Z-scores or SDs, it is usually clear which areas are abnormal and should be the focus of treatment. In addition, studies from adults with seizure, sleep and other disorders have shown the general value of SMR training for improvements in seizure thresholds, improved sleep, focused attention, on-task behavior and decreased motor hyperactivity.

Biofeedback treatment of enuresis, encopresis and constipation appears to be more straightforward and less complicated than other aspects of developmental disorders.

Neurofeedback and biofeedback interventions are often sought when other therapies have failed to produce desired or expected results. Neurotherapeutic successes with refractory seizure disorders and elimination disorders provide encouragement that the continued development of well-designed research will lead to additional successes for notoriously treatment-resistant developmental disorders.

REFERENCES

1. Bailey T. Beyond DSM: The role of auditory processing in attention and its disorders. *Appl Neuropsychol: Child.* 2012;1(2):112–120.
2. Butler MG, Youngs EL, Roberts JL, Hellings JA. Assessment and treatment in autism spectrum disorders: a focus on genetics and psychiatry. *Autism Res Treat.* 2012. http://dx.doi.org/10.1155/2012/242537
3. Willcutt EG, Pennington BF, Olson RK, DeFries JC. Understanding comorbidity: A twin study of reading disability and attention-deficit/hyperactivity disorder. *Am J Med Genet: Neuropsychiatry Genet.* 2007;144B:709–714.
4. Molina BS, Hinshaw SP, Swanson JM, et al. The MTA at 8 years: Prospective follow-up of children treated for combined-type ADHD in a multisite study. *J Am Acad Child Adolesc Psychiatry.* 2009;48:484–500.
5. Palombo J. *Learning Disorders and Disorders of the Self.* New York, NY: W.W. Norton & Company; 2001.
6. Surmeli T, Ertem A. Post WISC-R and TOVA improvement with qEEG guided neurofeedback training in mentally retarded: a clinical case series of behavioral problems. *Clin EEG Neurosci.* 2010;41(1):32–41.
7. Thompson L, Thompson M, Reid A. Neurofeedback outcomes in clients with Asperger's syndrome. *Appl Psychophysiol Biofeedback.* 2010;35:63–81.
8. Ewing-Cobbs L, Barnes MA, Fletcher JM. Early brain injury in children: development and reorganization of cognitive abilities. *Dev Neuropsychol.* 2003;24(2–3):669–704.
9. Grech R, Cassar T, Muscat J, et al. Review on solving the inverse problem in EEG source analysis. *J Neuroeng Rehabil.* 2008;5:25. http://dx.doi.org/10.1186/1743-0003-5-25
10. Canon R, Congedo M, Lubar J, Hutchens T. Differentiating a network of executive attention: LORETA neurofeedback in anterior cingulate and dorsolateral prefrontal cortices. *Int J Neurosci.* 2009;119:404–441.
11. Pascual-Marqui RD, Esslen M, Kochi K, Lehmann D. Functional imaging with low resolution electromagnetic tomography (LORETA): a review. *Methods Find Exp Clin Pharmacol.* 2002;24C:91–95.
12. American Psychiatric Association. Diagnostic and Statistical Manual-IV Text Revision. Washington, DC: 2000.
13. American Psychiatric Association. Diagnostic and Statistical Manual-5 Proposed Revisions. <http://www.dsm.5.org/proposedrevisions/pages/proposedrevision.aspx?rid=94#>2012.
14. Coben R. Connectivity-guided neurofeedback for autistic spectrum disorder. *Biofeedback.* 2007;35(4):131–135.
15. Coben R, Meyers TE. The relative efficacy of connectivity guided and symptom based EEG biofeedback for autistic disorders. *Appl Psychophysiol Biofeedback.* 2010;35:13–23.
16. Hammond DC. The need for individualization in neurofeedback: Heterogeneity in qEEG patterns associated with diagnoses and symptoms. *Appl Psychophysiol Biofeedback.* 2010;35:31–36.
17. Pineda JA, Juavinett A, Datko M. Self-regulation of brain oscillations as a treatment for aberrant brain connections in children with autism. *Medical Hypotheses.* 2012;79(6):790–798. epub ahead of print <http://dxdoi.org/10.1016/j.mehy.2012.08.031>.

18. Sterman MB, Kaiser DA. Comodulation: a new qEEG analysis metric for assessment of structural and functional disorders of the CNS. *J Neurotherapy*. 2001;4(3):73–83.
19. Thatcher RW. Cyclic cortical reorganization during early childhood. *Brain Cogn*. 1992;20:24–50.
20. Othmer S. *Assessment: EEG Spectrum Biofeedback Training Manual*. Encino, CA: EEG Spectrum, Inc; 1997.
21. Breteler MHM, Arns M, Peters Giepmans I, Verhoeven L. Improvements in spelling after qEEG-based neurofeedback in dyslexia: a randomized controlled treatment study. *Appl Psychophysiol Biofeedback*. 2010;35:5–11.
22. Kouijzer MEJ, de Moor JMH, Gerrits BJL, Buitelaar JK, van Schie HT. Long-term effects of neurofeedback treatment in autism. *Res Autism Spectr Discord*. 2009;3:496–501.
23. Kouijzer MEJ, de Moor JMH, Gerrits BJL, Congedo M, van Schie HT. Neurofeedback improves executive functioning in children with autism spectrum disorders. *Res Autism Spectr Discord*. 2009;3:145–162.
24. Pineda JA, Brang D, Hecht E, et al. Positive behavioral and electrophysiological changes following neurofeedback training in children with autism. *Res Autism Spectr Discord*. 2008;2:557–581.
25. van Leeuwen TH, Steinhausen HC, Overtoom CC, et al. The continuous performance test revisited with neuroelectric mapping: impaired orienting in children with attention deficits. *Behav Brain Res*. 1998;94(1):97–110.
26. Thornton KE, Carmody DP. Electroencephalogram biofeedback for reading disability and traumatic brain injury. *Child Adolesc Psychiatr Clin N Am*. 2005;14(1):137–162.
27. Sterman MB, Howe RD, Macdonald LR. Facilitation of spindle-burst sleep by conditioning of electroencephalographic activity while awake. *Science*. 1970;167:1146–1148.
28. Arns M, Kenemans JL. Neurofeedback in ADHD and insomnia: vigilance stabilization through sleep spindles and circadian networks. *Neurosci Biobeh Rev*. 2012. http://dx.doi.org/10.1016/j.neubiorev.2012.10.006
29. Courchesne E, Pierce K. Why the frontal cortex in autism might be talking only to itself: local over-connectivity but long-distance disconnection. *Curr Opin Neurobiol*. 2005;15:225–230.
30. Dennis M, Francis DJ, Cirino PT, Schachar R, Barnes MA, Fletcher JM. Why IQ is not a covariate in cognitive studies of neurodevelopmental disorders. *J Int Neuropsychol Soc*. 2009;15(3):331–343.
31. Sterman MB. EEG markers for attention deficit disorder: Pharmacological and neurofeedback applications. *Child Study J*. 2000;30(1):1–23.
32. Sterman, MB. Principles of Neurotherapy. *Proceedings of the Annual Conference, Int. Soc. for Neuronal Reg*. 2005;13:23.
33. Ramon C, Schimpf PH, Haueisen J. Influence of head models on EEG simulations and inverse source localizations. *Biomed Eng Online*. 2006;5:10. http://dx.doi.org/10.1186/1475-925X-5-10
34. Rice JK, Rorden C, Little JS, Parra LC. Subject position affect EEG magnitudes. *Neuroimage*. 2012. http://dx.doi.org/10.1016/j.neuroimage.2012.09.041
35. Bolton PF, Carcani-Rathwell I, Hutton J, Goode S, Howlin P, Rutten M. Epilepsy in autism: features and correlates. *Br J Psychiatry*. 2011;198(4):289–294.
36. Danielsson S, Gillberg IC, Billstedt E, Gillberg C, Olsson I. Epilepsy in young adults with autism: a prospective population-based follow-up study of 128 individuals diagnosed in childhood. *Epilepsia*. 2005;46(6):918–923.
37. Laoprasert P. *Atlas of Pediatric EEG*. New York, NY: McGraw-Hill Professional; 2011.
38. Cantor DS, Chabot qEEG studies in the assessment and treatment of childhood disorders. *Clin EEG Neurosci*. 2009;40(2):113–121.

39. Coben R, Linden M, Myers TE. Neurofeedback for autistic spectrum disorder: a review of the literature. *Appl Psychophysiol Biofeedback*. 2010;35:83–105.

40. Sterman MB. Biofeedback in the treatment of epilepsy. *Cleve Clin J Med*. 2010;77(suppl 3):S60–S67.

41. Ros T, Moseley MJ, Bloom PA, Benjamin L, Parkinson LA, Gruzelier JH. Optimizing microsurgical skills with EEG neurofeedback. *BMC Neurosci*. 2009;10:87. http://dx.doi.org/10.1186/1471–2202–10–87

42. Chan AS, Sze SL. Quantitative electroencephalographic profiles for children with autistic spectrum disorder. *Neuropsychology*. 2007;24(1):74–81.

43. Holtmann M, Steiner S, Hohmann S, Poustka L, Banaschewski T, Boelte S. Neurofeedback in autism spectrum disorders. *Dev Med Child Neurol*. 2011;53:986–993.

44. Coben R, Padolsky I. Assessment-guided neurofeedback for autistic spectrum disorder. *J Neurotherapy*. 2007;11(1):5–23.

45. Tan G, Thornby J, Hammond D. Meta-analysis of EEG biofeedback in treating epilepsy. *Clin EEG Neurosci*. 2009;40:173–179.

46. Thompson L, Thompson M, Reid A. Functional neuroanatomy and the rationale for using EEG biofeedback for clients with Asperger's syndrome. *Appl Psychophysiol Biofeedback*. 2010;35:39–61.

47. Sapolsky R. The Uniqueness of Humans. Class Day Lecture, Stanford University 2009; <http://www.youtube.com/watch?v=hrCVu25wQ5s> Minute markers 26: 31–30: 09.

48. Sterman MB, Kaiser DA, Veigel B. Spectral analysis of event-related EEG responses during short-term memory performance. *Brain Topogr*. 1996;9(1):21–30.

49. Niv Y. Cost, benefit, tonic, phasic; what do response rates tell us about dopamine and motivation? *Ann NY Acad Sci*. 2007;1104:357–376.

50. Leins U, Goth G, Hinterberger T, Klinger C, Rumpf N, Strehl U. Neurofeedback for children with ADHD: a comparison and SCP and theta/beta protocols. *Appl Psychophysiol Biofeedback*. 2007;32(2):73–88.

51. Sterman MB, Egner T. Foundation and practice of neurofeedback for the treatment of epilepsy. *Appl Psychophysiol Biofeedback*. 2006;31(1):21–35.

52. Talairach J, Tounoux P. *Co-planar stereotaxic atlas of the human brain: three dimensional proportional system*. Stuttgart, Germany: Georg Thieme; 1998.

53. Kayser J, Tenke CE. In search of the rosetta stone for scalp EEG: Converging on reference-free techniques. *Clin Neurophysiol*. 2010;121(12):1973–1975.

54. Barkhoudarian G, Hovda DA, Giza CC. The molecular pathophysiology of concussive brain injury. *Clin Sports Med*. 2011;30(1):33–48.

55. Sacco R, Curatol P, Manzi B, et al. Principal pathogenetic components and biological endophenotypes in autism spectrum disorders. *Autism Res*. 2010;3(5):237–252.

56. Schrieken M, Visser J, Oosterling I, et al. Head circumference and height abnormalities in autism revisited: the role of pre-and perinatal risk factors. *Eur Chil Adolesc Psychiatry*. 2012. 10.1007/s00787–012–0318–1

57. Corbett BA, Constantine LJ. Autism and attention deficit hyperactivity disorder: assessing attention and response control with the integrated visual and auditory continuous performance test. *Child Neuropsychol*. 2006;12:335–348.

58. Meltzer LJ, Johnson C, Crosette J, Ramos M, Mindell JA. Prevalence of diagnosed sleep disorders in pediatric primary care practices. *Pediatrics*. 2010;125(6):e1410–1418. http://dx.doi.org/10.1542/peds.2009–2725

59. Rimland B, Edelson SM. *Autism Treatment Evaluation Checklist (ATEC)*. San Diego: Autism Research Institute; 1999. revised 2005.

60. Roth SR, Sterman MB, Clemente CC. Comparison of EEG correlates of reinforcement, internal inhibition, and sleep. *Electroencephalorgr Clin Neurophysiol*. 1967;23:509–520.

61. Sterman Kaiser Imaging Laboratory, SKIL version 3.0. Los Angeles, CA.
62. Hammer BU, Colbert AP, Brown KA, Ilioi EC. Neurofeedback for insomnia: a pilot study of z-score SMR and individualized protocols. *Appl Psychophysiol Biofeedback*. 2011;36(4):251–264.
63. Bascom A, Penney T, Metcalfe M, et al. High risk of sleep disordered breathing in the enuresis population. *J Urol*. 2011;186(4 suppl):1710–1713.
64. Kibar Y, Ors O, Demir E, Kalman S, Sakallioglu O, Dayanc M. Results of biofeedback treatment on reflux resolution rates in children with dysfunctional voiding and vesi-couretal reflux. *Urology*. 2007;70(3):563–566.
65. de Jong TP, Klijn AJ, Vijverberg MA, de Kort LM, van Empelen R, Schoenmakers MA. Effect of biofeedback training on paradoxical pelvic floor movement in children with dysfunctional voiding. *Urology*. 2007;70(4):790–793.
66. Porena M, Costantini E, Rociola W, Mearini E. Biofeedback successfully cures detrusor-sphincter dyssynergia in pediatric patients. *J Urol*. 2000;163(6):1927–1931.
67. Khen-Dunlop N, van Egroo A, Bouteiller C, Biserte J, Besson R. Biofeedback therapy in the treatment of bladder overactivity, vesico-ureteral reflux and urinary tract infection. *J Pediatr Urol*. 2006;2(5):424–429.
68. Croffie JM, Ammar MS, Pfefferkorn MD, et al. Assessment of the effectiveness of biofeedback in children with dyssynergic defecation and recalcitrant constipation/encopresis; does home biofeedback improve long-term outcomes. *Clin Pediatr (Phila)*. 2005;44(1):63–71.

CHAPTER FOURTEEN

Nutrition for ADHD and Autism

Jacques Duff

This chapter presents the rationale that may explain why the incidence of attention deficit hyperactivity disorder (ADHD), autism, depression and modern diseases is relentlessly increasing, despite the billions of dollars invested in research and medications each year. This rationale leads to the need to investigate and treat the underlying genetic predispositions and the nutritional causes, rather than indiscriminately medicating our young at a time of their life when their vulnerable brains are still developing. Throughout this chapter reference is made to genes, enzymes, nutrients and lifestyle factors that affect mental health, including ADHD, autism, depression, anxiety and schizophrenia. It is common sense and good science to address these potential causal factors, in addition to addressing the dysfunctional neurophysiology with neurotherapy.

NUTRIGENOMICS, EPIGENETICS, NUTRIENTS AND LIFESTYLE

Through the processes of meiosis and mitosis a single fertilized egg differentiates into an embryo, and eventually into a unique baby on account of the genetic instructions in the DNA interacting with nutrients to form proteins and enzymes that catalyze biochemical reactions. These nutrigenomic interactions are responsible for the composition of our body tissues and carry out a multitude of functions in the circulatory, respiratory digestive, cardiovascular, endocrine, central and peripheral nervous systems. Some of these proteins and enzymes enable brain functions that make us uniquely human, such as the ability to talk, think abstract thoughts, plan ahead and organize our environment into complex systems to serve our needs and promote our survival.

Nutrigenomics is the study of the interaction between genes and nutrition. Research in this field has taught us that the nutrients in food have complex interactions with our DNA, affecting our health outcomes

357

and our disease risks. Everything we consume has some degree of impact on our DNA and has a consequence at a molecular level. Through the process of natural selection, our evolutionary ancestors adapted genetically to daily low-grade exercise, an organic diet and a clean environment. By the end of the Palaeolithic period, modern man had emerged as the result of an optimum balance between genes, environment, nutrition and the hunter–gatherer lifestyle. Today, we carry these genes and are genetically adapted to a Palaeolithic hunter–gatherer diet and lifestyle.[1,2]

Epigenetics is the study of changes in inherited gene expression or cellular phenotype caused by mechanisms other than changes in DNA nucleotide sequence. Epigenetics research has shown that our DNA is controlled by signals from outside the cell, and that environmental factors shape the development and function of cells. Recent scientific studies have revealed that we can influence our health outcomes through changes in lifestyle factors, nutrient uptake and the elimination of environmental and other toxins; even our thoughts and feelings can affect the expression of our genes.[3] Gene expression is altered by dietary transcription factors, such as low zinc status, or by exposure to toxic environmental substances, such as mercury or organophosphate pesticides. Studies have shown that gene expression patterns differ geographically between and within populations, suggesting that environmental factors are responsible. Such changes in gene expression can adversely affect neuronal plasticity, resulting in neurodevelopmental disorders such as ADHD, autism and mental retardation.[4]

Essential nutrients help maintain normal neuronal plasticity. Nutritional deficiencies, including deficiencies in the long-chain poly-unsaturated fatty acids eicosapentaenoic acid (EPA) and docosahexaenoic acid (DHA), the amino acid methionine, zinc and selenium, have been shown to affect neuronal plasticity and function and produce behavioral deficits in children, including those with ADHD.[5]

In 1998, Dean Ornish and colleagues demonstrated that improved nutrition, moderate exercise, stress management techniques and increased social support were associated with the expression of over 500 epigenetic genes being changed in only 3 months. These include upregulating or turning on disease-preventing genes and downregulating or turning off genes that promote heart disease, cancer, inflammation and oxidative stress.[6] Genetic screening for selected epigenetic gene polymorphisms that affect health outcomes is commercially available, suggesting that the future of healthcare may well be determined by personalized nutrigenomics and medicine. Some of these genes, when missing or mutated, can result in the complete absence of key enzymes responsible for liver detoxing, or in mild to dramatic reduction in the capacity of enzymes to carry out their functions. Hence, a one-size-fits-all diet and generic lifestyle recommendations no longer make sense in light of this emerging knowledge from epigenetics research.

Our highly processed modern diet, with its manmade *trans*-fatty acids, chemical additives, preservatives, colorings, added hormones and antibiotics, is affecting the delicate balance of nutrigenomic interactions and is affecting our genome. Genetic weaknesses, which previously did not seem to affect us, now interact with dietary nutritional deficiencies and environmental toxins to promote the modern diseases. It is not surprising that the rates of incidence of modern diseases, such as cancer, diabetes, heart disease, ADHD, autism, depression, anxiety, irritable bowel syndrome and inflammatory bowel disease, to name but a few, continue to rise despite the billions of dollars spent each year on research and pharmaceutical treatment, which for the most part are toxic to our genome and often carry unacceptable side effects.

A large part of my clinical practice consists of examining these genetic polymorphisms and recommending dietary and lifestyle changes and nutrient supplementation to modulate the expression of these genes, reduce toxicity and oxidative stress, modulate risk factors and promote optimum health. Throughout this chapter I shall be outlining the rationale for the need to test for genetic polymorphisms and nutrient levels, and for supplementing key nutrients to optimize the physical and mental health of patients, including children with ADHD and autism.

OMEGA-3 (n-3) AND OMEGA-6 (n-6) ESSENTIAL FATTY ACID (EFA) BALANCE

The body cannot manufacture EFAs; therefore they must be part of our diet. A number of studies have estimated that our modern diet provides around 20–40 times more n-6 and five to ten times less n-3 than the Palaeolithic hunter–gatherer diet.[1] Most of the n-6 in our diet comes from vegetable sources of linoleic acid (LA) such as nuts and vegetables; n-3 also comes from vegetable sources of alpha-linolenic acid (ALA), such as flaxseed oil and nuts such as walnuts. However, it is the consumption of polyunsaturated cooking oils and margarines in our modern diet that has caused the imbalance. These fatty acids are converted to longer-chain

EFAs by elongase and desaturase enzymes (Figure 14.1), and all play a crucial role in the body's composition and functions; human beings require the long-chain polyunsaturated fatty acids from fish for brain development and function.[1]

Polymorphisms in the desaturase encoding genes FADS1 and FADS2 have been associated with several n-6 and n-3 fatty acids. The relationship between FADS gene cluster polymorphisms and red blood cell (RBC) fatty acid levels in over 4000 pregnant women participating in the Avon Longitudinal Study of Parents and Children was analyzed. The study found that FADS polymorphisms influence maternal RBC n-3 DHA levels, which affected the baby's DHA supply during pregnancy.[7] Given the fundamental role of DHA in fetal neuronal development,[8] this finding is of particular concern. Animal studies have shown that an imbalance of high n-6:n-3 ratio early in life leads to irreversible changes in hypothalamic phospholipid composition, consistent with a dysfunction or downregulation of the conversion of ALA to DHA by the delta-6 desaturase enzyme (Figure 14.1). These two findings[7,9] suggest that FADS polymorphisms may lead to irreversible structural changes in brain cells, affecting their function; and that for those people with FADS polymorphisms, a higher lifetime consumption of fish and fish oils may be necessary to prevent deficiencies that affect brain function.

Arachidonic acid (AA), an n-6 fatty acid, is essential for cell membrane stability and also starts a cascade of inflammatory processes (thromboxins, leukotrienes and prostaglandins) for the defense of cells against antigens. EPA, an n-3 fatty acid, produces anti-inflammatory processes, protecting cells against free radical damage and from inflammatory cytokines.[10] The ratio of AA to EPA is ideally around 1.5–3.0, and this is achieved when a person limits his or her meat intake (a good source of AA) and consumes deep-sea cold-water fish four or five times a week, or has an adequate intake of fish oils as supplements. Too much AA leads to a propensity for excessive inflammation; too little adversely affects cell membrane stability and necessary inflammatory responses.[10]

Trans-fatty acids are manmade (usually resulting from heating polyunsaturated oils) and can displace EPA and DHA from cell membranes. This has two detrimental effects: first, the cell membrane becomes more permeable, allowing antigens to penetrate the cell and cause damage to intracellular mechanisms; second, as the RBC AA:EPA ratio rises, the propensity for inflammation increases. In addition, the decrease in DHA levels has a detrimental effect on neurodevelopment and mental health, as discussed next.

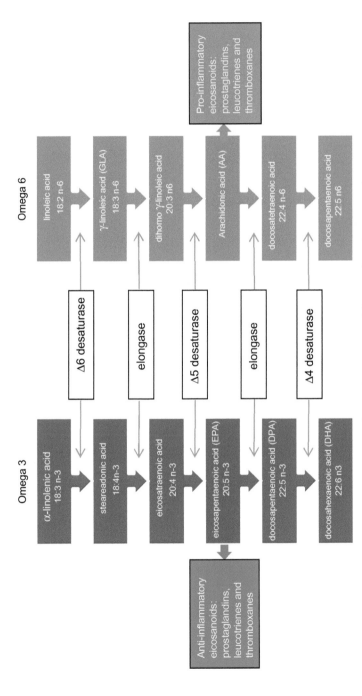

Figure 14.1 Conversion of dietary fatty acids to long-chain polyunsaturated fatty acids and eicosanoids.

The Role of DHA

DHA makes up around 25% of the dry volume of brain cells in all healthy mammals and concentrates in neuronal synapses,[11] where, in conjunction with proteins, it modulates the synthesis, transport and release of mono-amine neurotransmitters.[12] The results of a retrospective study examining the RBC EFAs in ADHD, autism and typically developing children are shown in Tables 14.1 and 14.2.[13] The Australian Twin Behavioural Rating Scales (revised) is a DSM-IV behavioral screening questionnaire for ADHD, and the Test of Variables of Attention (TOVA) is a computer-administered continuous performance task.

Note the dramatically low percentage of RBC DHA in children with autism compared to those with ADHD and typically developing controls. The optimum RBC DHA level is >6%, and is achievable with a diet high in fatty cold-water fish or fish oil supplementation. In addition, children with autism spectrum disorder (ASD) had very low RBC AA, suggesting impaired cell membrane integrity, and therefore vulnerability to damage from toxins and antigens.[13]

These results indicate that children with ASD had by far the worst EFA profile, and those with ADHD were lagging behind their typically developing peers. Given that DHA modulates the synthesis, transport and release of neurotransmitters in synapses, this is not surprising. However, many of the children with autism and ADHD had RBC DHA as low as 0.1%, while others had ratios around 4.0%. These large fluctuations suggest that whereas DHA deficiency may constitute a major part of the etiology of neurodevelopmental disorders, other factors are also at play. During treatment, optimum levels (>6.0%) are achieved by aggressive supplementation with high-quality fish oil concentrate. Maintenance after 12 months can be achieved by consuming oily fish four or more times a week. However, our experience has shown that this is applicable only for some children. Others seem to need to take fish oil supplements and nutrient cofactors permanently. This is probably a result of the irreversible down-regulation of desaturase stages, as previously discussed.[9] A comprehensive review of all the nutrients and enzyme cofactors involved in brain function is beyond the scope of this chapter. Therefore, only an overview of those that have been shown to be involved in the attentional system and in mood regulation is provided next.

Table 14.1 Means and Standard Deviations of Age, TOVA, ATBRS, CARS, EPA, DHA and AA Between Typically Developing, ADHD and ASD Groups

	Age	TOVA	ATBRS	CARS	% EPA	% DHA	% AA
TD (n = 81)	8.31 (2.53)	3.88 (1.69)	14.14 (7.49) ★★		1.82 (0.96)	4.70 (1.02)	10.46 (2.08)
ADHD (n = 401)	9.10 (3.58)	−3.78 (3.28)	42.43 (14.43)		0.89 (0.56)	2.28 (0.89)	9.73 (2.71)
ASD (n = 85)	5.32 (2.12)			40.71 (8.04)	0.56 (0.52)	0.85 (1.02)	6.24 (3.28)

EPA, eicosapentaenoic acid; DHA, docosahexaenoic acid; AA, arachidonic acid; ADHD, attention deficit hyperactivity disorder; ASD, autism spectrum disorder; TD, typically developing; TOVA, Test of Variables of Attention; ATBRS, Australian Twin Behaviour Rating Scales; CARS, Childhood Autism Rating Scale.
★★Parentheses denote SD.

Table 14.2 Independent Sample t-test Scores of EPA, DHA and AA in ADHD and ASD Groups Compared to a Typically Developing Sample

	EPA	DHA	AA
TD × ADHD	$t(480) = -11.91\star$	$t(480) = -21.84\star$	$t(480) = -2.30\star$
TD × ASD	$t(164) = -10.64\star$	$t(164) = -30.28\star$	$t(164) = -30.28\star$

EPA, eicosapentaenoic acid; DHA, docosahexaenoic acid; AA, arachidonic acid.
$\star$p < 0.05.

Monoamine Neurotransmission

There are five established biogenic amine neurotransmitters: the three cat-echolamines – dopamine, norepinephrine (noradrenaline) and epinephrine (adrenaline) – as well as serotonin and histamine. The main monoamine neurotransmitters, serotonin, dopamine and norepinephrine, are consid-ered brainstem neuromodulators, because their neurons have cell bodies in the brain stem and have projections to the limbic system and to the neo-cortex. Neuromodulation refers to the process of dynamic modulation of neuronal activity, at rest and during information processing. It includes (a) the manufacture of the neurotransmitters in brain synaptic vesicles from dietary amino acid precursors; (b) their transport in vesicles through the synaptic cleft; (c) their release into the synaptic gap; (d) their migration to receptor sites on the receiving neurons; (e) their effect on the receiving neurons; and finally (f) the reuptake of any residual neurotransmitter back into the transmitting neurons for recycling (Figure 14.2).

When a neurotransmitter is released into the synapse, it migrates to receptors located on dendrites, cell bodies and presynaptic termi-nals of second (receiving) neurons. Almost all monoamine receptors are G protein-coupled receptors that activate intracellular second-messenger molecules, such as inositol triphosphate. These molecules relay signals from surface receptors to target molecules inside the cell, amplifying the strength of the signal, and have an effect on the postsynaptic membranes on the receiving neuron.

Embedded among the monoamine neurotransmitter receptors are also G protein-coupled receptors for trace amines.[14] These amines are usually formed by the breakdown of proteins in foods. Some of the most com-mon are tyramine (from cheese), histamine (from wine) and phenylethyl-amine (found in chocolate). However, when the bowel environment has an acidic pH, some gut organisms, particularly lactic acid bacteria such as

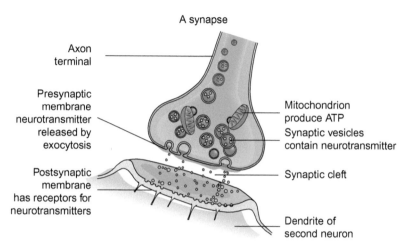

Figure 14.2 Synapse and neurotransmitters.

Bifidobacteria, overgrow and cleave proteins to produce large amount of amines, resulting in a much higher ratio of amines to amino acids than under neutral pH conditions.[15,16] In addition, the acidic gut conditions inhibit the growth of *Escherichia coli,* which is a major producer of the monoamine neurotransmitter precursors tryptophan, phenylalanine and tyrosine.[16] This reduces the amino acids available for neurotransmitter synthesis, whereas the amines key into amine receptors and scramble neurotransmission. Patients report a combination of symptoms, such as brain fog, poor concentration, muscle aches and pain, headaches, migraines and depression. It has been proposed that these biogenic amines may be involved in treatment–resistant depression.[17] In children the symptoms are feelings of unease, irritability, low frustration threshold, anger outbursts and poor concentration. Interestingly, a diet high in refined carbohydrates from cereal grains and dairy products is highly acid producing in the bowel and promotes the growth of lactic acid bacteria promoting amine production. These symptoms can easily be mistaken for those of ADHD. In our experience, symptoms improve or resolve with an alkaline-producing diet and nutrient supplementation.

Serotonin or 5-hydroxytryptamine (5HT)

Serotonin is both an excitatory and an inhibitory neurotransmitter. It is found in enteric neurons where it modulates peristalsis, and in the brain

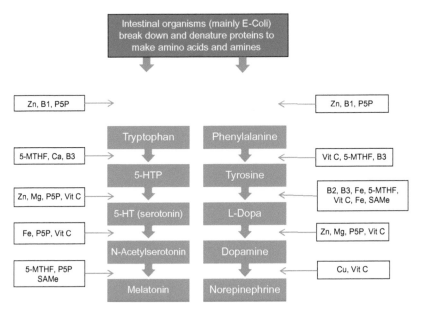

Figure 14.3 Neurotransmitter amino acid precursors and major nutrient enzyme cofactors.

where it modulates calmness and good feelings. Around 2% of the amino acid tryptophan in circulation is converted to 5-hydroxytryptophan (5HTP) by tryptophan hydroxylase, an enzyme that uses 5-MTHF (the active form of folate), iron, calcium and vitamin B3 as cofactors. 5-HTP is further converted to serotonin by the enzyme dopa decarboxylase, which uses magnesium, zinc, piridoxine-5-phosphate (P5P), the active form of vitamin B6 and vitamin C as cofactors. In the pineal gland and the retina, the enzyme N-acetyltransferase converts serotonin to N-acetyl serotonin, which in turn is converted to melatonin and released into the bloodstream and cerebrospinal fluid by the enzyme 5-hydroxyindole-O-transferase, a process requiring the active form of vitamin B6 (P5P) as cofactor. Melatonin promotes sleep, and its production is inhibited by daylight; even room lighting and television watching can inhibit melatonin production (Figure 14.3).

Suboptimal neuromodulation of brain serotonin has been linked to a variety of adverse behaviors and mental health issues, such as aggression, irritability, low frustration threshold, anger outbursts, depression, suicidality, obsessive–compulsive disorder, alcoholism, anxiety and affective disorders. Although these associations are known, the mechanism of action responsible remains largely unknown. In brain synapses the principal source of release of serotonin is from serotonin neurons, which have cell bodies originating in the raphe nuclei, in the brain stem. Their axons form a neurotransmitter system that enervates almost every part of the central nervous system.

The serotonin transporter (SERT) protein transports residual serotonin back into the synapse for recycling and ends the action of serotonin. This protein is the target of many antidepressant medications, particularly selective serotonin reuptake inhibitors, which block the action of SERT. Polymorphisms in the promoter arm of the SERT gene can affect serotonin neurotransmission, causing irritability and aggressiveness as well as an increased susceptibility to depression.[18] Nutritionally, people with this mutation require more aggressive supplementation with 5HTP, vitamin B6 (P5P) and vitamin C.

Effect of Diet on Serotonin and Health Outcomes

The large neutral amino acids (LNAA) such as tyrosine, valine, isoleucine, leucine, phenylalanine and lysine compete with tryptophan for transport through the blood–brain barrier. Hence, foods with a high ratio of tryptophan to LNAA may improve 5HT production in the brain. Meals typical of those consumed in the United States and Australia have been shown to cause substantial variations in the plasma tryptophan:LNAA and tyrosine:LNAA ratios, depending on the ratio of protein to carbohydrates. The differences between the ratios generated by a high-carbohydrate low-protein and high-protein breakfast can be >50% for tryptophan:LNAA and 30% for tyrosine:LNAA.[19] Hence, a western diet high in refined carbohydrates, wheat and cereals, and low in proteins can cause a rise in tryptophan, thereby increasing serotonin. Concurrently, such a diet also causes a rise in insulin, which is required to control blood sugar levels.[20] However, these dietary increases in serotonin and insulin are not in keeping with the homeostasis that existed during our evolutionary history, when meat proteins, fish, nuts, fruit and vegetables were our primary source of food.[1,2]

Chronically elevated insulin levels can cause hypoglycemia, insulin resistance, metabolic syndrome, polycystic ovarian syndrome, obesity and type 2 diabetes. Over time, insulin resistance can cause serotonin levels to drop, thereby predisposing to depression.[21] Exercise is known to activate hundreds of genes and builds up muscles through a process that uses many amino acids, with the exception of tryptophan. Consequently, people who exercise and build more muscle have more available trypto-phan and higher serotonin levels, thereby downregulating depression.[22]

E. coli, which accounts for 80–90% of the aerobic bacteria in the healthy large bowel, produces chorismate, which is a precursor to folic acid, coenzyme Q10, tryptophan, phenylalanine and tyrosine. Low bowel E. coli can result in lower tryptophan levels, and therefore lower serotonin production. This is associated with slow bowel transit time, constipation, irritability and depressed mood. In the past 12 years we have assessed the extended fecal microbiology of over 300 children through Bioscreen Medical at Melbourne University and examined their bacteria distribu-tion. Those children with low E. coli consistently display symptoms that include irritability, low frustration threshold, anger outbursts, poor sleep, moodiness and tantrums, and their Z-score quantitative electroencephalo-graph (qEEG) consistently shows low delta power. This is not surprising, because serotonin modulates delta frequencies. However, these children tick the boxes for ADHD and are often diagnosed as such, with a poor response to psychostimulants. Note that poor sleep quality is often caused by low serotonin, which is converted to melatonin to promote sleep.

Given that E. coli grows best in a neutral pH gut environment, it can be promoted with an alkalinizing diet, low in grains and dairy and rich in vegetables, legumes and pulses, and moderate meat intake. The diet should produce a first morning urine pH of 6.8–7.0. In addition, when delta power levels are low, 5HTP magnesium, zinc, vitamin B6 as P5P, and vitamin C can also be prescribed to promote serotonin and melatonin production.

The Role of Dopamine and Norepinephrine in the Attentional System

In order to understand ADHD and the effect of neurotherapy on the brain, an understanding of the attentional system is required. Tucker and Williamson reviewed the evidence for the underpinnings of the human attentional system, based on the biological mechanism of attention derived from animal dissections and studies carried out by Pribram and McGuinness.[23] They concluded that there was a self-regulating asymmet-rical neural control network linking a frontal, primarily left, dopaminer-gic system to a posterior, primarily right, noradrenergic system. The two linked systems were described as a "frontal tonic activation system" and a "posterior phasic arousal system."[24]

The "tonic activation system," centering on the forebrain basal gan-glia, was described as providing a state of tonic motor readiness for action.

This implied a state of alertness or vigilance, which Tucker and Williamson argued was mediated by two related dopaminergic systems: first, the primary nigrostriatal dopamine pathways, originating in the substantia nigra in the brain stem, enervating the caudate nucleus and putamen and handling sensorimotor integration. Increased dopamine modulation restricts the range of behaviors by increasing informational redundancy. In this context, redundancy refers to the processing of information of interest in related pathways, while simultaneously restricting the processing of other information. Thus increased redundancy not only increases reliability but also restricts alternative information from being processed. Second, a related dopamine pathway, the mesocortical or mesolimbic system, with cell bodies in the ventral tegmental bundle and connections to the nucleus accumbens, central amygdaloid nucleus and the lateral septal nuclei, supports controlled motivated interactions with the environment. They argued that this largely dopamine-mediated neural control system does not linearly increase activation but qualitatively facilitates vigilance, tight control of motor output and purposeful behaviors.

The "phasic arousal system" was described by Tucker and Williamson as a parietal noradrenergic system providing transient responses to changes in sensory information or novelty in sensory channels. They suggested that reiterative loops, which constantly compare new sensory channel patterns to previous ones, enable the detection of novelty. The primary noradrenergic pathway, from the dorsal tegmental bundle, originates in the pontine locus ceruleus and projects rostrally to the median forebrain bundle and the limbic system, including the amygdala, hippocampus, thalamus and neocortex. They proposed that norepinephrine does not linearly increase arousal, but "qualitatively" facilitates response to perceptual input from environmental novelty. Noradrenergic activity declines with repetitive input (habituation), inhibits neuronal discharge and reduces the spontaneous background activity of neurons. Thus norepinephrine may increase signal-to-noise ratio and augment the cell's evoked responses to stimuli, thereby increasing sensitivity to change.[24]

According to Tucker and Williamson,[24] the dopaminergic system appears to maintain the tonic level of neural activity by increasing the redundancy of the information (decreasing alternatives) in brain channels. This was demonstrated elegantly in the behavior of DAT-KO mice (mice with overstimulated dopamine pathways whose dopamine transporter was genetically knocked out).[25] In novel environments, the behaviors of DAT-KO mice became dominated by progressively fewer acts (repetitively exploring the same arm of the maze) with increasing frequency. Hence, tonic activation produces a redundancy bias, which restricts change and tightly controls or restricts motor output or behaviors. The qualitative regulatory effect of activation is thus opposite to that of arousal, which reduces redundancy. Yet for motor functions a redundancy bias applies a negative control, not unlike the negative feedback on perceptual responsiveness provided by arousal. Behavioral output therefore requires constant change in motor channels.[24]

Duff[26] supported this proposed explanation of the attentional system by demonstrating its elements in a study that examined changes in the electrical activity of boys with ADHD following neurotherapy. The study used steady state visually evoked potential (SSVEP) probe topography before and after neurotherapy while the boys with ADHD performed the CPT-AX computer-administered task. The cognitive attention task requires subjects to press a response button on the appearance of the letter X, only if the previous letter was an A. Figure 14.4 illustrates the changes in activation, from pre- to postneurotherapy. A reduction in normalized amplitude can be interpreted as increased neuronal activation, while an increase in amplitude can be interpreted as a reduction in activation.

Note the dynamic changes in activation following neurotherapy. It has been suggested that children with ADHD may have difficulties allocating attentional resources[27] and may inefficiently tie up prefrontal circuitry, which is needed for behavior control, instead of using presupplementary motor areas.[28] This suggestion is supported by findings from a study of suppression of BOLD response in functional magnetic resonance imaging while performing a reaction-time task, which found that increased visual response time in children with ADHD was associated with an inability to deactivate the ventromedial prefrontal cortex under increased reaction-time task demands.[29] Increased visual response time in ADHD has also been interpreted as suggestive of reduced perceptual sensitivity and response consistency, and was related to most ADHD symptoms.[30] The suggestions of inefficient allocation of attentional resources in ADHD, tying up prefrontal circuits instead of using presupplementary motor areas, leading to reduced perceptual sensitivity and response consistency, are consistent with Silberstein's[31] suggestion that cognitive proficiency is associated with efficient functional connectivity, i.e., the rapid recruitment and release of coherence between relevant brain areas contingent with task demands.

Whereas neurotherapy appears to help redress the inefficient allocation of dopamine and norepinephrine resources in the brains of children with ADHD, the nutritional precursors needed to synthesize these

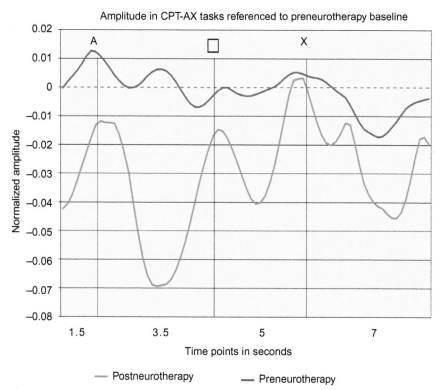

Figure 14.4 Steady-state visually evoked potential (SSVEP) amplitude during the target sequence in the CPT-AX task as a function of time in subjects with ADHD pre- and postneurotherapy. The dashed horizontal line represents the mean normalized amplitude for the baseline task, which was set to zero for both conditions. CPT-AX related amplitude changes are therefore expressed as differences from the baseline. The vertical lines represent the time points at which: the letter A is presented (A), the letter A disappears and the blanking interval commences (☐) and the letter X appears (X).

neurotransmitters in synapses and to facilitate their transport and release in the brain need to be optimal to facilitate neuromodulation. The following sections explain the role of gene polymorphisms, enzymes, nutrient cofactors and amino acids in this process.

ZINC AS AN ESSENTIAL NUTRIENT FOR HEALTH

Zinc compounds are found in soil and water, and in many foods. However, the soil in many countries is generally much lower in zinc than in countries that have a soil rich in volcanic minerals – so much so that one-third of the world's population has an inadequate intake of dietary zinc.[32] Zinc deficiency is one of the most prevalent nutritional deficiencies in the United States. Suboptimal zinc status has been noted in children of lower socioeconomic groups, low-birthweight infants, pregnant teenagers and some of the elderly.[33,34] In Australia, the Bureau of Statistics nutritional surveys have found that most of the population do not have the recommended daily intake of zinc. If too much zinc is consumed for the body's needs, less is absorbed and more is excreted in urine and feces; hence, zinc toxicity is rare. Individual requirements for dietary zinc are determined by the biological need to replace losses and maintain function, and the bioavailability of zinc from the foods consumed. The amount of dietary zinc required to replace tissue losses in individuals fully adapted to a diet low in zinc is considered the minimal zinc requirement and is often referred to as the recommended daily intake.[33,34] Blood serum zinc levels reflect recent dietary intake, are very variable and hence are poor indicators of tissue levels. RBC zinc is a better indicator of zinc status than serum zinc, because erythrocytes have a life of 3 months and RBC levels reflect the average level over that period. In one study, 31% of patients were found to have low RBC zinc levels, whereas only 10% had low plasma zinc.[35]

Zinc is an essential nutrient, involved in hundreds of biochemical pathways in the body, including many involved in neurotransmitter synthesis and synaptic function. Features of zinc deficiency are generally nonspecific, affecting the optimal function of a number of systems. In children deficiency may lead to poor appetite, a decreased sense of taste and smell, slow wound healing, skin lesions and decreased immune function. There is considerable evidence that maternal zinc deficiency has detrimental, possibly long-lasting, effects on fetal growth, neurodevelopment and immune system maturity. In the early 1970s a number of controlled studies of zinc supplementation in infants and toddlers in Colorado demonstrated the growth-limiting effect of zinc deficiency in otherwise healthy subjects. Zinc-supplemented children developed increased appetite and thrived compared to controls. These findings were replicated in studies from Ontario, and in school-aged children in Texas.[34]

Breast milk contains zinc citrate,[36] which animal studies have found to be twice as bioavailable as other forms, such as picolinate and sulfate.[37] Therefore, infants use the zinc in breast milk more efficiently than that in formula. During pregnancy, the fetus and other pregnancy tissue account for around 100 mg of zinc, which the expectant mother must provide,[4] and the additional zinc requirement occurs primarily in the last trimester, when fetal growth is most rapid.[34] This suggests that mothers should be advised to optimize their intake with zinc citrate supplementation, at least throughout pregnancy and breastfeeding.

Zinc, Brain Function and ADHD

Approximately 15% of the zinc in the brain is found in synaptic vesicles, from which it is released to the extraneuronal space during synaptic transmission. In the surroundings of the synapse, zinc acts upon a variety of neuronal receptors and ionic channels, playing a modulatory role that is not yet fully understood.[38] Within the vesicles, zinc is a cofactor for the production of dopamine from L-dopa, serotonin from 5HTP, and melatonin from serotonin (Figure 14.3). Hence, zinc is likely to be an important modulator of synaptic transmission.[38] Research suggests that zinc may regulate N-methyl-D-aspartate receptors,[39] and animal studies have shown that zinc is an important regulator of gamma-aminobutyric acid receptors, affects the excitability of hippocampal glutamatergic neurons, and may play an important role in cerebellar function.[40] Indeed, recent studies have shown evidence for a significant reduction of the combined glutamate/glutamine to creatine ratio in the right anterior cingulate cortex in patients with ADHD,[41] and striatal glutamate, glutamate/glutamine and creatine concentrations were higher in ADHD subjects than in controls, providing evidence of a striatal creatine/glutamatergic dysregulation in ADHD.[42]

Several studies have associated low zinc status with symptoms of ADHD.[43–50] Children with the inattentive type of ADHD have been shown to have significantly lower levels of zinc and ferritin than controls, but not magnesium and copper. Children with the hyperactive type had significantly lower levels of zinc, ferritin and magnesium than controls, and no significant difference with regard to copper. Children with the combined type of ADHD had significantly lower levels of zinc and magnesium than controls, but not ferritin and copper levels.[44]

It has been observed in vitro that the dopamine transporter contains a high-affinity zinc-binding site on its extracellular face that modulates its function. Hence, it has been suggested that in ADHD patients with low zinc status, zinc supplementation may improve the binding status of insufficiently occupied zinc binding sites.[45] This is supported by a number of studies suggesting that response to stimulant medication is reduced in zinc-deficient ADHD patients and improved by zinc supplementation, resulting in lower medication dosages.[51–56] A double-blind placebo-controlled study of zinc supplementation in ADHD has found that zinc sulfate was statistically superior to placebo in reducing symptoms of hyperactivity, impulsivity and impaired socialization, but not in reducing attention deficits. Zinc supplementation appears to be a useful adjunct in the treatment for some children with ADHD and low levels of zinc and fatty acids.[57]

Zinc and Thyroid Dysfunction

It has been suggested that children with ADHD and developmental learning disabilities should be checked for optimum thyroid function as a possible mediating factor for their difficulties.[58] Zinc in plasma and RBCs has been found to be lower in both hypothyroidism and hyperthyroidism. In one study, RBC zinc in hyperthyroidism was inversely related to plasma thyroxine concentration. The hyperthyroid group excreted significantly greater amounts of zinc than controls, indicating a catabolic process. This provides evidence for marked alterations in zinc homeostasis in persons with thyroid problems.[59] Thyroid problems have been found in some children with ADHD: one study found that thyroxine concentrations were associated with mood symptoms and unusual behaviors, but were less strongly related to attentional functioning and not related to hyperactivity.[60]

Zinc, Histidine and Histamine

The enzyme histidine decarboxylase produces histamine from the amino acid histidine. Histamine is best known for its release from mast cells as a response to allergic reactions or tissue damage. However, more importantly for the treatment of ADHD, histamine is found in high concentrations in neurons in the hypothalamus, from where it mediates arousal and attention. Pfeiffer and colleagues[61] found that approximately 50% of their outpatient schizophrenics were "histapenic" (low in blood histamine) and high in blood serum copper, and 20% were histadelic (high in blood histamine) and normal in serum copper. They also found that either group may be low in serum zinc and/or manganese. Zinc is needed by mast cell and hippocampus terminal vesicles to store histamine. Without adequate zinc, histaminergic neurotransmission may be impaired. These two suggested categories, histapenia and histadelia, accounted for around 70% of the schizophrenias in Pfeiffer's patients.[61]

Zinc, Vitamin B6 and Pyroluria

The remaining group of Pfeiffer's patients had normal blood histamine and serum copper levels. This group had excessive urine excretion of "kryptopyrroles," also referred to as the "mauve factor." The pyrroles combine with pyridoxal (vitamin B6) and then complexes with zinc, producing symptoms of vitamin B6 and zinc deficiency. They found that these patients responded to large supplementary doses of vitamin B6, zinc and manganese.[61] Such individuals have very low RBC zinc and require heavy supplementation of zinc and vitamin B6. Pyrolurics can exhibit severe behavioral disorders, have a low frustration threshold and lose their temper easily. The disorder is familial and is responsible for the high incidence of behavioral disorders and schizophrenia in families, with an incidence of 30–40% in schizophrenics and only 5–10% in the normal population.[61] Kryptopyrroles increase in the blood during stress, and zinc and B6 rapidly become unavailable for neurotransmitter synthesis.

We have found that a number of children diagnosed with ADHD have very low RBC zinc, the levels of which are resistant to moderate supplementation. These children can be extremely unreasonable, have erratic moods, can easily lose control when stressed, and often have disruptive behavioral disorders. We typically test for RBC zinc and copper as well as serum histamine. In addition, we test for mauve factor in urine, which, when elevated, is indicative of pyroluria. When we aggressively add zinc citrate, vitamin B6 (P5P) and manganese to their supplementation regimen, their urinary kryptopyrrole excretion reduces significantly and in most cases behavioral symptoms improve significantly. However, symptoms return rapidly when supplementation is stopped.

MAGNESIUM

Magnesium is found in the soil and is present in vegetables. In the hunter–gatherer diet, magnesium-containing foods were common, but in the last 100 years or so industrialization of food sources, processing of cereal grains and changing diets have diminished dietary intakes of magnesium and other micronutrients.[2,62,63] The magnesium content of vegetables has declined by 25–80% compared to prior to 1950, and food refining processes remove most of the available magnesium from grains and cereals.[63] Consequently, the average American diet affords just over half of the conservative recommended daily allowance for magnesium.[64,65] National Health and Nutrition Examination Survey data show that a large percentage of North Americans fail to meet the recommendations for optimal calcium, magnesium and vitamin D intake.[66]

Intestinal interactions between vitamin D, magnesium and calcium have been demonstrated in both humans and animals.[67] The low levels of vitamin D commonly seen in western society may be a cause for concern, given that animal studies have shown that severe vitamin D deficiency during lactation produces marked osteomalacia and secondary hyperparathyroidism in both mothers and their offspring. Vitamin D treatment during lactation reversed the mineral, hormonal and skeletal abnormalities in mothers, but not in offspring.[68] Although a substantial amount of magnesium absorption occurs independent of vitamin D status, there is evidence that pharmacological doses of vitamin D increase magnesium absorption in both vitamin D-deficient and vitamin D-replete animals.[67]

The diet of Palaeolithic hunter–gatherers and pre-agricultural societies contained more vegetables, fruit legumes and pulses than meats, and produced alkaline potential renal acid load values. In contrast, today's western diet contains high amounts of animal proteins, grains and dairy products and produces highly acidic potential renal acid load values.[69–72] Therefore, to buffer the acid and maintain normal blood pH, the blood's homeostatic system uses the base minerals such as magnesium, calcium, sodium and potassium. This leaching of these base minerals leads to a condition known as latent acidosis, associated with low availability of base minerals for biochemistry, including brain function.[71] Figure 14.3 illustrates the importance of magnesium and calcium as cofactors in neurotransmitter synthesis. Hence, deficiencies in base minerals are likely to have an impact on monoamine neurotransmitter synthesis and are expected to manifest as attention deficits and mood disorders.

Magnesium works synergistically with calcium to relax the nervous system, and symptoms of deficiency include irritability, restlessness, fidgetiness, muscle cramps and twitches. Kozielec and Starobrat-Hermelin[73] measured hair, plasma and RBC magnesium in 116 children (94 boys and 20 girls) aged 9–12 years with ADHD. Magnesium deficiency was found in 95% of the cohort, 77.6% in hair, 58.65% in RBC and 33.6% in serum. Further analysis indicated an inverse correlation between levels of magnesium and the Freedom from Distractibility Index. Several studies have identified magnesium deficiency in the RBCs of children with ADHD.[73–77]

Magnesium supplementation has been shown to reduce excitability and improve concentration in children with low serum and RBC magnesium levels.[74–76] Forty children with ADHD and 36 controls participated in a magnesium and vitamin B6 supplementation study. At baseline the children from the ADHD group showed significantly lower RBC magnesium values than controls. Magnesium and vitamin B6 were supplemented for at least 8 weeks. Symptoms of ADHD, including hyperactivity, mood, aggressiveness and lack of attention at school, were scored from 0 to 4 at different times, and RBC magnesium and ionized calcium levels were monitored. The supplementation regimen significantly increased RBC magnesium values, and in almost all cases significantly reduced the clinical symptoms of ADHD. Hyperactivity, mood and aggressiveness were reduced, and attention at school improved. However, when the supplementation was stopped, clinical symptoms reappeared within a few weeks along with a decrease in RBC magnesium.[78,79] This study suggests that children with ADHD frequently have low magnesium levels, which is associated with their symptoms, and that supplementation improves those symptoms.

EVIDENCE-BASED PRESCRIBING OF NUTRIENTS

In order to maximize brain function, the nutrient cofactors necessary for neurotransmitter synthesis, including those of the enzymes involved in the conversion stages, must also be optimized. This is particularly important if the genes that encode these enzymes have polymorphisms that reduce their effectiveness, requiring more of the cofactors to upregulate the enzyme activity. Given what we know about how poor our western diet is at providing these nutrients, it makes sense for informed health practitioners to test these in blood and supplement deficiencies. The following is a list of biomedical tests frequently used at the Behavioural Neurotherapy Clinic for clients with ADHD: (a) RBC EFAs; (b) RBC zinc, copper, magnesium, manganese, selenium (in the United States these are available as a RBC minerals test); (c) serum: vitamin D3, homocysteine, iron studies; (d) extended fecal microbiology analysis from Bioscreen Medical; (e) SMART DNA genetic screen; and of course a TOVA and a qEEG analyzed through Neuroguide. Although useful, RBC magnesium is a poor indicator of tissue levels and needs. Each laboratory reference range for blood nutrients is determined from a statistical analysis of patients' blood test results in a population low in minerals and is therefore skewed toward abnormally low ranges. We generally supplement fish oils, magnesium, zinc, iron, selenium (as Brazil nuts) and vitamin B complex, and aim for RBC levels that are well into the highest quartile of the range. We use the SMART DNA test as an indicator of which genes are mutated and how aggressively we may need to supplement, and we use homocysteine levels as a rough guide for the need for methionine and S-adenosyl methionine, P5P, methylcobalamine, folinic acid and tri-methyl glycine supplementation. The improvements observed in the TOVA, qEEG and behavioral measures are often outstanding.

REFERENCES

1. Eaton SB, Cordain L. Evolutionary aspects of diet: old genes, new fuels. Nutritional changes since agriculture. *World Rev Nutr Diet.* 1997;81:26–37.
2. Eaton SB, Eaton III SB, Konner MJ. Paleolithic nutrition revisited: a twelve-year retrospective on its nature and implications. *Eur J Clin Nutr.* 1997;51(4):207–216.
3. Lipton B. *The Biology of Belief: Unleashing the Power of Consciousness, Matter, & Miracles.* New York, NY: Hay House; 2005.
4. Dufault R, Lukiw WJ, Crider R, Schnoll R, Wallinga D, Deth R. A macroepigenetic approach to identify factors responsible for the autism epidemic in the United States. *Clin Epigenetics.* 2012;4(1):6.
5. Dufault R, Schnoll R, Lukiw WJ, et al. Mercury exposure, nutritional deficiencies and metabolic disruptions may affect learning in children. *Behav Brain Funct.* 2009;5:44.
6. Ornish D, Lin J, Daubenmier J, et al. Increased telomerase activity and comprehensive lifestyle changes: a pilot study. *Lancet Oncol.* 2008;9(11):1048–1057.
7. Koletzko B, Lattka E, Zeilinger S, Illig T, Steer C. Genetic variants of the fatty acid desaturase gene cluster predict amounts of red blood cell docosahexaenoic and other polyunsaturated fatty acids in pregnant women: findings from the avon longitudinal study of parents and children. *Am J Clin Nutr.* 2011;93(1):211–219.
8. Innis SM. Perinatal biochemistry and physiology of long-chain polyunsaturated fatty acids. *J Pediatr.* 2003;143(4 suppl):S1–S8.
9. Li D, Weisinger HS, Weisinger RS, et al. Omega 6 to omega 3 fatty acid imbalance early in life leads to persistent reductions in DHA levels in glycerophospholipids in rat hypothalamus even after long-term omega 3 fatty acid repletion. *Prostaglandins Leukot Essent Fatty Acids.* 2006;74(6):391–399.
10. Tassoni D, Kaur G, Weisinger RS, Sinclair AJ. The role of eicosanoids in the brain. *Asia Pac J Clin Nutr.* 2008;17(suppl 1):220–228.
11. Bradbury J. Docosahexaenoic acid (DHA): an ancient nutrient for the modern human brain. *Nutrients.* 2011;3(5):529–554.
12. Rohrbough J, Broadie K. Lipid regulation of the synaptic vesicle cycle. *Nat Rev Neurosci.* 2005;6(2):139–150.
13. Duff J. Essential fatty acid profiles of children with autism, ADHD and typically developing controls. in Transpacific Autism Conference. 2011. Perth.
14. Borowsky B, Adham N, Jones KA, et al. Trace amines: identification of a family of mammalian G protein-coupled receptors. *Proc Natl Acad Sci U S A.* 2001;98(16):8966–8971.
15. Lorencová E, Bunková L, Matoulková, et al. Production of biogenic amines by lactic acid bacteria and bifidobacteria isolated from dairy products and beer. *Int J Food Sci Technol.* 2012;47(10):2086–2091.
16. Smith EA, Macfarlane GT. Studies of amine production in the human colon: enumeration of amine forming bacteria and physiological effects of carbohydrate and pH. *Anaerobe ecol.* 1996;2:285–297.
17. Parker G, Watkins T. Treatment-resistant depression: when antidepressant drug intolerance may indicate food intolerance. *Aust N Z J Psychiatry.* 2002;36(2):263–265.
18. Caspi A, Sugden K, Moffitt TE, et al. Influence of life stress on depression: moderation by a polymorphism in the 5-HTT gene. *Science.* 2003;301(5631):386–389.

19. Wurtman RJ, Wurtman JJ, Regan MM, McDermott JM, Tsay RH, Breu JJ. Effects of normal meals rich in carbohydrates or proteins on plasma tryptophan and tyrosine ratios. *Am J Clin Nutr.* 2003;77(1):128–132.

20. Young SN. How to increase serotonin in the human brain without drugs. *J Psychiatry Neurosci.* 2007;32(6):394–399.

21. Kelly GS. Insulin resistance: lifestyle and nutritional interventions. *Altern Med Rev.* 2000;5(2):109–132.

22. Grossman MH, Hart CR. *The Feel-Good Diet.* New York, NY: McGraw-Hill; 2008.

23. Pribram K, McGuinness D. Arousal, activation and effort in the control of attention. *Psychol Rev.* 1975;82(2):116–149.

24. Tucker DM, Williamson PA. Asymmetric neural control systems in human self-regulation. *Psychol Rev.* 1984;91:185–215.

25. Gainetdinov RR, Wetsel WC, Jones SR, Levin ED, Jaber M, Caron MG. Role of serotonin in the paradoxical calming effect of psychostimulants on hyperactivity. *Science.* 1999;283(5400):397–401.

26. Duff J. *Changes in brain electrical activity of boys with ADHD following neurotherapy*, in Brain Sciences Institute 2010, Swinburne University: Melbourne. p. 348.

27. Holcomb PJ, Ackerman PT, Dykman RA. Cognitive event-related brain potentials in children with attention and reading deficits. *Psychophysiology.* 1985;22(6):656–667.

28. Simmonds DJ, Fotedar SG, Suskauer SJ, Pekar JJ, Denckla MB, Mostofsky SH. Functional brain correlates of response time variability in children. *Neuropsychologia.* 2007;45(9):2147–2157.

29. Fassbender C, Zhang H, Buzy WM, et al. A lack of default network suppression is linked to increased distractibility in ADHD. *Brain Res.* 2009;1273:114–128.

30. Epstein JN, Erkanli A, Conners CK, Klaric J, Costello JE, Angoid A. Relations between continuous performance test performance measures and ADHD behaviors. *J Abnorm Child Psychol.* 2003;31(5):543–554.

31. Silberstein RB. Dynamic sculpting of brain functional connectivity and mental rotation aptitude. *Prog Brain Res.* 2006;vol. 159:63–76.

32. Alloway BJ. Soil factors associated with zinc deficiency in crops and humans. *Environ Geochem Health.* 2009;31(5):537–548.

33. Costello RB, Grumstrup-Scott J. Zinc: what role might supplements play? *J Am Diet Assoc.* 2000;100(3):371–375.

34. Hambridge M. Overview: essentiality of zinc. In: Costello B, Marriott M, eds. *Conference on Zinc: What Role Might Supplements Play?* Bethesda, MD: NIH Office of Dietary Supplements; 1998.

35. Akanli L, Lowenthal DB, Gjonaj S, Dozor AJ. Plasma and red blood cell zinc in cystic fibrosis. *Pediatr Pulmonol.* 2003;35(1):2–7.

36. Michalke B, Munch DC, Schramel P. Contribution to Zn-speciation in human breast milk: fractionation of organic compounds by HPLC and subsequent Zn-determination by DCP-AES. *J Trace Elem Electrolytes Health Dis.* 1991;5(4):251–258.

37. Roth HP, Kirchgessner M. Effect of different concentrations of various zinc complexes (picolinate, citrate, 8-hydroxyquinolate) in comparison with sulfate on zinc supply status in rats. *Z Ernahrungswiss.* 1983;22(1):34–44.

38. López-García C, Molowny A, Ponsoda X, Nácher J, Sancho-Bielsa F. Synaptic zinc in the central nervous system. *Rev Neurol.* 2001;33(4):341–347.

39. Li YV, Hough CJ, Sarvey JM. Do we need zinc to think? *Sci STKE.* 2003;2003(182):19.

40. Schmid G, Chittolini R, Raiteri L, Bonanno G. Differential effects of zinc on native GABA(A) receptor function in rat hippocampus and cerebellum. *Neurochem Int.* 1999;34(5):399–405.

41. Perlov E, Philipsen A, Hesslinger B, et al. Reduced cingulate glutamate/glutamine-to-creatine ratios in adult patients with attention deficit/hyperactivity disorder – a magnet resonance spectroscopy study. *J Psychiatr Res.* 2007;4(111):934–941.

42. Carrey NJ, MacMaster FP, Gaudet L, Schmidt MH. Striatal creatine and glutamate/glutamine in attention-deficit/hyperactivity disorder. *J Child Adolesc Psychopharmacol.* 2007;17(1):11–17.

43. Scassellati C, Bonvicini C, Faraone SV, Gennarelli M. Biomarkers and attention-deficit/hyperactivity disorder: a systematic review and meta-analyses. *J Am Acad Child Adolesc Psychiatry.* 2012;51(10):1003–1019. e20.

44. Mahmoud MM, El-Mazary AA, Maher RM, Saber MM. Zinc, ferritin, magnesium and copper in a group of Egyptian children with attention deficit hyperactivity disorder. *Ital J Pediatr.* 2011;37:60.

45. Lepping P, Huber M. Role of zinc in the pathogenesis of attention-deficit hyperactivity disorder: implications for research and treatment. *CNS Drugs.* 2010;24(9):721–728.

46. Kiddie JY, Weiss MD, Kitts DD, Levy-Milne R, Wasdell MB. Nutritional status of children with attention deficit hyperactivity disorder: a pilot study. *Int J Pediatr.* 2010;2010:767318.

47. Oner O, Oner P, Bozkurt OH, et al. Effects of zinc and ferritin levels on parent and teacher reported symptom scores in attention deficit hyperactivity disorder. *Child Psychiatry Hum Dev.* 2010;41(4):441–447.

48. Arnold LE, Bozzolo H, Hollway J, et al. Serum zinc correlates with parent- and teacher- rated inattention in children with attention-deficit/hyperactivity disorder. *J Child Adolesc Psychopharmacol.* 2005;15(4):628–636.

49. Arnold LE, DiSilvestro RA. Zinc in attention-deficit/hyperactivity disorder. *J Child Adolesc Psychopharmacol.* 2005;15(4):619–627.

50. Yorbik O, Olgun A, Kirmizigül P, Akman S. Plasma zinc and copper levels in boys with oppositional defiant disorder. *Turk Psikiyatri Derg.* 2004;15(4):276–281.

51. Zamora J, Velásquez A, Troncoso L, Barra P, Guajardo K, Castillo-Duran C. Zinc in the therapy of the attention-deficit/hyperactivity disorder in children. A preliminary randomized controlled trial. *Arch Latinoam Nutr.* 2011;61(3):242–246.

52. Arnold LE, Disilvestro RA, Bozzolo D, et al. Zinc for attention-deficit/hyperactivity disorder: placebo-controlled double-blind pilot trial alone and combined with amphetamine. *J Child Adolesc Psychopharmacol.* 2011;2(11):1–19.

53. Uckardes Y, Ozmert EN, Unal F, Yurdakök K. Effects of zinc supplementation on parent and teacher behaviour rating scores in low socioeconomic level Turkish primary school children. *Acta Paediatr.* 2009;98(4):731–736.

54. Dodig-Curkovic K, Dovhanj J, Curkovic M, Dodig-Radic J, Degmecic D. The role of zinc in the treatment of hyperactivity disorder in children. *Acta Med Croatica.* 2009;63(4):307–313.

55. Yorbik O, Ozgad MF, Olgun A, Senol MG, Bek S, Akman S. Potential effects of zinc on information processing in boys with attention deficit hyperactivity disorder. *Prog Neuropsychopharmacol Biol Psychiatry.* 2008;32(3):662–667.

56. Akhondzadeh S, Mohammadi MR, Khademi M. Zinc sulfate as an adjunct to methylphenidate for the treatment of attention deficit hyperactivity disorder in children: a double blind and randomized trial [ISRCTN64132371]. *BMC Psychiatry.* 2004;4:9.

57. Bilici M, Yildirim F, Kandil S, et al. Double-blind, placebo-controlled study of zinc sulfate in the treatment of attention deficit hyperactivity disorder. *Prog Neuropsychopharmacol Biol Psychiatry.* 2004;28(1):181–190.

58. Suresh PA, Sebastian S, George A, Radhakrishnan K. Subclinical hyperthyroidism and hyperkinetic behavior in children. *Pediatr Neurol.* 1999;20(3):192–194.

59. Dolev E, Deuster PA, Solomon B, Trostmann UH, Wartofsky L, Burman KD. Alterations in magnesium and zinc metabolism in thyroid disease. *Metabolism.* 1988;37(1):61–67.

60. Stein MA, Weiss RE. Thyroid function tests and neurocognitive functioning in children referred for attention deficit/hyperactivity disorder. *Psychoneuroendocrinology*. 2003;28(3):304–316.

61. Pfeiffer CC, Sohler A, Jenney CH, Iliev V. Treatment of pyroluric schizophrenia (Malvaria) with large doses of pyridoxine and a dietary supplement of zinc. *Orthomolecular Psychiatry*. 1974;3(4):292–300.

62. Dickinson N, Macpherson G, Hursthouse AS, Atkinson J. Micronutrient deficiencies in maternity and child health: a review of environmental and social context and implications for Malawi. *Environ Geochem Health*. 2009;31(2):253–272.

63. Dreosti IE. Trace elements in nutrition. *Med J Aust*. 1980;2(3):117–123.

64. Medicine IO. *Dietary Reference Intakes for Calcium, Phosphorous, Magnesium, Vitamin D, and Fluoride*. Washington, DC: National Academy Press; 1997.

65. Marier JR. Magnesium content of the food supply in the modern-day world. *Magnesium*. 1986;5(1):1–8.

66. Moshfegh A. What We Eat in America, NHANES 2005–2006: Usual Nutrient Intakes from Food and Water Compared to 1997 Dietary Reference Intakes for Vitamin D, Calcium, Phosphorus, and Magnesium. U.S. Department of Agriculture, Agricultural Research Service, 2009.

67. Hardwick LL, Jones MR, Brautbar N, Lee DB. Magnesium absorption: mechanisms and the influence of vitamin D, calcium and phosphate. *J Nutr*. 1991;12(11):13–23.

68. Cancela L, Marie PJ, Le Boulch N, Miravet L. Influence of vitamin D on mineral metabolism, hormonal status and bone histology in lactating rats and their pups. *J Endocrinol*. 1985;105(3):303–309.

69. Eaton SB, Eaton III SB. Paleolithic vs. modern diets–selected pathophysiological implications. *Eur J Nutr*. 2000;39(2):67–70.

70. Pigoli G, Dorizzi RM, Ferrari F. Variations of the urinary pH values in a population of 13.000 patients addressing to the National Health System. *Minerva Ginecol*. 2010;6(22):85–90.

71. Eaton SB, Konner MJ, Cordain L. Diet-dependent acid load, Paleolithic [corrected] nutrition, and evolutionary health promotion. *Am J Clin Nutr*. 2010;91(2):295–297.

72. Strohle A, Hahn A, Sebastian A. Estimation of the diet-dependent net acid load in 229 worldwide historically studied hunter-gatherer societies. *Am J Clin Nutr*. 2010;91(2):406–412.

73. Kozielec T, Starobrat-Hermelin B. Assessment of magnesium levels in children with attention deficit hyperactivity disorder (ADHD). *Magnes Res*. 1997;10(2):143–148.

74. Starobrat-Hermelin B. The effect of deficiency of selected bioelements on hyperactivity in children with certain specified mental disorders. *Ann Acad Med Stetin*. 1998;44:297–314.

75. Starobrat-Hermelin B, Kozielec T. The effects of magnesium physiological supplementation on hyperactivity in children with attention deficit hyperactivity disorder (ADHD). Positive response to magnesium oral loading test. *Magnes Res*. 1997;10(2):149–156.

76. Dubovický M, Kovacovsky P, Ujhazy E, Navarová J, Brucknerová I, Mach M. Evaluation of developmental neurotoxicity: some important issues focused on neurobehavioral development. *Interdiscip Toxicol*. 2008;1:206–210.

77. Nogovitsina OR, Levitina EV. Neurological aspect of clinical symptoms, pathophysiology and correction in attention deficit hyperactivity disorder. *Zh Nevrol Psikhiatr Im S S Korsakova*. 2006;106(2):17–20.

78. Mousain-Bosc M, Roche M, Polge A, Pradal-Prat D, Rapin J, Bali JP. Improvement of neurobehavioral disorders in children supplemented with magnesium-vitamin B6. I. Attention deficit hyperactivity disorders. *Magnes Res*. 2006;19(1):46–52.

79. Mousain-Bosc M, Roche M, Rapin J, Bali JP. Magnesium vitB6 intake reduces central nervous system hyperexcitability in children. *J Am Coll Nutr*. 2004;23(5):545S–548S.

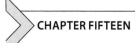

CHAPTER FIFTEEN

Vision Therapy as a Complementary Procedure During Neurotherapy

John K. Nash

INTRODUCTION

Neurofeedback, a form of biofeedback, can be used to signal a therapist and a client when a shift toward a desirable brain state has occurred. When this is done for therapeutic effect to treat particular psychological or neurological disorders, we call it neurotherapy. This shift toward a more desirable brain state can be operationalized as a change in the behavior of neuronal networks, as reflected in alterations in a specific electroencephalographic (EEG) parameter (e.g., power within a defined frequency band, the coherence of electrical rhythms between two recording sites, etc.). Further, this shift can be measured and its duration timed, i.e., one can operationalize a shift toward improved attention as a change in the theta/beta power ratio, or a drop in theta and/or alpha power for a discrete amount of time. The neurofeedback signal then represents one requirement for operant conditioning: an observable, measurable behavior occurs.

The momentary state of the brain can be thought of as a behavior that would ordinarily be invisible, but which can be made visible with modern digital EEG equipment and software. Therefore, one can reward (usually with verbal praise, or the switching on of a movie, or awarding a point) small "operants of alertness," for example, as one does with attention deficit hyperactivity disorder (ADHD) clients. One can reward on a brain level brief "operants of connectivity" with brain-injured clients or "operants of stillness" with anxious or hyperactive clients. Clients can (and should) be taught to self-reward, e.g., "smile at yourself inside," tell yourself "you're doing great" when the desired shift happens. As in any form of operant conditioning, one can shape, i.e., gradually extend the length of time the desirable state is held. With practice, the client becomes able

Clinical Neurotherapy.
Doi: http://dx.doi.org/10.1016/B978-0-12-396988-0.00015-5

to exercise more voluntary control over his or her attention, or state of calm, or whatever state is being trained. There are also very much unconscious effects that accrue. This is perhaps best illustrated by the early study by Sterman and Shouse[1] on epilepsy that showed not only a reduction in seizures and a relative normalization of the background EEG during the waking state, but – perhaps most importantly – a normalization of the sleeping background EEG. The study was a single-blind double-crossover ABA design. This indicates that a systemic change is occurring as a result of neurotherapy, and that the changes are not simply voluntary, because they occurred during sleep. Additionally, many epileptic patients also developed the ability to "head off" seizures voluntarily.

Many therapists have found it useful to include various cognitive tasks as part of the neurotherapy session. The value of this is immediately seen if one records EEG (typically from 19 channels), studies it visually, quantifies it and compares the results to a normative database, not only during eyes closed and eyes open resting conditions, but during "activation" tasks such as reading, listening, drawing, math and writing. In our clinic we routinely record during each of these activation conditions. For all conditions one must be careful with using a normative database, and remember you are averaging across the time of the recording. Although this is interesting and useful for some purposes, the averaging process can obscure significant intermittent failures of attention. Understanding the raw EEG signal visually is critical to being able to understand the client's experience.

Often we see that abnormalities observed during resting recordings are present during all the tasks. With other clients, however, we may see poor activation (e.g., intermittent failure of alpha blocking in parietal/occipital regions, or the emergence of excessive frontal/prefrontal theta or alpha) during a task such as listening, although there may be relatively normal EEG during other tasks. Generally we will incorporate the tasks during neurotherapy in which we have seen notable failures of brain activation or connectivity. For example, while giving an auditory neurofeedback signal, we will read to the person who has trouble sustaining alpha blocking while listening. The feedback tone lets the person and the therapist know when efficient attention is occurring. Similarly, we will use auditory feedback and have a person read or write if he or she has trouble sustaining a focused brain state during these tasks.

Failures of normal activation and brain resource allocation may be very regional. People with math difficulties may, for example, have very poor alpha blocking over the right parietal and/or low and variable coherence around this region. A person who gets very anxious while doing a task may develop strong over-activation – usually seen as excessive high-frequency beta or sometimes as excessive alpha blocking – over parietal, central or frontal/central regions. With such a person one might want to train for less high-frequency beta or even a little more intermittent alpha (usually "high-band alpha", 10–12 Hz) during the task.

VISION TRAINING

One of the most unique and activating tasks I have used during neurofeedback is binocular vision training. I learned about this from a developmental optometrist who had been doing it for 40 years, Clayton O. Johnson (now deceased). He confronted me after a talk I gave on ADHD and neurotherapy, saying "this ADHD is nothing but a visual disorder." Because I am an inherently curious person, I asked him to explain what he meant. The claim did not make sense to me, because obviously people with ADHD have trouble listening, organizing and staying motivated to tasks – and not just visual tasks. He later showed me a series of graded binocular stimuli, the Bernell Fixed Demand Tranaglyphs (Figure 15.1).

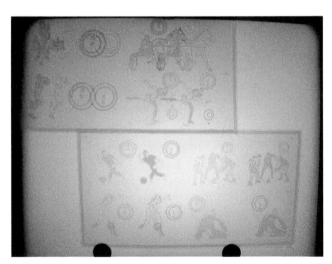

Figure 15.1 The first two Bernell Tranaglyphs arranged on a lightbox. The images at the lower right are separated by 10 prism diopters when viewed from 40 cm. When set in this direction (the red images on the right) the person must converge the images to fuse them. This task trains near-point convergence, which is needed for fast, accurate and comfortable reading. Flipping the cards over turns this into a divergent task for training divergent fusion (distance depth perception).

These are red/green anaglyphs in which the duplicate images are separated by increasing degrees of separation, measured in "prism diopters." The person observes these stimuli from a standard distance of 40 cm between the eye and the card. Variable demand cards are also available that are easier to use for people with very poor binocular control, because the vergences (the amount the eyes have to tip in or out to allow binocular fusion) are continuously variable instead of having "jumps" of increased demand (1–2–3–4–6–8–10…30 prism diopters, pd) for each successive stimulus. I looked at the cards through red/green glasses that allow the "3D" effect and could easily "pull" 30 prism diopters of convergent fusion (necessary for long periods of fast, accurate reading or other close work). He then flipped the cards over and I could pull 18 pd divergent fusion (necessary for good depth perception). He said, "Ah hah! You've got 30 and 18!", and I said, "So what?" His response was that every MD or PhD he had tested could pull 30/18; this is the optimal convergent and divergent fusion. He explained that if you could not do that there was no way you could read enough and remember enough to get an MD or PhD degree! I thought that was interesting, but whether it is always true or not was another matter. I have since seen a number of highly educated people with suboptimal binocular control. However, they tend either to be very diligent but somewhat slow readers, or complain of eye strain and headaches, or may essentially read with one eye as the result of amblyopia – the extreme favoring of data from one eye over data from the other.

I had learned about binocular fusion and stereopsis, the primary binocular disparity cue to depth, and all the secondary and tertiary cues to depth in my graduate perception and psychophysics seminar. However, I was never told that this does not develop in everyone, or that traumatic brain injury (TBI) invariably compromises this complex and distributed neurological system that affords accurate eye "teaming."

I proved to Clayton that ADHD was more than just a visual disorder by testing six of his "finished" clients. Half were (1) normal on the integrated visual and auditory (IVA) continuous performance test; and (2) their parents had no further complaints. I believe they had in fact been misdiagnosed with ADHD (by psychologists or pediatricians) and actually had "nothing but a visual disorder." When the visual disorder (usually "convergence insufficiency" and "intermittent exotropia") was corrected with vision therapy (operant conditioning of successive approximations to normal binocular control), the "ADHD" went away. The other half did much better with reading but continued to have clinically significant symptoms of ADHD and performed poorly on the IVA. This discovery was very interesting to me and to Clayton. I invited him into my practice, and we set up an eye clinic alongside my psychology practice.

We began doing visual binocular testing and vision therapy. I coupled this with auditory neurofeedback using the Lexicor systems, typically single channel. We found that by dedicating only about 10 minutes of each 30-minute session to binocular vision training coupled with auditory neurofeedback, we were able to normalize about 80% of the patients with binocular visual disorders The neurofeedback protocol used was individualized and based generally on the Neuroguide Z-scores. Often this was decreasing theta/alpha frontally, although we addressed coherence abnormalities when they were prominent and likely related to symptoms. Anecdotally we found that Biolex "synch" training across the premotor areas, e.g., F4–C4 seemed very effective, causing rapid acquisition of binocular control. The other 20% of patients required much more intensive eye interventions, which Clayton addressed. I continue to use the basic vision therapy coupled with neurofeedback, referring for standard eye examinations and later for vision therapy with an expert optometrist when the case is complex.

How We Do Basic Vision Therapy

The process of vision therapy that we use is one of reinforcing successive approximations to optimal levels of binocular fusion in both the converging and diverging directions. Using stimuli with gradually increasing binocular separation ("demand"), the person's visual system learns to acquire stronger convergence and divergence. One can fuse images more easily in peripheral than in foveal vision, so you "pick up" the next more difficult stimulus in your peripheral vision first. Also, because it is easier to fuse binocular images when not moving your eyes (or the stimulus), the therapist starts with static fusion, and then has the client gradually begin moving his or her head, or the stimulus, to create truly powerful dynamic fusion. This dynamic fusion is particularly important for sports performance and often is sold to athletes as "sports vision training." With the typical uncomplicated cases of poor convergent/divergent control, we usually accomplish normalized binocular vision (30 pd convergent/18 pd divergent on the fixed demand Bernell Tranaglyphs over the course of 20–40 neurotherapy sessions.

The reader should develop at least a basic vocabulary that will allow meaningful communication with an optometrist or ophthalmologist, so here are definitions of common terms regarding vision. Many more terms can be seen at http://eyeglossary.net/, which excerpts the *Dictionary of Eye Terminology*.[2]

- *Accommodation.* This refers to the focusing of the eyes to near or far points. Accommodation is accomplished by the ciliary muscles around the lens of the eye contracting or relaxing, thereby changing the shape of the lens and hence the focus plane of the eye. People with poor binocular fusion often will have accommodative problems, including accommodative spasm. I have seen little on what is thought to cause this, but it is likely that the failure of accurate aiming at near or far objects confuses the focusing mechanism.

- *Acuity.* This is a measure of visual clarity at far and near points. The familiar "20/20" vision means, for example, that one's vision is as clear at 20 feet as it normally is at 20 feet, and is measured by the eye charts one is familiar with from visits to the eye doctor.

- *Amblyopia.* This term describes a person who shows full suppression of the imaging from one eye. This results in a loss of 3D perception and is difficult, but not impossible, to correct. This is typically called "lazy eye" and represents a profound lack of binocular coordination.

- *Anisomatropia.* This is a condition in which one eye requires a vastly different acuity correction than the other eye. For example, one eye may need a minor correction for acuity, say −1.25 diopters. The other eye might require a very strong correction to achieve clarity, say −4.50 diopters. This would result in the retinal image of the weaker eye being very much smaller than that of the eye requiring less correction. When the disparity in retinal images is large enough, binocular fusion will be impossible. Sometimes the Lasix procedure can get the two eyes close enough in acuity to make vision therapy possible, but this is difficult. Patients with significant anisomatropia usually will suffer amblyopia.

- *Binocular fusion.* This is the brain function that brings the images from the two eyes together. It is a "software" function of the brain that in effect "slides" the images from the two eyes together, within a certain distance. You will notice that if you look at your finger at reading distance, objects in the far background will be doubled. Conversely, if you look across the room but hold your finger in your line of sight, you will see two somewhat transparent and out of focus images of your finger. That happens when the objects you perceive are too far from each other. There is a range within which objects will all appear single and in "3D".

- *Convergence insufficiency.* Poor convergence makes it difficult to aim the eyes consistently at near objects. This problem is worsened with small objects, like text. The common complaint of people with convergence insufficiency is that they skip words, have to re-read passages a lot, and that their eyes get dry and sore during extended reading. There is also often compromised depth perception at near point, and this can result in bumping into things and spilling drinks.
- *Diplopia.* This is the subjective complaint of "seeing double."
- *Divergence insufficiency.* Poor divergence compromises distance depth perception. This usually results in poor coordination and a self-perception of "clumsiness." People with inadequate divergent fusion will often note (once you ask them) that they cannot catch a ball or (in adults) that they absolutely cannot parallel park. Correcting this problem dramatically improves distance depth perception, and, along with it, sports performance and confidence. Relevant to this, I once successfully eliminated "escalator phobia" in a woman who had been treated with standard desensitization techniques and had made no progress. She had no distance depth perception. Once this was normalized with vision therapy, she could easily get on escalators because she became able to see the shape of the steps. Previously she saw only vertical and horizontal lines. I also helped put a national downhill slalom skier in the winner's circle for the very first time by normalizing her distance depth perception. After her treatment she came back having placed fourth, second and then first in three successive races. She exclaimed "I could *see* the shape of the snow in the gates!" Strangely enough, I have not seen "divergence insufficiency" diagnosed, only "convergence insufficiency". Perhaps this is because of our culture's emphasis on reading.
- *Esophoria.* The tendency of the eyes to cross at a neutral distance. When this is extreme "cross-eyedness" or "strabismus" is diagnosed.
- *Exophoria.* The tendency of the eyes to splay outward. There is a normal amount of exophoria at a given distance.
- *Intermittent exophoria.* This is a common diagnosis by developmental optometrists indicating that the person's eyes periodically break near-point fusion and splay outward.
- *Stereopsis.* This is the ability to "see space," i.e., the perception of the "3D" effect that is produced when binocular fusion occurs as a result of accurate converging or diverging. It is the brain's aligning of images that

have slightly different degrees of "binocular disparity" that makes the "3D" effect happen. I emphasize that this is a brain function, not having to do with eye muscles.

- *Suppression.* This is a brain phenomenon in which the data stream from one eye is suppressed to varying degrees. It typically happens with smaller objects, which are easier to suppress than larger stimuli. This happens when binocular fusion is poor, and it represents a compensation tactic of the brain to avoid seeing double.

- *Vergences.* This refers to the degree to which one's eye/brain systems automatically *converge* on objects that are close and *diverge* to objects that are further away. Vergences are measured in many different ways. We use the Bernell Fixed Demand Tranaglyph cards (Bernell Corporation, 2012), which provide red/green images at increasing separations.

- *Vision therapy.* This term denotes the treatment of convergence and binocular fusion with training and sometimes with prisms; this is sometimes called "orthoptics" or orthoptic vision therapy. It is largely practiced by "orthoptists," who usually also are optometrists. Some ophthalmological practices (medical eye doctors) offer this as well. This should not be confused with visual perceptual training, which does not involve 3D perception, or with the use of colored filters, or with simple techniques such as "pencil push-ups" (repeatedly focusing near to far, near to far, in the hope of improving converging and diverging. At some point true vision therapy will always involve "3D" stimuli seen through polarized or red/green glasses.

OPTOMETRIC RESEARCH

There has been one multicenter randomized placebo-controlled study by Scheiman and colleagues[3] demonstrating that office-based vision therapy improves symptoms of convergence insufficiency. The authors used a survey form to assess the level of symptoms from carefully measured convergence problems in 221 patients 9–17 years of age. The study compared the effects of home-based "pencil push-ups" (focusing on the letters on a pencil up close, then looking far away, going back and forth as quickly as possible), home-based computer vergence/accommodative therapy plus pencil push-ups, office-based vergence/accommodative therapy with home reinforcement, and office-based placebo therapy. The results showed greater effectiveness of office-based vision therapy in reducing symptoms of convergence insufficiency. The same group of collaborators also had published two previous randomized and placebo-controlled pilot studies, and a 1-year follow-up found that gains were sustained in 87.5% of the office-treated group, thereby demonstrating long-term efficacy.[4]

Although earlier studies of the treatment of convergence insufficiency were less rigorous, a review by Grisham[5] at the University of California, Berkeley School of Optometry, had found that optometric vision therapy corrected problems in 72% of cases. A more recent review by Shainberg[6] states: "Concrete evidence in the mainstream literature supports the positive effects of eye exercises in patients with convergence insufficiency and yoked prisms in patients with neurologic deficits." An important follow-up on the Scheiman et al. studies showed academic improvement from convergence insufficiency treatment, at least according to parent ratings of fewer school reading and homework problems after the treatment.[7]

CONTROVERSY

The medical community continues to be only somewhat supportive of optometric vision therapy. The American Academy of Pediatrics (AAP) website[8] states: "While vision problems can interfere with the process of learning, vision problems are not the cause of dyslexia or learning disabilities. There is no scientific evidence to support the use of eye exercises, vision therapy, tinted lenses or filters to directly or indirectly treat learning disabilities, and such therapies are not recommended or endorsed. There is no valid evidence that children participating in vision therapy are more responsive to educational instruction than children who do not participate." The AAP does not describe which vision problems *may* interfere with learning, although one may speculate that they are thinking primarily of the child getting corrective lenses. The reader should be clear that correcting acuity does not ameliorate a basic deficit of binocular control and binocular fusion. If the eyes are not aiming steadily at the same word or phrase, one would expect a confusing signal to reach the brain. Personally, I have seen over 1500 cases in which developing consistent binocular fusion has resulted in reports of more rapid, accurate reading and increased pleasure in the reading process.

A number of developmental/behavioral optometrists have made claims that visual disorders cause "dyslexia" and ADHD. This sort of claim creates further problems. I continue to see material from some optometrists (as with my old friend Clayton) stating that "ADHD is nothing but a visual disorder." Clearly, ADHD is a lot more than a problem with the teaming of the eyes. Similarly, there is general agreement today that "real" dyslexia is a disorder of central processing involving areas of the brain separate from the regions that control visual processing and eye movement.[9] However, what I think has happened is that some children have been misdiagnosed with ADHD or dyslexia by pediatricians, psychologists and psychiatrists. Children who cannot converge or diverge properly are not going to pay much attention to books or desk work, and may not be able to readily look at the board or their teacher. Doubtless some of these children have shown up at an optometrist's office, and the parent has told the eye doctor the child has been diagnosed with ADHD or dyslexia. Then, after vision therapy, the symptoms go away. So the doctor and the parent may have assumed that the "ADHD" or "dyslexia" was eliminated; hence the claim of ADHD being "nothing but" a visual disorder, or that dyslexia can be treated with vision therapy. In fact, what was going on was that the visual disorder was creating symptoms that mimicked ADHD, or was creating slow, unreliable and unpleasant reading. I have seen this with both ADHD and "dyslexia."

SUGGESTIONS FOR CLINICAL PRACTICE

Vision problems are common among persons with ADHD and those with TBIs. Stroke can also cause eye movement impairment that will result in reading problems.[10] There has apparently been little work examining the effects of brain injury on oculomotor function, although a study by Heitger et al.[11] reported deficits in oculomotor control in 30 mild TBI patients compared to a noninjured control group. O'Shanick and O'Shanick[12] note that in TBI there may be disruptions of visual tracking, figure-ground awareness, visual organization and 3D perception. The organization and recognition of visual percepts is far beyond the scope of this chapter, but it is clear that true 3D perception will not happen in the absence of binocular fusion, which creates the binocular disparity cue necessary for real "3D" perception. The widespread disruption of cortical connectivity that occurs in even mild brain injury should be expected to produce problems with the precision tuning of the binocular control system. In practice, I have seldom seen someone with a claim of mild TBI who did not show a moderate to severe impairment of infusion and stereopsis, with concomitant symptoms such as slowed, inaccurate reading,

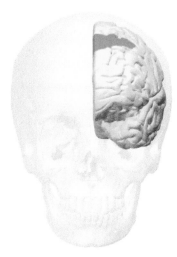

Figure 15.2 Illustration of Brodman area 8, which incorporates the frontal eye fields. From BodyParts3D, The Database Center for Life Science licensed under CC Attribution-Share Alike 2.1 Japan.

clumsiness and headaches from eye strain. This is not surprising, given the complexity of the visual control system and the fact that "the frontal eye fields" (FEF) that serve to coordinate eye movements (Brodman area 8) are in the front of the brain, an area most commonly affected in closed head injuries (Figure 15.2).

Even more important than the frontocortical location of the FEF is the fact of their truly extensive connectivity with and regulation by other parts of the visual system. This connectivity will be disrupted by the shearing and tearing that occurs in mild brain injury. The connectivity of the FEF is illustrated in Figure 15.3.

For those able to do low-resolution electromagnetic tomography analysis, it may be interesting to note whether Brodman area 8 (prefrontal region with lateral supplemental motor area) is indicated, because this area has been identified with the FEF, and the functional magnetic resonance imaging literature shows overlapping effects on executive functions,[13] attention,[14] memory[15,16] and motor functions.[17] One should always ask patients with these diagnoses about their experiences with reading and depth perception. People with poor binocular fusion almost never say they read for pleasure. They frequently complain of skipping words or whole lines of print, and of having to re-read paragraphs. While this might be a sign of ADHD or of impaired primary attention caused by a brain injury,

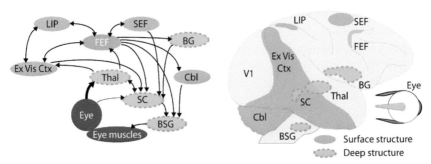

Figure 15.3 The connectivity and anatomical locations of the frontal eye field (FEF) and other structures within the visual and oculomotor systems of the rhesus macaque monkey brain. Left panel, diagram of the connectivity of the FEF with other visual and oculomotor structures. Some connections that do not directly involve the FEF are omitted. Right panel, locations of the brain regions pictured in the left panel shown in the lateral view of the monkey brain. In both panels, surface structures other than the FEF are coloured darker blue. Deep structures are illustrated as lighter blue with a dashed outline. BG, basal ganglia; BSG, brain-stem saccade generator; Cbl, cerebellum; Ex Vis Ctx, extrastriate visual cortex; LIP, lateral intraparietal area; SC, superior colliculus; SEF, supplementary eye field; Thal, thalamus; V1, primary visual cortex. (*From Ryan Fox Squire et al. (2012) Frontal eye field. Scholarpedia, 7(10): 5341, revision#128240.*)

re-reading also is a sign of poor eye tracking and poor binocular control. These patients also commonly complain of light sensitivity. When this is severe they often come to the office with a baseball cap low over their eyes, and sometimes wear sunglasses indoors. They also commonly experience motion sickness while riding. For such clients, a referral for a thorough visual examination that includes assessment of binocular control and possible vision therapy is recommended.

One should not attempt to do vision therapy without proper training. I was trained by a developmental/behavioral optometrist in the orthoptic methods for 3 years, and submitted records of this to the Board of Psychology with a request that screening and basic binocular vision therapy be listed as one of my Areas of Competence. This was accepted by the Board. Basically, vision therapy involves detailed behavior modification of the visual control systems. Perception and psychophysics have been part of psychology since the late 19th century, so this is a natural extension of behavior therapy if you get proper training and supervision from an eye doctor. I always require the involvement of an eye doctor to ensure eye health, proper correction of eyesight and correct diagnosis of any complex eye problems. Further illustrating the importance of this, I once saw a patient with all the typical complaints of someone with binocular control problems. On referral it was discovered the patient had a separation of the retina that was apparently caused by a recent automobile accident. This was successfully repaired with laser surgery, and the symptoms were largely ameliorated. I treat vision therapy simply as one of the tasks we do during a session, like listening, reading, or using various cognitive rehabilitation computer games: it is a basic part of many of my neurotherapy training sessions. If you do not learn to properly and legally administer vision therapy yourself, find referral sources among local optometrists or ophthalmologists who assess and treat binocular problems. One also could question them about screening methods that could be used to identify clients likely to be candidates for referral to a vision specialist.

REFERENCES

1. Sterman MB, Shouse MN. Quantitative analysis of training, sleep EEG and clinical response to EEG operant conditioning in epileptics. *Electroencephalogr Clin Neurophysiol*. 1980;49:558–576.
2. Cassin B, Rubin ML. *Dictionary of Eye Terminology*. 6th ed. Gainesville, FL: Triad Publishing; 2007.
3. Scheiman M, Cotter S, Mitchell GL, et al. Vision therapy/orthoptics for symptomatic convergence insufficiency in children: treatment kinetics. *Optom Vis Sci*. 2010;87(8):593–603.
4. Borsting E, Mitchell GL, Kulp MT. Long-term effectiveness of treatments for symptomatic convergence insufficiency in children. *Optom Vis Sci*. 2009;86(9):1096–1103.
5. Grisham JD. Visual therapy results for convergence insufficiency: a literature review. *Am J Optom Physiol Opt*. 1988;65(6):448–454.
6. Shainberg MJ. Vision therapy and orthoptics. *Am Orthopt J*. 2010;60:28–32.
7. Borsting E, Mitchell GL, Kulp MT, et al. Improvement in academic behaviors after successful treatment of convergence insufficiency. *Optom Vis Sci*. 2012;89(1):12–18.
8. American Academy of Pediatrics. <http://www.aap.org/en-us/about-the-aap/aap-press-room/Pages/AAP-Policy-Vision-Problems-Do-Not-Cause-Dyslexia.aspx>; 2012.
9. Rapcsak SZ, Beeson PM, Henry ML, et al. Phonological dyslexia and dysgraphia: cognitive mechanisms and neural substrates. *Cortex*. 2009;45(5):575–591.
10. Rowe F, Wright D, Brand D, et al. Reading difficulty after stroke: ocular and nonocular causes. *Int J Stroke*. 2011;6(5):404–411.
11. Heitger MH, Anderson TJ, Jones RD, Dalrymple-Alford JC, Frampton CM, Ardagh MW. Eye movement and visuomotor arm movement deficits following mild closed head injury. *Brain*. 2004;127(Pt 3):575–590.
12. O'Shanick GJ, O'Shanick AM. Personality and intellectual changes. In: Silver JM, Yudofsky SD, Hales RE, eds. *Neuropsychiatry of Traumatic Brain Injury*. Washington, DC: American Psychiatric Press; 1994:180.
13. Kübler A, Dixon V, Garavan H. Automaticity and reestablishment of executive control-an fMRI study. *J Cogn Neurosci*. 2006;18(8):1331–1342.

14. Cheng K, Fujita H, Kanno I, Miura S, Tanaka K. Human cortical regions activated by wide-field visual motion: an H2(15)O PET study. *J Neurophysiol*. 1995;74(1):413–427.

15. Babiloni C, Ferretti A, Del Gratta C, et al. Human cortical responses during one-bit delayed-response tasks: an fMRI study. *Brain Res Bull*. 2005;65(5):383–390.

16. Rugg MD, Fletcher PC, Frith CD, Frackowiak RS, Dolan RJ. Differential activation of the prefrontal cortex in successful and unsuccessful memory retrieval. *Brain*. 1996;119(Pt 6):2073–2083.

17. Inoue K, Kawashima R, Satoh K, et al. A PET study of visuomotor learning under optical rotation. *Neuroimage*. 2000;11(5 Pt 15 1):505–516.

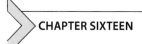

CHAPTER SIXTEEN

Future Considerations

Thomas F. Collura

INTRODUCTION

This book has provided perspectives on a broad range of issues related to neurotherapy, including function and behavior, clinical and pharmaceutical concerns, and applications to various clinical conditions. The purpose of this chapter is to examine potential developments in technologies that will play increasing roles in the field, and put them in context. In addition, other areas of engineering and neuroscience may become incorporated, and introduce important new capabilities.

When considering the future of neurotherapy, several divergent perspectives are helpful. One is a view of the past, tracing an evolution that dates from the earliest studies of electroencephalography (EEG), and takes its earliest recognizable form in the 1960s and 1970s. During its heady beginnings, EEG biofeedback comprised a mixture of diligent scientific studies, as well as popularized devices and methods. While the former were characterized by respected names such as Kamiya, Sterman and Lubar using high standards of scientific rigor and laboratory quality instrumentation, the latter have included a host of over-the-counter devices and their respective "gurus" heralding a new age of "mind machines." It is understandable that the water was perceived as murky, if not muddy, and the controversy and some of the discord have persisted into the present day. Currently, depending on whom one manages to contact, the newcomer to neurotherapy may encounter anything ranging from a solid, sound, research-based set of clinical practices to a distilled, broad-based "one size fits all" compendium of systems and practices proffered by self-styled entrepreneurs and promoters.

A second useful perspective is a snapshot of the present. Neurotherapy has maintained its dualistic nature until today. Although there are increasing numbers of responsible, evidence-based researchers and practitioners introducing new methods and studies, there persists a body of less rigorous, more commercially oriented providers, and these may attract

Clinical Neurotherapy.
Doi: http://dx.doi.org/10.1016/B978-0-12-396988-0.00016-7

attention. This produces the potential for a popular perception of the field as less than thorough, which detracts from the possibility for acceptance and growth. As a result, a current emphasis in neurotherapy is the development of evidence-based models and techniques with demonstrated efficacy, and the ability to articulate the operational principles and mechanisms of action.

A third perspective is to peer into the future and speculate as to what can happen, what should happen, and what can be done today to optimize future developments. Neurotherapy is undergoing an acceleration of interest and change, corresponding with increased awareness of the relevance of the brain to mental health science, as well as significant technical and clinical advances. Dominant themes are increasingly sophisticated techniques and instrumentation, combined with more structured approaches and ease of use. However, our view of the future tends to be distorted in general. In the 1950s we envisioned jet-packs, hovercraft, wrist-radios and talking appliances. We have yet to see these as mainstream products, yet are well beyond them in other ways, such as hybrid cars and ubiquitous computers and smart devices. We never envisioned the internet, smartphones, video game consoles, or the PC-based quantitative EEG (qEEG) machine. What becomes useful in the future may be somewhat unrecognizable according to our current view.

The future is both made possible, but is also limited, by the present. We carry tools forward, but we also carry biases, misunderstandings and conventional "truths." Neurotherapy may well become something quite different from what we currently envision, much the way the iPad seemingly came out of nowhere and transformed an entire generation of wireless information consumers. Hopefully, future developments will not be hampered by current limitations, in the way that the QWERTY keyboard has continued to endure, despite its deliberately designed clumsiness and inefficiency. A top-down look at neurofeedback that is free of conventions or parochialisms may help to provide a vision of possible futures.

CLASSIFICATION OF NEUROTHERAPY SYSTEMS

When considering the broad range of neurotherapeutic approaches, it is useful to distinguish between volitional and nonvolitional approaches. Volitional methods necessarily incorporate contingency of the feedback and consequent learning, and operate through some volitional mechanism on the part of the client. The client does not necessarily need to "try" to learn and may not even be aware of learning. However, the process of learning involves goal-seeking mechanisms such as homeostasis and allostasis, and tends to produce lasting change. It is the brain that learns, as distinguished from the "person" or the "mind." Such learned behaviors may be reversed by extinction or reverse conditioning, and may also fade over time. However, as is often the case with learned responses, some learning is generally retained for the future.

Nonvolitional approaches differ in that the system produces some change in the client through an active mechanism, and the client's volition is not necessarily a part of the learning process. Nonvolitional systems may be thought of as "doing something to" the client, in contrast to having the client learn "to do something." Nonvolitional approaches may use a contingent stimulus or a noncontingent stimulus. It is further possible to distinguish those that provide a perceptible suprathreshold feedback signal from those that would provide an imperceptible, subthreshold signal. These latter systems may elicit neural change, but presumably not through the same mechanisms associated with overt feedback signals such as computer displays, sounds, flashing lights, or suitably sized electromagnetic currents or fields. In suprathreshold systems either the client is aware of the feedback signal (light, sound, vibration, etc.), or the signal produces an expected and measurable change in the client's neuronal activity, generally visible in the form of overt changes in the EEG. The effects of a nonvolitional intervention may disappear when the intervention is removed, as when an evoked potential disappears when a light is turned off. However, other more lasting changes, such as with activation, metabolism or even connectivity, may be produced by the active agent.

Table 16.1 shows the currently recognizable neurotherapeutic approaches according to this classification. Systems that record some aspect of the EEG and present a visible or audible feedback signal are all considered volitional suprathreshold systems. There may be debate regarding the nature or even the validity of the measured variables, but all such systems still provide a tone or visual feedback signal, of which the client is made aware. Another group are the nonvolitional suprathreshold systems, including all types of stimulators and light/sound machines that influence the brain through known psychosensory or bioelectric mechanisms. When such systems are controlled by EEG signals, they become nonvolitional suprathreshold, of which several examples exist.

Since the beginning, neurotherapists have incorporated methods other than "traditional" operant learning based on the principle of

Table 16.1 Classifications and Examples of Neurotherapeutic Interventions

Mode	Mechanism	Subthreshold	Suprathreshold
Volitional (always contingent)	Operant (instrumental) learning		Neurofeedback: conventional, qEEG-based, Z-score, LORETA, SCP, Infra-Slow/Infra-Low, HEG
Nonvolitional Noncontingent	Entrainment or disentrainment; electromagnetic; metabolic	Neurofield, pRoshi Magstim	CES, rTMS, rDCS, pEMF, ECT, DBS, AVS, pRoshi
Nonvolitional Contingent	Selective disentrainment, classical conditioning	EEG-driven microstimulation, LENS	EEG-driven AVS, Roshi I, Roshi II

contingent reinforcement of a brain rhythm. These have included the use of auditory–visual entrainment (AVE) delivered by lights or speakers, and direct stimulation using electrical connections or magnetic devices. There is currently a considerable amount of divergence as well as advancement. AVE systems subscribe to different paradigms and principles for the precise control of stimulus timing and possible contingency. Science fiction movies of the 1950s were enamored with the possibility of a strobe-light being used to control or condition someone's mind. This vision has been realized somewhat with the systematic development of devices that elicit relaxation or other desirable effects, based on frequency, color and other stimulus parameters. EEG-driven stimulation has also been employed with benefits and has led as well to subthreshold EEG-driven methods. More recently, approaches have moved beyond the basic fixing or sequencing of frequencies and now use methods that consider entropy or stability as design considerations.

In the area of electrical stimulation, devices range from low-level DC stimulation (of the order of 1 V), through medium- and high-intensity devices providing cranioelectrotherapy stimulation (CES) that operate using up to 9 V, up to ECT (hundreds of volts) and DB systems (direct brain stimulation) that produce overt immediate neuronal responses by causing (or extinguishing) action potentials. However, there may be broader applicability in neurotherapy when working at lower levels. Transcranial direct current stimulation (typically 1 V or less) operates in this regime, in that it has an influence on, but is not an immediate cause of, changes in neuronal activation, and the client cannot typically feel it.

Electromagnetic devices also fall into a range of strengths, but the traditional approach has to use large enough levels of energy to produce overt neuronal responses. The levels necessary for this require equipment that is relatively costly and less accessible than typical neurofeedback equipment. It is not possible, for example, to power such devices with batteries. However, magnetic stimulation, or pulsed electromagnetic fields (pEMF), can operate at significantly lower levels, also with clinical effectiveness. There is an increasing interest in systems operating at extremely low levels, at or below 100 milliGauss. These can be regarded as "subthreshold" devices. While they may not necessarily produce significant immediate overt EEG responses, they can nonetheless produce shifts in transmembrane potentials that affect population behavior. It is not hard to understand that an intervention that can systematically alter the postsynaptic potential by even a few millivolts can affect how populations will behave. When this potential is viewed as a statistical distribution, a shift of a few percent can alter the likelihood of many affected neurons to reach (or not reach) their action potential threshold. Thus, depending on the location and specifics of the stimulation, such systems can be expected to have effects including excitatory and inhibitory, and also depend on neuronal locations and geometries, in determining clinical effects.

The evident absence of a volitional subthreshold system bears note. This would imply an approach that implements instrumental learning, but during which the client is not aware of any feedback. While this may seem contradictory, an example exists of just such learning in which the subject was not aware of the goal or the learning process. This is the often-cited case of the college professor whose students conditioned him to stay on one side of the room, by subtly changing their behavior depending on his position.[1] This illustrates that a client does not have to be consciously aware of a cue, in order to respond to it. This leads to the general question of whether we in fact respond to things of which we are not aware, on a routine basis. Without going into the arcane realm of subtle energy medicine or "psychic fields," it can safely be posited that we likely respond to external phenomena of which we are consciously unaware, but which affect our feelings and actions in a direct manner. These may include minute electrical fields or very weak chemical signals that escape everyday detection. Therefore, it is not unreasonable to speculate that a neurofeedback system that provides subthreshold or subliminal information contingent on EEG activity could produce instrumental learning and subsequent change. It may even be argued that a system such as the LENS implements such as strategy, even though the precise mechanism has yet to be identified and articulated.

Future systems will need to incorporate consideration of all of these design elements, while avoiding limitations or barriers derived from categorical approaches. One can anticipate increasingly EEG-driven systems, as well as built-in assessments of state and state change. Devices that present increasingly specific feedback information with precise contingency on EEG parameters have the potential to provide an increasing level of specificity, further potentiating the learning process. EEG parameters can include amplitude and frequency, but also phase, coherence, entropy, and other measures relevant to brain function. By tying feedback to immediate function rather than global parameters, the brain can be provided with more detailed information regarding its own state.

INDIVIDUALIZED ASSESSMENT AND TREATMENT

If the purpose of neurotherapy is to help a client get from point A to point B, it should be emphasized that not only is point A different for each individual, but point B is also individualized. Despite the importance and clinical success associated with the use of standardized, normative databases, it is still a fact that every individual has unique set points within the population continuum. This is evident from the simple reality that even the normative database contains individuals with EEG values that reside 1, 2 or even 3 standard deviations from the mean, yet do not have reported abnormalities. When these individuals are encountered, the decision whether to move them toward the population average must be justified by clinical judgment, not a wholesale subscription to normal for everyone.

Even if it is argued that the proper target is the population mean, it does not follow that normalizing the EEG is the solution to the client's problems. A clean map is not necessarily the answer to the relevant clinical questions. The EEG has deviated for a compendium of reasons and simply setting it straight does not mean that everything is solved. This point of view may be an adaptation of the pharmaceutical model to neurotherapy, but it does not address the core issues. Normalizing the EEG does not cancel out the experiences, learning, cognitive and behavioral dynamics, or physiological underpinnings that constitute the client's condition. It also does not change the environment or the reward system in which the client functions. Neurotherapy is part of a process of change and recovery, and must be applied within that context.

A second consideration relative to normative databases is that the widespread use of Fourier Transform methods leads to misleading information when EEG components are not purely sinusoidal. Fourier Transforms will necessarily introduce the appearance of higher frequencies, whenever the shape of a rhythm is not a simple sinewave. However, nature has no reason to restrict EEG waves to being pure sinewaves, and various configurations, such as squared-off waves, pointed waves or even wicket-shaped waves, can be observed in the EEG. Any deviation from a perfect sinewave introduces frequencies at integer harmonics of the fundamental, producing the illusion in frequency plots of beta or higher rhythms, whereas no such generators actually exist in the brain. Methods such as independent components analysis and principal component analysis can effectively address these components in a mathematically sound manner, so that they can be separated in time as well as in space. Real-time implementation of these approaches could engender a new type of feedback based more upon brain processes than on the presence or absence of a frequency band. It is also likely that alternate transforms, such as the Wavelet Transform, the Hilbert–Huang Transform, or other morphologically informed methods, will become useful in this regard.

In cases such as EEGs that deviate from normal in a "good" way, neurotherapy to produce a normal EEG may not be clinically indicated. For example, when a large, fast posterior alpha rhythm is present, the EEG findings can easily produce a report showing "excess beta," and may also show "excess high beta" because of the presence of the first harmonic of the alpha wave, producing energy in the vicinity of twice the dominant frequency, for the reason described. Z-scores are highly sensitive to small elevations in this range and can easily suggest that deviations from normal exist, leading to the possibility that they will be interpreted as something to be treated. In such cases, simply noting that the client has "fast posterior alpha" provides more information than a collection of maps and graphs showing various features that are not relevant to the core issues.

What these considerations point to is the need for individualized assessment and treatment planning, plus a move away from a simple use of qEEG frequency analysis in this process. Despite the precision and rigor offered by mathematical analysis, automated processing of the EEG neglects certain key considerations. One of these is the fact that Fourier-based methods are

useful only in the context of an assumed repetitive, sinusoidal set of waveforms, and this abstraction neglects significant detail that is evident in the
EEG. Among the aspects that are opaque to frequency analysis are the morphology of the EEG, the directed sequence of time events, the information
content of the EEG signal, and relationships between brain locations with
regard to communication and control.

An important aspect of future automated analysis will be an emphasis
on recognizing higher-level properties of the EEG, and in classifying and
clustering individual EEGs in meaningful terms. The recognition of EEG
phenotypes is an important element of sound clinical practice and has a
growing evidence base.[2] Although qEEG analysis can help to uncover some
phenotypes, this type of classification requires an informed eye to inspect the
raw waveforms. Certain key phenotypes, such as "spindling beta," may not
stand out in a qEEG analysis, whereas others, such as "mixed fast and slow,"
might. There is no substitute for the visual inspection of EEG waveforms
and classification based on experience and clinical judgment. Arns et al.[3-6]
have shown, for example, that neurofeedback treatment as well as pharmaceutical treatment of children with attention/deficit disorder/attention
deficit hyperactivity disorder based on EEG phenotypes led to an improved
outcome. Phenotypes introduce a "big picture" that resides above a detailed
analysis of metrics and provides an overarching set of principles explaining
how a particular EEG may lean in one or more directions as part of an individualized profile. In this case, rather than a picture being worth a thousand
words, a few words can be worth many pictures.

INTEGRATION AND EASE OF USE

Ease of use is a critical factor. Neurotherapy is integrated into practice as part of a process, and this places demands on simplicity and repeat-
ability in clinical use. Users will naturally gravitate toward the simplest
and most direct approaches, even if they do not produce optimal results.
The extra effort required to ensure a thorough assessment and individualized treatment is hard to justify when the alternative is a pill that can be
administered in seconds, and without special training. However, a certain
amount of flexibility is important, and this implies options and choices
that the practitioner must make. Simplicity may imply inflexibility and
singleness of purpose, and thereby limit potential overall clinical effectiveness. Simple to use implies fewer options when tailoring the system to a
particular client. Although a standardized approach may suffice as an entry,

it may wind up on the shelf or being sold or traded by users who wish to evolve toward more flexibility and power. An optimal approach will incorporate flexibility, yet default to behavior that provides a suitable starting point from which to grow and develop.

Even though technology and protocols become more sophisticated, the simple yet effective approaches are not going to disappear. The use of one-channel EEG is likely to remain an important element, particularly as the sophistication of signal processing and interpretation continue to evolve. It is likely that small-channel systems will continue to reduce in size and move further toward wireless, lightweight, head-mounted devices with built-in sensor quality checking and dry or near-dry electrodes. We may see a return to the self-contained architecture once dominant in analog systems, in this case incorporating digital as well as analog components in increasingly smaller packages.

In the long term, minimum-contact – or even contactless – sensors would be ideal. In the fullness of time, perhaps a room-temperature method for achieving magnetic signals from the brain could facilitate a headset that does not require direct scalp connections. Until there is a simple, clean, rapid and dependable electrode system, the use of EEG in neurotherapy will remain associated with some levels of gooiness, inconvenience or cost.

The ability to address the connections between symptoms and functions and EEG activity is a key strength of neurotherapy. Neurotherapy can take a point of view that is more fundamental than diagnosis, and even more fundamental than symptoms. By identifying functional concerns, it can address requisite brain activity without regard for how the behavior or disorder is classified. Designs that incorporate symptom checklists or questionnaires and other relevant information can help ensure that neurotherapeutic interventions take into account the client's limitations and strengths, as well as address clinical goals in a directed fashion. Davidson and Begley,[7] for example, describe a method that provides 60 specific questions and then leads to information related to likely levels of brain activity in specific regions. This information is applicable to self-awareness and clinical approaches in general, but has particular potential value in relation to neurotherapy that modulates the activity of the relevant areas.

Technical innovation can further strengthen this approach by providing functional information related to performance and event-related activity. The more sophisticated techniques and databases become, the more systems can approach the goal of being a true brain monitor/trainer that operates according to sound and relevant principles of brain function and plasticity. These considerations will likely move us away from a conventional linear, clockwork-based model, to a fuller appreciation of brain dynamics as nonlinear and goal-oriented, organized around change, not stasis. Theoretical development will also be incorporated into technical development, as new metrics and methods emerge from evolving points of view.

With regard to assessment, one important trend will be the divergence from the "roll your own" style of acquiring and interpreting EEGs, or even sending records out for third-party evaluation, toward the use of built-in programs, structured services and web-based utilities. In much the same way that clinics routinely send blood or urine to nationally recognized laboratories for analysis, EEGs will be increasingly uploaded for screening, review and correlation with symptoms. Recommendations can be generated and relative to medications, nutrition, supplements, diet or neurofeedback protocols (CNS Response, BRC, New Mind). Such approaches can also incorporate the practice model as they produce analyses, summaries and follow-up assessment and interpretation. Generally, the integration of assessment and treatment will enable the process to be more cyclical and repetitive, rather than comprising a series of distinct steps.

A blurring of the distinction between qEEG and neurofeedback is already evident. One important factor is the provision of qEEG-based methods into 1, 2, and 4-channel systems in the form of mini-assessments and reports, live Z-score capabilities and live low-resolution electromagnetic tomography analysis (LORETA)-based approaches. It is now possible to acquire qEEG data on the fly during training without resorting to a sequential process of qEEG–train–qEEG as separate operations. Live Z-score training methods essentially encapsulate a portion of the qEEG process into the live environment, thus providing a simultaneous integration of assessment and training as a combined process. By watching live Z-score maps, for example, a client can actually see his or her qEEG change in real time and guide the brain as precisely as one can use a global positioning system to find the local hardware store.

One area that will likely grow in importance is that of very low-frequency work, including slow cortical potentials, and also infra-slow work $<0.01\,Hz$.[8,9] The theoretical models applicable to these modalities are not well understood and also not without controversy. Whereas the mechanisms of low-frequency rhythms likely involve nonneuronal mechanisms, including glial activity as well as respiratory, cardiac and other somatic rhythms combined with skin and sensor effects, the various contributions of these factors to biofeedback are not clear. Nonetheless, clinical experience has driven the move toward lower frequencies as a heuristic method driven by client and clinician experience. This does present a move from the concept of "rhythms" to that of "shifts." When the EEG filters are set for very low values, <0.01 Hz, the salient property is no longer its ability to filter a repetitive, periodic wave. Rather, the time-constant inherent in the low-frequency cutoff dominates the response. The effect of such low filters appears to be one of primarily selecting the magnitude and duration of a transient shift in the EEG baseline, not detecting a wave that has a fixed periodicity. This approach is therefore more event-related than it is state-related.

LOCALIZATION AND CONNECTIVITY-BASED METHODS

The ability to recover localized brain activity data in real time is a significant advancement. Rather than providing information related to scalp EEG from one sensor or from sensors or the whole head, live localization provides the ability to reflect the activity of specific locations, such as the cingulate gyrus, dorsolateral or mesiotemporal frontal lobes, insula, the limbic system, or other regions of interest. Because the scalp signals are spatially smeared from the brain distribution, controlling scalp EEG requires a broader scope of change than if one is focusing on changing one region. Live localization training of a particular region changes the client's experience from one of receiving rather more muddled feedback, to receiving clear information related to a particular anatomic and functional area. In addition to the use of live images as direct feedback, localization data can be fed back as power in specific bands, connectivity between regions of interest, or advanced properties such as dipole orientation and stability. Watching an accurate and rapid depiction of brain activity is an alternative to the typical bargraph, game or video, and provides a type of brain/mind link that is unprecedented either in the laboratory or in the clinic.

The best-known localization technique is LORETA and its derivatives, sLORETA, eLORETA, and VARETA.[10–12] However, this is not the only method of performing the mathematical transforms and is but one set of examples of the general idea of brain electrical activity localization. Live localization cuts through the blurring of EEG signals as they are transferred from the cortex to the scalp and provides a new window of clarity. It can be applied with either conventional approaches, such as training theta or beta up or down in the anterior cingulate, or with approaches such as live Z-scores or region of interest-based connectivity training. Localization is an approach in itself and should be applicable in broad areas such as multivariate assessment and feedback, DC, slow cortical potentials and infra-slow/infra-low frequency work.

Techniques based on brain activity localization have the potential to take advantage of emerging technology providing three-dimensional (3D), even holographic, displays. An ultimate realization would present the client's brain activity directly in a 3D form, appropriately encoded using color and graphics, and in real time. This would lead to a unique type of virtual reality environment in which the environment becomes the brain, and the client experiences the inner world as a vivid representation in the outer world. Neurofeedback has benefited from advancements in gaming, media and consumer electronics technology. This trend will continue, as more rapid, vivid and informative displays and sounds are produced in conjunction with brain monitoring.

Live localization also provides a level of noise reduction that is relevant to event-related potential work. A significant reason that event-related potentials must be averages is that the responses are buried in so much extraneous EEG, regarded as noise. A considerable amount of this "noise" is volume-conducted from widespread areas of the brain. Live localization-based methods capture the activity of the regions of interest and separate it from extraneous noise, as part of the localization process. Therefore, these approaches have the potential to provide immediate data that are relevant to short-term changes in brain function.

An area of significant potential is that of localization-driven subthreshold feedback. A system integrating live brain region imaging or training with a precisely timed subthreshold method would be expected to affect brain function efficiently, directly and rapidly. This approach provides the ability to present the brain with information related to specific activity in specific regions at a specific time. This becomes a form of event-related feedback, in which the events are those detected in the brain, rather than external events.

Increased attention has been focused on brain imaging technologies such as functional magnetic resonance imaging, positron emission tomography, magnetoencephalography and related methods. Although these are invaluable in basic science and medical applications, it is not clear that they will have significant impact on neurotherapy. They are among the most costly and slowest methods available for operant learning and related paradigms. Given the speed, cost-effectiveness and physiological relevance of EEG-based neurofeedback, it can be expected to remain the method of choice for clinical assessments and interventions in fields related to mental health.

One area in which materials and fabrication sciences will likely make a strong impact is in the creation of a suitable electrode cap or helmet that is free of paste or gel, easy and rapid to apply, and readily cleanable or reusable. No existing system satisfies all of these needs, and those that approach these are generally costly. An elastic or otherwise adjustable cap made of an advanced material, integrated with active sensors and a dry or semi-dry skin contact method, would provide suitable signals, if the 10–20 sites locations can be assured. An additional benefit would be wireless operation, but this requires more significant headgear and a source of battery power, thereby adding weight. There have been many attempts at electrode caps, some successful and some not, but the perfect electrode cap has yet to be designed. The small size of the market limits the interest of entities that could develop such a device; unless the market suddenly expands, demand for electrode caps will remain modest. However, a more perfect electrode system would go a long way toward increasing acceptance and broadening into other, larger markets.

INTEGRATED SYSTEMS

It is not uncommon for clinicians to accumulate a collection of equipment suited to diverse needs, and to integrate their use into a personal clinical model. Such approaches often take the form of a sequence of operations alternating the use of different interventions. A typical process might include an intake and qEEG, then a stimulation, low-energy or infra-low frequency procedure, followed by a directed neurofeedback session using live Z-scores or localization-based training. The cost for all the equipment necessary for such a process can exceed $30,000, which is out of the reach of many clinicians. Given the commonality of many of the systems and software, there is no reason why economies cannot be achieved through integrated designs and methodologies. Single-purpose parochially oriented systems will likely give way to newer cohesive designs, in much the same way that the personal computer displaced diverse systems such as word processors, data terminals and communications devices with more economical and more versatile solutions. Standardization will be an important influence. The recent standardization effort by the Institute of Electrical and Electronics Engineers will likely have a positive impact on future developers looking for guidelines for quality, and to meet user expectations.

A further level of integration that will be of value is that of incorporating continuous performance tests, educational and cognitive development or rehabilitation systems, virtual reality and other emerging approaches. Neurofeedback integrated with task-based systems derives further benefits from the aforementioned blurring between qEEG and neurofeedback therapy. A system can put a participant through various mental exercises, evaluate performance and incorporate real-time brain activation data into the administration as well as the interpretation of results. When combined with localization-based event-related brain activity monitoring, it becomes possible to create systems that literally see the brain in action, interact with it, and produce a real-time assessment of brain function concurrent with specific interventions. It may become possible to capture the moment that a client, for example, "zones out" and misses a cue, and condition the brain to maintain focus at critical instants, thereby improving efficiency and performance. The supplementation of power and connectivity-based methods with event-related and phase-based approaches can be expected to further improve the ability to identify key neuronal events and respond accordingly.

EXTERNAL FACTORS AFFECTING NEUROTHERAPY

Technology can only go so far in ensuring the success of neurotherapy. Even the most perfectly advanced and effective systems will not proliferate in the absence of acceptance, education and reimbursement. The factors that are important in this regard are more in the area of external influences and forces, rather than those qualities or capabilities embodied in the equipment itself. Neurofeedback is not a replacement for medication, but it may be viewed as such. A mindset that puts a pill as one option and neurotherapy as another option may miss the distinct advantages as well as demands posed by an approach based on brain plasticity.

The progress of neurotherapy hinges in part on education and training. The growth of university-based training and degree programs is essential to acceptance and reimbursement. One important theme that will shape future evolution is the importance of "training the trainers." In contrast to pharmaceutical approaches, neurotherapy has a significant element of art as well as science. It does not take much training to learn how to administer a pill, or even to give an injection. Even the task of selecting medications is based primarily on a review of client symptoms and diagnoses, and following a predefined plan or protocol. Neurotherapy, on the other hand, can be a highly individualized process in which myriad factors are taken into account, and the treatment can be very specific to each client. This requires a paradigm that is different from either the "talk therapy" approach on one hand, or the pharmaceutical approach on the other. It combines the thought and content of the client's mental processes, and also affects the brain in a physiologically relevant manner. It is empowering in that it can combine the best of both worlds. The difficulty largely entails conveying this understanding to a generation of practitioners who may not be oriented by training or mindset to accept its tenets.

The areas of regulatory control and insurance reimbursement will require significant progress if neurofeedback is to proliferate. These are separate but related issues. The Food and Drug Administration still does not recognize neurofeedback for any application other than "relaxation and re-education." Until specific clinical trials are conducted with specific devices, this situation will not change. The resources necessary to produce a study supporting a premarket approval (PMA) are out of reach of most institutions. The European authorities take a different approach and allow the citation of controlled studies with equivalent devices, to support claims of efficacy for particular disorders. Insurance reimbursers look to these registrations and approvals to justify paying for specific interventions. Clinicians are understandably hesitant to adopt new methods if they are not reimbursed. Global acceptance and reimbursement of neurofeedback as a valid clinical intervention is a requisite for its increased growth and widespread use. The role that technology can play in this evolution is by providing sound, evidence-based methods that will satisfy those with a financial stake in the client's wellbeing. Research-oriented tools and software will also provide a valuable capability, so that systems can deliver the evidence required to assess their effectiveness, as part of the routine clinical operations.

Technology does not evolve in isolation. Clinical utility is not based solely on feature sets and performance specifications. Usefulness is a function of addressing a clear need and purpose, with a focused design intent. Neurotherapy will not progress optimally if it pursues a deterministic model of fixing a problem by relieving symptoms. Rather, the functionally based approach looks at neuronal processes and events viewed in the context of the client's needs and capabilities. Interventions can thus address the "what is happening" and "why it is happening" of the client's brain activity, not just "how much" or "when" a given process is evident.

The question being increasingly asked is "when will neurotherapy become mainstreamed?" An alternate question is, "why should neurotherapy become mainstreamed?" Ultimately, the future of neurotherapy will likely depend less on equipment and software, and more on its role in mental health care. Neurotherapy is poised to revolutionize psychology, counseling and even medicine itself. It has the potential to enlighten practitioners as well as clients, and in doing so to empower those who are receptive to its methods and approaches. At some point, a new generation of systems has to break the mold and rethink the entire process.

REFERENCES

1. Sabado SM. Basic Principles of Operant Conditioning. Out of Print: Retrieved from <http://www.scribd.com/doc/28687783/Basic-Principles-of-Operant-Conditioning>; 1970.
2. Johnstone J, Gunkelman J, Lunt J. Clinical database development: characterization of EEG phenotypes. *Clin EEG Neurosci.* 2005;3(2):99–107.
3. Arns M, Gunkelman J, Breteler M, Spronk D. EEG phenotypes predict treatment outcome to stimulants in children with ADHD. *J Integr Neurosci.* 2008;7(3):421–438.
4. Arns M, de Ridder S, Strehl U, Breteler M, Coenen A. Efficacy of neurofeedback treatment in ADHD: the effects on inattention, impulsivity and hyperactivity: a meta-analysis. *Clin EEG Neurosci.* 2009;40(3):180–189.
5. Arns M, Gunkelman J, Olbrich S, Sander C, Hegerl U. EEG vigilance and phenotypes in neuropsychiatry: implications for intervention. In: Coben R, Evans J, eds. *Neurofeedback and Neuromodulation Techniques and Applications.* Amsterdam, The Netherlands: Elsevier; 2011.
6. Arns M, Drinkenburg W, Kenemans JL. The effects of qEEG-informed neurofeedback in ADHD: an open-label pilot study. *Appl Psychophysiol Biofeedback.* 2012;37(3):171–180.
7. Davidson R, Begley S. *The Emotional Life of Your Brain.* London, England: Hodder & Stoughton; 2012.
8. Othmer S, Othmer SF. Infra-low frequency training. Retrieved from <http://www.eeginfo.com/research/articles/Infra-LowFrequencyTraining.pdf> 2008.
9. Othmer S. Introduction to Infra-low frequency training. Retrieved from <http://www.eeginfo.com/newsletter/?p=523> 2010.
10. Pascual-Marqui RD. Review of methods for solving the EEG inverse problem. *Int J Bioelectromagnetism.* 1999;1(1).
11. Pascual-Marqui RD. The human brain resting state networks based on high time resolution EEG: comparison to metabolism-based networks. Proceedings of the Annual Meeting of the International Society for Neurofeedback & Research, Keynote Presentation. <http://www.isnr.org>; 2011.
12. Pascual-Marqui RD, Michel CM, Lehmann D. Low resolution electromagnetic tomography: a new method for localizing electrical activity in the brain. *Int J Psychophysiol.* 1994;18:49–65.

BIBLIOGRAPHY

Collura TF. Neuronal dynamics in relation to normative electroencephalography assessment and training. *Biofeedback.* 2009;36(4):134–139.
Collura TF, Guan J, Tarrant J, Bailey J, Starr F. EEG biofeedback case studies using live Z-score training (LZT) and a normative database. *J Neurother.* 2010;14(2):22–46.
Collura TF, Thatcher RW, Smioth ML, Lambos WA, Stark CR. EEG biofeedback training using Z-scores and a normative database. In: Evans W, Budzynski T, Budzynski H, Arbanal A, eds. *Introduction to qEEG and Neurofeedback: Advanced Theory and Applications.* 2nd ed. New York, NY: Elsevier; 2009.

Index

Note: Page numbers followed by "*f*" and "*t*" refers to figures and tables respectively.